# LABOR

## CLINICAL EVALUATION AND MANAGEMENT

# LABOR

# CLINICAL EVALUATION

# AND MANAGEMENT

SECOND EDITION

Emanuel A. Friedman, M.D., Med. Sc.D.
Professor of Obstetrics and Gynecology
Harvard Medical School
Obstetrician-Gynecologist-in-Chief
Beth Israel Hospital
Boston, Massachusetts

APPLETON-CENTURY-CROFTS/New York

78 79 80 81 82 / 10 9 8 7 6 5 4 3 2

Prentice-Hall International, Inc., London
Prentice-Hall of Australia, Pty. Ltd., Sydney
Prentice-Hall of India Private Limited, New Delhi
Prentice-Hall of Japan, Inc., Tokyo
Prentice-Hall of Southeast Asia (Pte.) Ltd., Singapore
Whitehall Books Ltd., Wellington, New Zealand

LIBRARY OF CONGRESS CATALOGING IN PUBLICATION DATA
Friedman, Emanuel A.
Labor.

Bibliography: p.
Includes index.
1. Labor (Obstetrics) I. Title.
[DNLM: 1. Labor. 2. Labor complications.
W0300 F911L]
RG651.F7 1978 616.4 77-25883
ISBN 0-8385-5580-2

Text design: Meryl Sussman Levavi
Cover design: Kristin Herzog

PRINTED IN THE UNITED STATES OF AMERICA

*Dedicated to the premise that the hazards of parturition can be minimized through understanding and ingenuity, through acquired knowledge and its application*

# Contents

# Preface

Twenty-five years have elapsed since I first undertook objective clinical studies to elucidate the evolution of cervical dilatation and fetal descent, and it is now ten years since publication of the first edition of this book summarizing those investigations for purposes of direct application to clinical obstetric practice. My objective in this edition is to present in a lucid, easily assimilable manner those pertinent aspects of normal and abnormal labor that have been learned through the study of the patterns of cervical dilatation and fetal descent. It is not my intention to display all the documented clinical knowledge that is available concerning labor, but rather to limit the scope of this book to areas of relevance to both the practicing clinician and the investigative physiologist.

The graphic approach to observing and analyzing the course of labors in progress is now familiar to clinicians everywhere. Indeed, its acceptance around the world has been very gratifying. However, universal acceptance and application are still far from complete. Recent simplifying modifications have contributed much to a resurgence of interest in this area with resulting wider dissemination. Nevertheless, major barriers to the fullest possible diffusion are recognized to exist. These take the form primarily of a reluctance on the part of obstetric attendants to objectify observations and, more often, an abhorrance of the quantitation that is involved. The need for any form of mathematical calculation has been eliminated, for all practical purposes, by one or more of the currently available techniques that are described here.

While such nonarithmetical means were primarily designed for health-related paraprofessional and nonprofessional personnel, it must be emphasized that it is essential for every physician who uses these methods to understand the underlying concepts that form their basis. Failing such comprehension, one risks practicing without rational justification for one's own automatic reflexive responses. Thus, one cannot readily incorporate new information into the armamentarium of practice as new data and concepts are evolved in this dynamic discipline, nor can one serve adequately in the important role of indoctrinating peers, students, or assistants.

I have been prevailed upon to update this book in order to satisfy perceived needs in this area. In doing so, I have made a major effort to revise it extensively to incorporate all newly developed material, formulated by the continuing and expanded data collection and analyses completed during the decade since the first edition was published. In addition, I felt the pressures to relieve some of the admittedly overindulgent grandiloquence of the original work. My problem with regard to the latter objective was to ensure that I would not deprive the devoted, inquiring scholar of the full panoply of the data base upon which the thesis was conceived and subsequently developed.

I have tried to accomplish both objectives—that is, to provide a book for obstetric clinicians to help them assimilate meaningful principles and acceptable practices quickly, and at the same time to display investigational information and analytic complexities for the clinical scientist. Where appropriate, chapters include a relatively concise, readable portion that is clinically oriented and a more explicitly detailed part in which experimental aspects are summarized.

I have been candid in presenting material, particularly emphasizing those areas where I felt a need existed for distinguishing between fact and fancy. I have adhered tenaciously to this principle, stating objective data as uncovered despite wide and unchallenged acceptance of some rather poorly founded clinical dogma to the contrary. Much has been questioned and a great deal left unanswered, as befits our continuing state of limited knowledge. There are no panaceas and no shortcuts to help us understand the mechanisms of labor or the mysteries of myometrial function. Even after a lifetime of study in this area, I frankly accept the fact that very little is actually known as to why specific labor patterns evolve in response to (more correctly, in association with) certain adverse conditions. The material presented is empirical. While objectivity is stressed, emphasis should nonetheless be placed on the fact that the primary approach to the parturient as a patient is still largely an art.

The book has been divided into four parts. The first deals with normal labor and the development of the clinical methods of approach to its study, reviewing known physiologic material and demonstrating the value and limitations of method. The second part details the analyses of varieties of abnormal labor, concentrating on definition, etiology, therapy, and prognosis. The effects of endogenous and exogenous factors on the course of labor are dealt with in the third section. Finally, the concluding portion presents practical programs of management of the several labor abberations based on all the foregoing material. This last section has been greatly expanded so as to provide the clinician with as much insight into his or her analysis of individual labors in progress as possible. The material should be especially useful for application to daily practice.

It is hoped that the changes in format, style, emphasis, and scope will prove acceptable to a wider range of readers, thereby making this volume worthy to serve as a vehicle for communication and dispersion. I believe the material to be valuable to clinicians—experienced and novice alike, those in practice as well as those in training—and to academicians, to students of medicine and nursing, and to obstetric assistants. Its message should be carried to all those who are or who may be called upon to care for laboring patients. Having acquired the fundamental working knowledge in this important discipline, these critical people will have thus been endowed with the essential wherewithal to comprehend the nuances of the clinical labor phenomena and to conduct the management of parturients so as to recognize abnormalities promptly and to treat them appropriately and expeditiously. In this way, they should be able to optimize maternal and fetal results.

# Normal Labor

## PART I

# Introduction

## CHAPTER 1

The phenomenon of labor is dynamic. In order for the clinician to be able to comprehend its dynamism and translate this comprehension into practical terms for purposes of evaluation and management, objective details are essential. It is not my intention here to give a stereotyped, textbook-style review of the classic, accepted concepts of the mechanisms of labor, nor to deal with the pelvic and fetal diameters and anatomic configurations and the forces involved; nor even to discuss routine management of the parturient. For extensive discussions of such matters, the reader is referred to any one of several excellent textbooks that are currently available. Adequate fundamental background in these areas is essential if the reader is to benefit from the material to be presented. This should represent a supplement to the standard obstetric textbook presentations on labor.

Studies begun a quarter of a century ago showed the limitations of isolated, static observations in labor, no matter how elaborately they were obtained. Those early investigations demonstrated the intrinsic value of serial observations related in a meaningful way to elapsed time. Although they dealt only with changing cervical dilatation and fetal station, they helped to clarify some of our clouded concepts of clinical labor. Previously, labor was regarded in a vague, nebulous way. It was defined as a physiologic process that expels the products of conception at or near term. Traditionally, labor was characterized by progressive increases in frequency, intensity, and duration of uterine contractions, progressive effacement and dilatation of the cervix, and the progressive descent of the fetus through the birth canal.

The progressive changes called for by such definitions, however, were never adequately specified. The niceties of judgment necessary for assessing labor were attainable only as a consequence of long clinical experience. The mark of the authorities in such matters was the subtle nuances of their ill-defined pronouncements. These, of course, were usually accepted on faith. Dispassionate belief, unencumbered by facts, paved a straight pathway to practical learning.

Of course, one cannot deny that strong intuitive feelings develop with experience. Nevertheless, such concepts are difficult to characterize clearly. Despite this limitation, these insights are useful and meaningful in attacking many clinical situations faced in practice. The real problem comes when one tries to verbalize them for the purposes of teaching, clinical justification, or consultative rationalization.

Notwithstanding the thorough grounding we may acquire in our clinical training with particular reference to labor, many find serious defects in understanding. This comment is not meant to denigrate our postdoctoral residency training programs, but rather to reflect on our current limited state of knowledge. It applies especially to our approach to the extremes of variability in the labor patterns that we encounter in our daily clinical experience. At one extreme, for example, we accept as normal the multipara with clinically poor labor, whose contractions are mild, weak, of short duration, and relatively infrequent or even irregular, yet who progresses rapidly in cervical dilatation and in descent of the fetal presenting part. She may

*Table 1. TERMS IN CURRENT USE TO DESCRIBE LABOR VARIANTS*

| | |
|---|---|
| Aberrant labor | Hypotonic uterine dysfunction |
| Abnormal labor | Idiopathic functional dystocia |
| Arrested labor | Idiopathic inertia |
| Asymmetrical uterine action | Incoordinate labor |
| Bony dystocia | Incoordinate uterine action |
| Cervical achalasia | Inefficient uterine action |
| Cervical dystocia | Inert labor |
| Cervical rigidity | Inertial dystocia |
| Cervical spasm | Mechanical dystocia |
| Colicky labor | Myometrial dysfunction |
| Constriction ring dystocia | Obstructed labor |
| Desultory labor | Pathologic labor |
| Difficult labor | Pelvic dystocia |
| Dilatory labor | Positional dystocia |
| Discoordinate labor | Presentational dystocia |
| Disordered labor | Primary dysfunctional labor |
| Disordered uterine inertia | Primary inertia |
| Dysfunctional inertia | Primary uterine inertia |
| Dysfunctional labor | Prolonged labor |
| Dyskinetic dystocia | Protracted labor |
| Dystocia dyspituitary syndrome | Secondary inertia |
| Dystocic inertia | Secondary uterine dysfunction |
| Dystocic labor | Secondary uterine inertia |
| Failed labor | Soft tissue dystocia |
| Failure to progress | True uterine inertia |
| Faulty labor | Underaction of uterus |
| Fetal dystocia | Uterine asynchrony |
| Functional dystocia | Uterine dysfunction |
| Functional inertia | Uterine dystocia |
| Hypertonic incoordinate labor | Uterine exhaustion |
| Hypertonic inertia | Uterine fibrillation |
| Hypertonic lower uterine segment | Uterine inertia |
| Hypotonic inertia | |

even deliver precipitately in bed while we debate the question of whether or not she is actually in labor. At the same time, at the other extreme of the spectrum of clinical pictures of labor, we may also label as normal the labor of the nullipara with "booming" contractions, characterized as long, frequent, and of strong intensity, whose cervix dilates slowly and whose fetus descends almost imperceptibly over long periods of time through the birth canal. Between these extremes lies the entire spectrum of normal labor, consisting of myriads of variations.

If we recognize and accept the limitations of our clinical knowledge and diagnostic acumen, we must concede that there is a vast, ill-defined gray zone between the obviously normal and the clearly abnormal case. Without objective criteria, therefore, we cannot expect that we will be able to understand labor and its variants fully. This is cogently illustrated when we examine the wide range of terms used to describe abnormal labor. The 65 terms listed in Table 1 are a partial compilation, limited to the English language only. The breadth of variations of labor patterns that we see has made detailed and critical evaluation very difficult indeed. It is perhaps impossible to characterize the individual labor objectively if we wish to consider all its features at once. The presentation of material in this monograph, however, will show that the situation is not so hopeless as would appear to be the case at first. We will deal with the relationships of cervical dilatation against elapsed time in labor and the comparable patterns of fetal descent with elapsed time as practical clinical tools for assessing individual labors in progress. Moreover, they will serve as useful means for detecting abnormalities as they arise. Further, they will be shown to be valuable for purposes of studying the factors that may affect labor and for teaching important and pertinent principles of obstetric practice.

# Historical Background

## CHAPTER 2

The literature dealing with the clinical evaluation of the individual labor is extensive. Most reports are concerned with management and with the influence of certain procedures and medications upon labor. Extensive review of this material is well beyond our scope here. However, it must be stressed that foregoing studies based almost entirely on comparisons of the duration of labor or the duration of the first stage lack much of the sophistication that is available today.

Some of the clinical research that has been undertaken over the years in pursuit of useful knowledge concerning labor will be outlined. The desire to rise above mere clinical impression is apparent in those reports that define, document, and categorize the observable features of clinical labor. Such observations seek methods for analyzing labors in progress, with the ultimate objective of determining when abnormalities exist.

Among the substantive developments in the study of uterine function are the techniques for objective measurement through the application of increasingly sensitive bioelectronic devices. The approach of early investigators seems now to have been rather crude. Nonetheless, it represented an attempt to examine the features of labor objectively, acknowledging the obvious limitations then existing in knowledge and in the available tools for experimentation.

### *CLINICAL RESEARCH*

Calkins and his co-workers (1930, 1931, 1934, 1941, 1944) presented a growing mass of objective data bearing on variations in the length of the stages of labor. Careful retrospective studies attempted to demonstrate the effect on labor of such factors as maternal age, height, weight, parity, length of gestation, size of pelvis, and fetal weight. Parity was found to have a clearly defined effect on the duration of both the first and second stages of labor. Shortening with increasing parity was encountered. In multiparas, none of the clinical factors that were studied seemed to affect the length of either the first or second stage of labor, except fetal presentation. Occiput posterior positions, at first thought to prolong the first stage somewhat, were later found to have no influence. In the nullipara, large fetal size prolonged the first and second stages somewhat, whereas advancing maternal age (more than 30 years) influenced only the second-stage duration in a similar manner.

Calkins was convinced that accurate observations of the resistance of the cervix and of the pelvic floor, together with determinations of the effectiveness of the uterine contractions, would ultimately be useful in determining why there were such extreme variations in the length of labor. He felt that such critical observations of the factors of force and counteracting resistance should enable one to predetermine the probable duration of labor, and serve to reduce the high rate of operative interference. To this end, Calkins suggested that the consistency of the cervix, the thickness of its wall, and the length of its canal should be accurately determined and recorded just before labor begins or as early in labor as possible, together with observations on the effectiveness of labor contractions, when established.

In 1941, Calkins' work culminated in a report detailing the factors relevant to prediction of the length of the first stage. Analysis of information pertaining to the consistency of the cervix at the onset of labor and the motive force of uterine contractility as evaluated at the onset of active dilatation yielded information useful for purposes of predicting when delivery should occur. He showed that it was possible to predict the approximate length of the normal first stage on the basis of the intensity of the contractions, the degree of cervical effacement, softening of the cervix, and engagement of the fetal presenting part. For nulliparas, for example, if the cervix was soft and effaced and the fetal head engaged, good contractions completed the first stage in 3 hours, fair contractions in 6 hours, and poor contractions in 12 hours. If the cervix was firm, 3 hours was added to each of these estimates; if the head unengaged, 1 hour was added; if the cervix uneffaced, 3 more hours were added.

Admittedly a coarse technique, Calkins' scheme for predicting first-stage duration never enjoyed extensive acceptance. It required a degree of subjective uniformity in order to be effective. Such uniformity is not usually obtainable for meaningful, reproducible clinical evaluations of cervical resistance and of motive force. The resistance of the cervix in his hands was graded according to effacement, dilatation, and softness at the onset of labor; the uterine contractility, according to intensity and frequency at the onset of active dilatation. Additionally, the wide range of variations in the length of otherwise normal labors could not always be completely explained by this method.

Calkins presented a similar approach to the evaluation of the second stage of labor in 1944. He paid particular attention to the number of contractions it took to evolve the descent process. He emphasized the sequence of contractions rather than the elapsed or total time in labor. Duration of labor to that time was considered almost to the exclusion of all other factors in assessing labor progress. Calkins' approach represented a revival of a once-popular method.

The Wehenzahlen (pain count) technique, developed and popularized by Frey in 1929, proved to have limited usefulness as a graphic method for studying labor as a function of duration and the number of contractions necessary for its evolution. Frey felt that labor would not evolve without a predetermined given number of sufficiently strong contractions and that this number was more important than the time factor. His graphic method consisted of half-hourly notations of the accumulated number, the average duration, and the character of the contractions, together with information on the fetal heart rate, fetal presentation, cervical effacement and dilatation, and the gross degree of engagement. He found that nulliparas seldom required more than 300 contractions after the rupture of the membranes to deliver, and multiparas, rarely more than 200 (cited by Geisendorf, 1937). The consistent point of departure, namely, rupture of the membranes, should be noted in passing.

It is clear that, despite its obvious shortcomings, this method was the forerunner of more recent techniques that summate the number and the intensity of uterine contractions in a similar sequential manner. The much more meaningful uses of the so-called Montevideo units by Caldeyro-Barcia and his group (1958) are dealt with below. Unfortunately, neither the Wehenzahlen technique nor the approach used by Calkins provided any means for accurate evaluation of a labor in progress. Both directed attention to overall summation of the factors bearing on total duration. They left much unresolved with regard to the individual labor in progress.

Wolf (1946) recognized the need for exact and timely registration of the progress of cervical dilatation in 1930, and he accomplished the first such reported observations in modern times. Previously, only total labor time or the total time of rupture of the membranes was treated as a matter of pertinent interest. Wolf first portrayed his concept of Teileröffnungszeiten (fractional cervical dilatation time) in a graphic manner. This illustrated the dynamic aspects of the labor phenomenon, which he termed Bewegungsvorgang (motion process). It was represented diagrammatically in a retrospective fashion, with cervical dilatation plotted against the number of hours prior to delivery. It was obvious that the curve could not be constructed until delivery had taken place, since the delivery was used as the primary point of reference. Wolf implied that the course of the curve could provide significant insight into the operation of the biologic forces of labor, but his sole publication related only to rupture of the membranes and its effect on labor.

Zimmer revived interest in this subject in 1951. He presented studies using a Wegzeit-Diagramm (course-time graph) modified from the earlier work of Wolf. Here, too, the rupture of membranes was the central theme. Extensive statistical analysis of the curves yielded interesting information. For example, cervical dilatation was seen to progress faster in multiparas than in nulliparas. Similarly, maternal age seemed to have no influence on the pattern, except for some slight retardation in older multiparas. The curve was the same whether or not bony disproportion existed. The time of amniotomy also did not appear to alter it.

The course of the average normal curve showed an accelerated bend at 3- to 4-cm cervical dilatation. It was expressed as a pattern consisting of two straight lines meeting at this point of acceleration. The curve of labor progress was thought to be the result of change in the consistency of cervical tissue. The magnitude of the biologic forces that brought about these changes was felt to be determinable only when the degree of progressive change in the frequency of the contractions was taken into consideration. Again, one sees the prominence of the concept of contraction frequency and number in the obstetric thought processes of the day.

The curves were essentially hyperbolic in pattern. Their sigmoid characteristics were entirely overlooked. Although the major change in the slope was recognized to occur normally at or beyond 3 or 4 cm, no finite interval of transition was expected, and pure linearity was insisted upon. The influence of obstructive phenomena or of other conditions as they relate to changes in the curve was neither considered nor recognized. Variations in the pattern, both quantitative and qualitative, were not described. The device was used only in its academic role and strictly on a retrospective basis.

Independently at the same time, Koller (1948) described a graphic representation of the course of labor to facilitate practical control of the entire labor process and aid in its scientific study. His Partogramm consisted of a coordinate record, with zero time representing the point at which the membranes ruptured. Cervical dilatation was presented on an irregular scale with unequal divisions. Several steps in the cervical dilatation and the delivery process were used, namely, the diameters of a 1–2-franc coin, a 5-franc coin, a small palm, a palm, complete dilatation, and delivery of the baby and of the placenta.

Superimposing curves aligned at the time of rupture of the membranes, Koller demonstrated that dispersion of the patterns before and after this event was different. The curves indicating progress of labor tended to be less steeply inclined prior to amniotomy; labor progressed more rapidly following it. He concluded, therefore, that the effect seen was the result of the event of amniotomy. He felt that the amniotomy influences the duration of the total period of dilatation and the duration of the period of expulsion. Since the length of labor was likely to affect maternal and fetal prognosis, the diagram was felt to be valuable in that it gave one the option to try to maintain the duration within favorable limits. The continuous Partogramm was used extensively in the obstetric units at Basel with apparent success.

Koller and Abt (1950, 1952) reported that the curve begins horizontally and then changes progressively according to the degree of dilatation. The curve reflects the progress of labor by the angle of steepness. The greater the inclination, the faster the labor. When it is more flattened, the labor is slower. It is perfectly horizontal in arrested labors. An index of labor was devised by which the curve could be expressed simply. To obtain the index, one divided the duration preceding or following amniotomy by the number of phases that had transpired. The index obtained prior to amniotomy was expressed arbitrarily with a minus sign; after rupture of membranes, as a positive number. The sign had no apparent mathematical significance, merely indicating the status of the membranes.

These same investigators claimed that the establishment of the continuous Partogramm and the calculation of the indices gave a complete view of the progress of labor. We can take issue with this assertion from several points of view. The graphs were not actually true representations of progressive change because the scale was nonlinear and represented irregular increments of dilatation. This particular problem was a matter of contention for many years. Liepmann had made a strong plea for standardization of the cervical dilatation nomenclature in 1921. He stressed the practical need for expressing dilatation uniformly in centimeters.

Another deficiency of the Partogramm was the technique of centering the curve at the time of rupture of the membranes. Additionally, linear change was assumed to exist throughout. Analysis was solely concerned with average slope and with maximum delivery time. These measures provided only a rough picture of the course of labor and almost no ongoing means for evaluating a labor in progress.

In many of these early investigations, the prime focus was the effect of amniotomy on labor. Despite the intense effort expended by these studies, they essentially ignored objective study for purposes of (1) defining the complex phenomenon of labor, (2) establishing norms for its course with which comparisons might be made more accurately and more profitably, and (3) determining meaningful limits of normal. In retrospect, such serious shortcomings nullified a good deal of the value of these foregoing studies. Nevertheless, they have played an important role, serving to form the foundation for many more recent investigations.

## *LABORATORY RESEARCH*

Foregoing investigations dealing with human labor have been arbitrarily divided into clinical and laboratory segments here. Many objective clinical observations and studies have experimental laboratory overtones; by the same token, laboratory-type investigations using the human animal are often clinical in context. Nevertheless, we can distinguish approaches that employ the observer's inborn senses and learned skills from those which utilize mechanical contrivances of various kinds to document and delineate physical alterations of both qualitative and quantitative nature. We can show the value of purely clinical observations when properly interrelated. At the same time, we can recognize the limitations of the most sensitive instruments when employed to study the highly variable clinical course of the labor phenomenon.

Such tools may sometimes actually be too sensitive to provide a correct overall picture of labor, even though they may give accurate, detailed information concerning its intimate features. One might draw an analogy to the study of a large variegated structure with a magnifying glass or a microscope. Although the lens gives fine close-up details, it cannot be expected to help synthesize the entire organism easily.

Reynolds (1951) summarized the three basic mechanisms for the physiologic evaluation of the phenomenon of labor, encompassing morphologic, physical, and biochemical aspects. The first two of these refer to organ and tissue changes, with special reference to the anatomic variations of growth, increase in thickness, alteration on muscle distribution, vascular change, cervical softening and effacement, and many others. In addition, they involve the biophysical effects resulting from these changes. The morphologic changes that occur in pregnancy were described by him in such great detail (Reynolds, 1965) that they need not be recounted here.

Biochemical alterations include those cellular and subcellular changes involving the active contractile protein of muscle, actomyosin, its hormonal control, and the energy relationships prevailing. Csapo (1955) demonstrated the rapid increases in actomyosin, myosin, and adenosinetriphosphate (ATP) activity in myometrium with advancing pregnancy. He investigated the complex interrelationships between these substances, creatine-phosphate, the high-energy phosphate linkages binding the phosphate adenosine–ribose radical of the ATP, the ovarian steroid hormones, ion concentrations, and cell membrane potential. In this way Csapo helped to elucidate the biochemical mechanisms of the process.

Such studies have uncovered the superficiality of our earlier understanding. The underlying mechanisms by which skeletal muscle functions are not fully known, and skeletal muscle has been studied far more extensively than myometrium. This provides us with tangible evidence that much remains to be learned. For more detailed expositions of the biochemical aspects of uterine muscle contraction, the reader is referred to the extensive reviews written by Carston (1968) and by Vorherr (1972).

Among the biophysical parameters, research activities have largely concentrated upon the measurement of the expulsive forces and the electrical potential produced by the uterine muscle during contraction. Study of the physical aspects of myometrial activity—that is, the energy, force, work, and power of the uterine contractions generated in labor—has been based on in vivo measurement of pressure gradients.

A century of research on uterine contractility in pregnancy was surveyed by Harris and Gillespie (1950) and by Reynolds, Harris, and Kaiser (1954). These excellent reviews trace the technical growth in this field. Table 2 provides a superficial overview and is acknowledged to be incomplete at best.

Significant among these advances are the monumental works by Murphy (1947), Reynolds (1965), Caldeyro-Barcia (1961), and Csapo (1955). Murphy's exhaustive studies demonstrated the extent to which the Lorand tocograph could be applied. Of pertinent interest was his inability to distinguish

*Table 2. STUDIES ON HUMAN LABOR*

| | | |
|---|---|---|
| Kristeller | 1861 | Spring measuring device in forceps handle |
| Schatz | 1872 | Intrauterine balloon, 80-ml capacity |
| Haughton | 1873 | Polar orientation of uterine contraction theorized |
| Poullet | 1878 | Intrarectal balloon, multiple balloon systems |
| Polaillon | 1880 | Marey tambour modification |
| Westermark | 1880 | Semimicroballoon, 2-ml capacity |
| Schäffer | 1896 | External tocography introduced; air-hood |
| Bukömsky | 1896 | External tocograph with Marey tambour |
| Fabre | 1913 | Tocograph with steel spring device |
| Rübsamen | 1920 | Tocograph with suspended weight |
| Liepmann | 1921 | Standardized dilatation nomenclature |
| Rucker | 1925 | Voorhees bag pressure sensing |
| Crödel | 1927 | Direct reading tocograph |
| Wieloch | 1927 | Transabdominal cannulation |
| Frey | 1929 | Pain count techniques |
| Calkins et al | 1930 | Clinical predictors of length of labor |
| Wolf | 1930 | Cervical dilatation graphed |
| Bode | 1931 | Electrical activity recorded (electrohysterograph, EHG) |
| Dodek | 1932 | Self-contained tocograph |
| Frey | 1933 | Revolving disc recording tocograph |
| Lorand | 1933 | Single-unit, compact recording tocograph |
| Clason | 1934 | EHG with plate electrodes |
| Rech | 1934 | Tocograph with remote electrical recording device |
| Moir | 1936 | Pressure sensing via umbilical cord of first twin |
| Woodbury, Hamilton, and Torpin | 1938 | Multiple differential manometers |
| Karlson | 1944 | Carbon receptor pressure sensing |
| Dill and Maiden | 1946 | Rapid alternating and slow direct current EHG |
| Reynolds | 1947 | Multichannel strain gauge tocodynamometer |
| Alvarez and Caldeyro-Barcia | 1948 | Intrauterine hydrostatic pressure graphed |
| Koller | 1948 | Labor course graphed |
| Alvarez and Caldeyro-Barcia | 1950 | Intravesical catheter abdominal pressure sensing |
| Steer and Hertsch | 1950 | Multichannel EHG |
| Zimmer | 1950 | Labor course graphed |
| Wolf | 1951 | Induction coil cervimeter |
| Williams and Stallworthy | 1952 | Intraamniotic catheter |
| Alvarez and Caldeyro-Barcia | 1952 | Intramyometrial microballoon |
| Holliday and Heyns | 1952 | EHG with Ag–AgCl electrodes |
| Friedman | 1953 | Cervical dilatation–time function defined |
| Smyth | 1954 | Guard ring tocograph |
| Smyth | 1954 | Transformer coil cervimeter |
| Ingelman-Sundberg and Lindgren | 1955 | Intrauterine strain gauge sensing |

*Table 2. STUDIES ON HUMAN LABOR (cont.)*

| | | |
|---|---|---|
| Friedman | 1956 | Mechanical cervimeter |
| Siener | 1956 | Cervimeter with pneumatic recording device |
| Nixon and Smyth | 1957 | Transcervical extraamniotic balloon |
| Hendricks et al | 1959 | Intervillous space pressure measurement |
| Lindgren and Smyth | 1961 | Measurement of forces applied to cervix |
| Kelly and Schleifer | 1962 | Intrauterine extraamniotic strain gauge |
| Kornmesser and Nyboer | 1962 | Impedance plethysmography |
| Csapo and Takeda | 1963 | Implanted EHG microelectrodes |
| Friedman and Von Micsky | 1963 | Electromechanical recording cervimeter |
| Siener | 1963 | Cervimeter with potentiometric sensing |
| Csapo | 1964 | Intrauterine extraamniotic microballoon |
| Cordey and Stander | 1964 | Modified Malmström pressurized transducer |
| Siener | 1964 | Cervical dynamometer |
| Friedman | 1965 | Descent pattern defined |
| Stander | 1966 | Planimetric quantitation of contractions |
| Borell and Fernström | 1967 | Mechanisms of labor defined radiographically |
| Myers, Krapohl, and Varner | 1967 | Fourier series analysis of contraction wave |
| Lingren and Holmlund | 1969 | Utero-fetal frictional coefficient measured |
| Effer et al | 1969 | Uterine arrhythmia quantitated |
| Hogaki | 1969 | Labor simulation by mathematical model |
| Curran et al | 1969 | Ballistocardiographic study |
| Nyboer and Kornmesser | 1970 | Electrical impedance hysterography |
| Neuman et al | 1970 | Radiotelemetric pressure monitoring |
| Wolfs and Rottinghuis | 1970 | Internal bipolar electromyography |
| Sakaguchi and Nakajima | 1970 | Transcervical needle electrodes |
| Persianinov and Davydov | 1971 | Radiotelemetric intrauterine pressure recording |
| Hon and Paul | 1973 | On-line quantitation of contraction area |
| Sokol et al | 1973 | On-line interactive program for labor diagnosis |
| Smyth | 1973 | Ultrasonography of contractions |
| Lindgren | 1973 | Dilatation and contractility pattern correlated |
| Daels | 1974 | Differential contractility of myometrial zones |
| Chik et al | 1974 | Contractility data characterized temporally |
| Zador et al | 1974 | Cervimeter with ultrasound transducer |
| Kepka et al | 1975 | Computerized quantitation of contractility parameters |
| Seitchik and Chatkoff | 1975 | Pressure wave form characterized |
| Miller et al | 1976 | Contractility and progression correlated |

tocographically between the contractions of true and false labor. Despite this, the instrument was said to be able to distinguish primary from secondary inertia. Unfortunately, the use of single-channel instruments did not provide for study of coordination of uterine activity. This proved to be a serious shortcoming of the technique.

Revivals of various modifications of external tocography have been attempted from time to time (LaCroix, 1968). Although increasingly greater precision has been possible, such instrumentation does not permit precise physiologically meaningful documentation of the magnitude of the contractions or the resting tonus of the uterus between contractions. The use of distorted detection and recording systems provide data that are not reliable. They cannot provide information concerning coordination or propagation of myometrial activity.

Even the study of the pressure generated within the amniotic sac by the uterine contraction (see below) does not necessarily portray the overall picture of the labor process as it evolves. Reliance on such means stems from the widely held assumption that progress in labor must directly reflect the amplitude and frequency of uterine contractions. Despite the fact that this may seem reasonable and overtly logical on the basis of currently limited knowledge of uterine physiology, one should be wary of drawing untenable conclusions about clinical phenomena solely from this type of limited evidence. We should be cognizant of the relatively small degree of clinical validity with which we can assess uterine activity, even with the aid of sophisticated tocodynamometric techniques. Only in conjunction with other measures of labor progress can the efficacy of contractility be weighed (Friedman, 1968).

With the multichannel tocodynamometer, Reynolds expanded the vista in this area. His monograph (1965) detailing extensive studies will serve for many years as a starting point for any relevant physiologic undertaking. It is beyond our scope here to review this material, but it is important to emphasize that many of the concepts of uterine action that we hold today are well founded in his work. Of special interest are his clear demonstrations of fundal dominance and the relationship between myometrial structure and the tensile forces that develop during pregnancy and labor.

Caldeyro-Barcia (1958, 1959) studied the aspects of labor relating to isometric pressure produced during myometrial contractions. He used intra-amniotic polyethylene catheters connected to a pressure transducer for recording amniotic pressure. A convenient unitage was devised, incorporating intensity and frequency of contractions. The intensity was measured by the amplitude of the intrauterine pressure above the basal tonus; the frequency was the number of contractions for each 10-minute interval. This was expressed as Montevideo units in millimeters of mercury per 10 minutes. In practice, it is merely necessary to summate the peak contractile amplitudes of contractions occurring within a given 10-minute interval to obtain the relevant unitage. It is unnecessary duplication to obtain the average amplitude first (summation of amplitudes divided by the number of contractions) and then multiply that value by the number of contractions in the interval under consideration.

By this method, only peak pressures are taken into account. No consideration is given to the duration of the contractions, the area under the curve, or the potential influence of any alteration in the basal tonus. Despite these minor shortcomings, this method of study is of considerable value and has contributed a great deal to our understanding of the physiology of labor.

The cumulated pressures have been described for the different stages of pregnancy and for labor as well. Tracings have been correlated with clinical information. The apparent origin of the contractile wave in the cornual region of the uterus, ostensibly from a pacemaker site, has been defined by using multiple intramyometrial microballoons. It should be noted that no specific conducting structures comparable to those in the heart have as yet been demonstrated. Moreover, frequency–curve analytic studies by Schulman and Romney (1970) yielded data incompatible with the concept of a focal pacemaker site; they felt that uterine contractions appeared to obey the uniform probability law instead.

A triple descending gradient has been described: the musculature at the fundus of the uterus undergoes stronger contractions that occur earlier and are of longer duration than those of the lower uterus. These descending gradients of propagation, duration, and intensity are said to be essential for the production of cervical dilatation. Coordination of the contractile waves has also been described. More pertinently, incoordination in the form of asynchrony was demonstrated. The end results of such abnormal contractile patterns are slowed or arrested progress in labor.

The functional kinetic characteristics of the myometrium in vitro have been detailed by Csapo (1955) with regard to (1) the factors that determine the maximum tensile strength that the muscle is capable of developing, (2) the relationship between muscle length and tension, (3) the correlation between the strength of electrical stimulation and the duration of the resulting contractions, and (4) the relationship between the speed of muscle shortening and the weight of the load that is applied. He found that the principles of myometrial contraction are entirely comparable to those of skeletal muscle, but that there were significant differences in the kinetics of their reaction. In relative terms, skeletal muscle fibers manifest small forces over long distances at high velocities; by contrast, the smooth muscle fibers of the myometrium exert large forces over short distances at low speed. While the contractile mechanism appears to be the same as in skeletal muscle, our knowledge must be considered very fragmentary.

Disparities exist between the data obtained by all these very sensitive techniques and the course of clinical labor. It has been shown, for example, that only small increases in amplitude and frequency of uterine contractions occur as labor advances. Despite this, the pattern of cervical dilatation undergoes marked change. Very slow progress occurs early in the first stage, and usually there is very rapid progress subsequently. One can infer from this that a great deal of energy is dissipated in preparing the cervix early in labor, but much smaller increments of activity are needed to produce the rapid cervical dilatation that occurs near the end of the first stage (Burnhill, Danezis, and Cohen, 1962; Miller et al, 1976). Moreover, the rates of normal cervical dilatation do not appear to be related to either rhythmical or nonrhythmical uterine action (Schulman and Romney, 1970). No change in the index of uterine arrhythmia was encountered in association with labor progression (Effer et al, 1969). Similarly, neither basal tonus nor duration of contractions was correlated (Krapohl et al, 1970), although amplitude was somewhat related to labor progression.

Other examples of the dissociation between uterine contractility patterns and the work produced by such contractions will be presented later. For now, it is important to bear in mind that contractility per se does not necessarily give one a clear idea of labor progression. This holds no matter how precisely the contractility is measured. To date, moreover, there is literally no objective way to distinguish between contractions of normal labor, disordered labor, false labor, or nonlabor.

The basic limitations of internal tocography in current common use today are as follows: (1) The intrauterine balloon, bag, catheter, or strain gauge acts as a foreign body, thus altering the normal physiology that is being studied; (2) limited, damped, or otherwise distorted detection and recording systems provide reproducible data that may or may not reflect what is actually taking place; (3) the use of a single modality or limited modalities of observation do not provide information concerning coordination or propagation; (4) study of a single parameter, such as the pressure generated isometrically within the amniotic sac by uterine contraction, does not necessarily give an accurate overall picture of the labor process as it evolves. Recent engineering improvements have overcome some of these objections, but the techniques still face serious limitations. For an impressive review of the diagnostic use of intrauterine pressure measurement and its limitations in current practice, the reader is referred to Csapo (1970).

Most of these modalities of study have contributed to the expansion of the frontiers of obstetric research. They may in the future provide us with greater insights into the physiology and physiopathology of the uterus than we have today. Nevertheless, for all their accuracy and reproducibility, these techniques involve cumbersome, expensive, and delicate equipment as well as degrees of technical knowledge generally not possessed by the average practicing obstetrician. Moreover, they require time, competence, and the inclination to apply. These modalities of study are becoming more widely available, however, as necessary concomitants of fetal heart rate monitoring. In view of their limited value for assessing labor, it is reasonable to try to provide more practical and usable tools for the study of individual labors in progress by obstetricians who do not have the advantages available in teaching and research institutions.

# Hypothetical Considerations

## CHAPTER 3

Except for cervical dilatation and fetal descent, none of the clinical features of the parturient patient appears to be useful in assessing labor progression. A conceptual model of the labor phenomenon, employing the two relevant markers of dilatation and descent, is outlined. A simple method for implementing this concept is introduced for purposes of clinical quantitation.

The clinical features of uterine contractions—namely, frequency, intensity, and duration—cannot be relied upon as measures of progression in labor nor as indices of normality. Normal uterine contractile patterns encompass a broad range, from negligible to tumultuous activity. At the same time, abnormal forms of labor may be associated with patterns that are entirely indistinguishable from normal labor in all its features.

Of course, we cannot summarily dismiss the factor of contractility as meaningless. Contractions are essential for evolving the process of labor. Nevertheless, we should be cognizant of the relatively small amount of useful clinical information that is provided by an assessment of uterine activity. It is only in conjunction with other measures of progress that the efficacy of contractility can be weighed. These other measures include cervical effacement, cervical dilatation, and descent of the fetal presenting part through the birth canal. These constitute the work output of the gravid uterus and are the end results of all the forces of labor acting on the uterine contents and on the maternal soft tissues.

Effacement is the passive reduction in length of the cervical canal. It reflects intrinsic changes that have taken place within the cervix itself, affecting stromal connective tissue, blood vessels, collagen, fluid content, and other components. Effacement is a response to the forces of uterine contraction transmitted to the cervix from the active contractile portion of the upper uterus by way of the lower uterine segment. While basically considered a passive response, Danforth et al (1974) have shown that collagen and glycoprotein destruction, with simultaneous synthesis of unidentified glycosaminoglycans, suggests an active dynamic process is taking place during cervical dilatation.

However, the value of effacement is very limited in the assessment of labor. This is so because the process is generally completed before labor begins in most nulliparas, and it may not take place in many multiparas until late in the first stage. There is no question that effacement, softening, and the beginning of dilatation are integral phenomena of late pregnancy and the early portion of the first stage. They often take place during a major increment of time elapsed in labor. Effacement can neither be relied upon to give the clinician a realistic picture of progress, nor does it necessarily indicate normalcy.

This leaves us with only two observable and clinically useful features of labor that can be used profitably for assessing labor with any degree of reliability; namely, cervical dilatation and fetal descent. It is of critical concern, therefore, that we attempt to characterize the normal progressive course of both of these variables as indices of what should be expected in labor. If such information were available, we would have in hand a critical means for assessing normality and for diagnosing abnormality.

Although a somewhat oversimplified viewpoint, it is appropriate to consider the patient in labor as a complex machine. Accepting our limited understanding of the mechanisms involved in uterine activity, we can study energy input, work output, and factors that affect both. The two components of the inherent work demanded of the gravid patient are cervical dilatation and fetal descent. Dilatation of the cervix is essential for purposes of overcoming the barrier to empty the uterine contents. Descent merely reflects the sequence of events involved in the evacuation itself.

The energy sources acting to accomplish these objectives are uterine contractions on the one hand, and the expulsive efforts of the abdominal and diaphragmatic muscles on the other. By analogy, a lever can serve to elucidate the interrelationship between the energy input and the work output (Fig. 1). At the lower end, the box representing the work to be accomplished (cervical dilatation and fetal descent) may be considered as being filled with heavy objects to be lifted. In order to lift the work output box (that is, to accomplish dilatation and descent), the empty energy input counterweight on the upper arm of the lever must be filled. The filling material consists of effective uterine contractions and strong expulsive efforts.

The mechanistic concept of the balance of forces and resistances at play during the course of labor may be readily clarified in this way. It permits us to consider factors that can enhance or diminish the efficacy of uterine contractility; similarly, we can discuss those factors that increase or decrease the burden of the work that has to be accomplished. For example, the driving force of the uterine contractions may be enhanced by the use of uterotonic agents, or may be attenuated by a variety of factors, including anxiety states, uterine anomalies, overdistention by multiple pregnancy or hydramnios,

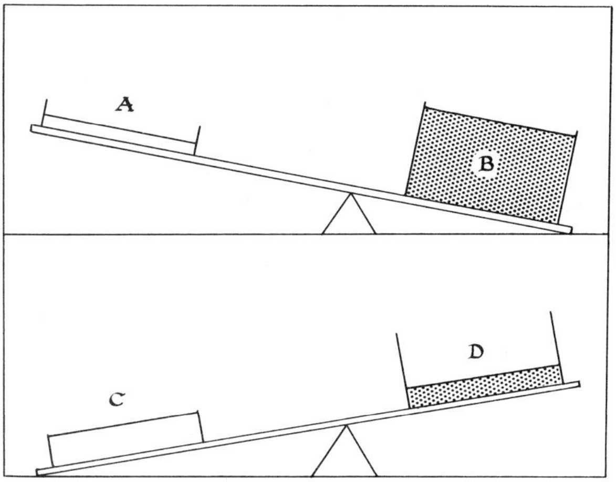


*Fig. 1.* Lever concept to represent energy input in the form of uterine and abdominal expulsive forces (A,C) needed to achieve work output in overcoming soft tissue and bony resistance (B,D) to accomplish cervical dilatation and fetal descent in labor. Poor contractions (A), perhaps caused by anxiety, high parity, debilitation, uterine anomaly, or overdistention by multiple pregnancy or hydramnios, may fail to achieve the work objective. Similarly, increased resistance (B), due to poor prelabor preparation, inelasticity, scarring, disproportion, malpresentation, tumor obstruction, or contraction ring, may impede effective progress. By contrast, strong contractile and expulsive forces (C) coupled with increased elasticity and decreased resistance (D) yield good labor performance.

leiomyomata uteri, high parity, and various debilitating disorders. Additionally, inhibitory pharmacologic agents may also adversely affect contractility, thereby reducing its influence on work output.

The burden of work that the pregnant uterus must achieve is reduced significantly if maternal soft tissues have been adequately prepared prior to labor, that is, by increasing their elasticity and decreasing the resistance to dilatation. This is a recognized characteristic of women who have had prior vaginal deliveries. An extreme variant of decreased resistance is the situation prevailing in the gravida with cervical incompetence; excessive prelabor soft tissue preparation offers essentially no resistance to dilatation and descent under these circumstances. The work requirement is considerably enhanced, on the other hand, by increased resistance and inelasticity, as in patients whose labors begin with the cervix long, closed, rigid, and unyielding. Factors that impose additional problems in this regard include fetopelvic disproportion, tumor obstruction, malpresentation, and malposition; these increase the work to be accomplished considerably.

Such a simple, mechanistic concept of the labor phenomenon allows us to consider separately those factors relating to energy resources and those contributing to or alleviating work requirements. Furthermore, the two component ends of the lever diagram can also be interrelated. The physics of this relationship between energy input and work output is well defined: the ratio of one to the other is a measure of the efficiency of the mechanical device under study. This is usually represented by the equation

$$\text{efficiency} = \frac{\text{work output}}{\text{energy input}}$$

The degree of efficiency of any device can be ascertained only when both the energy input and work output are quantifiable. When both are measurable, the level of efficiency can serve for the purpose of determining when the machine is malfunctioning.

The components of the efficiency equation for the laboring patient consist of the summation of contractile and expulsive forces counterbalanced by the composite resistance of maternal tissues to dilatation and descent. Whereas the driving forces are readily measurable in great detail by available means today (Chapter 2), we have no way to measure resistance accurately. Therefore, a direct quantitation of efficiency is not obtainable. A more indirect approach, however, is at hand. The end results of all the forces of labor are apparent in the essential work that must be accomplished in order for labor to terminate normally; namely, progressive cervical dilatation and progressive descent of the fetal presenting part. Both must occur in the normal course of labor. As we shall see below, examination of the rates at which these events take place, particularly at their maxima, will provide an indirect measure of the efficiency of the labor process. For our purposes, it will serve adequately for assessing normality.

Measurement of cervical dilatation has long been used as a guide for evaluating labor. Comparable objective measurement of fetal station by the vaginal or rectal route is of more recent vintage. Isolated observations, however, present a static concept in that they represent only momentary observations within the framework of a process that is continually changing. The picture of the entire process of labor that is portrayed by such isolated observations is wholly inadequate. These observations may provide a false or distorted view. Nonetheless, determinations of the cervical dilatation and the fetal station are the most readily available means at our disposal for studying labor. When properly employed and correlated with other available information, these determinations may be of inestimable aid in elucidating the proper management of the parturient. The objectives of study, development, utilization, and extensive application have been to accumulate information and to translate it into valuable and practical principles.

Among the major observable clinical features of labor, as we have seen, only cervical dilatation and fetal descent seem utilitarian because they mirror overall progress. This applies to all but the initial portion of the first stage. Analogous to an only door in a windowless room, the cervix represents the major impediment to the passage of the conceptus from the uterus. It is apparent that the cervix must open and descent of the fetus must take place for the uterine contents to be ejected. Looking at the situation from the mechanistic point of view, we can see that the cervix plays essentially a passive role as an innocent obstruction and is acted upon by all the forces of labor. From this vantage point, as stated earlier, its dilatation is the resultant of all the driving forces of uterine contraction acting against passive tissue resistance. Thus, dilatation of the cervix is one of the effective end results of these forces, and in this role it serves to reflect the progress of labor. The same can be said about the station of the fetal presenting part in later progress in labor. Late in the first stage and during the second stage of labor, when the cervix has been fully dilated and retracted out of reach, the fetal station subserves the same role as an index of progression, as cervical dilatation did earlier.

Even if we accept that changing dilatation of the cervix and descent of the fetus represent progress and reflect degrees of normalcy, we are still lacking any significant means for quantitation. Ephemeral concepts are widely held about what constitutes normal progress. In some quarters, rapid change is expected and somewhat less rapid change is accepted. In other areas, even the most dilatory progress is considered normal as long as some progress is being made. At either extreme, errors in judgment are evident. The great sensitivity of the former approach categorizes many normal labors as abnormal; at the other extreme, the narrow selectivity causes many cases that are probably abnormal to be included in the normal group. Thus, sensitivity and selectivity are at odds. This is precisely the kind of dilemma faced in any biologic phenomenon that encompasses a wide spectrum.

How then might one quantitate progress in labor? Historically, we sought the answer to this practical question in the early 1950s. At that time, great interest was being generated in the effect of conduction anesthesia on labor. It soon became evident that we had no satisfactory means for assessing progress in labor or for determining the short-term effect on the course of labor of the anesthesia that was being administered. Although studies could be performed for measuring contractile patterns (Hallet, 1953) or the total duration of labor, these did not give us the information we desired. Contractility studies were much too sensitive and did not truly reflect overall progressive change; total labor duration was far too insensitive to reflect the transient effects that the anesthesia might have brought about.

A simple, objective, reproducible, clinically available tool was needed for this purpose. Evaluation of progress in labor—previously synonymous with a nebulous degree of change—had to be made available in terms of specific rate of change. This was conceived as a possible solution to our dilemma. Without prior knowledge of foregoing work in this area, a method was devised whereby the rate of change in cervical dilatation could be related to elapsed time. Careful study has since revealed that the rate of change is essentially specific for each patient. This refers to the increments of cervical dilatation per unit of time as well as to the rate of change in fetal station, within the limits of acceptable error. Further, the rate of change could be shown to undergo predictable changes during the course of normal labor. By this technique, a new dimension was introduced to us. This early seed of discovery and invention resulted from necessity. Since then, many tangential explorations have been possible, and much has been learned about labor.

Very simply, the method consists of inscribing multiple isolated observations of cervical dilatation and fetal station on simple *xy* coordinates, using square-ruled graph paper. The abscissa is the elapsed time in hours from the onset of labor, and the ordinate is cervical dilatation in centimeters, or the station in centimeters above (negative values) or below (positive values) the plane of the ischial spines (or zero station). A degree of uniformity was obtained by timing labor from the onset of regular uterine contractions. This retrospective historical concept of onset was recognized to have certain limitations because it depended upon the patient's subjective perception of her contractility. The time of onset was based upon simple inquiry of when the contractions had begun with regularity. If the response to this question left the issue unresolved, the patient was asked when the contractions had changed to their current character. At best, this information was subjective in nature and prone to error, but acceptable for our purposes, since nothing else comparable was available.

Some difficulty has been encountered in correlating our data with those of laboratory-oriented physiologists, because they prefer to consider the onset of labor as that point in time when 2 cm of cervical dilatation has been reached after the onset of uterine contractions. Similarly, there are those who are concerned only with that part of labor beginning with hospital admission (Hendricks et al, 1970; Philpott and Castle, 1972a, b; Studd, 1973). This categorically ignores the rather important interval from the onset of contractions to actively progressive dilatation, an interval that we now call the latent phase. Since one cannot distinguish the contractile pattern of prelabor from that of the latent phase of early labor by the most sensitive instruments, this portion of labor is thereby conveniently overlooked by physiologists. To the practicing clinician, however, it is sometimes rather important; to the patient and her offspring, it is often very significant.

An attempt was made to ensure uniformity with regard to estimating cervical dilatation and fetal station. Occasional discrepancies existed between measurements obtained during contraction and during the quiescent interval between contractions. It was felt that the estimation of dilatation (or station) at the height of a contraction would not only be more reliably accurate, but would also be more realistic as a measure of the effective dilatation (or descent) that had been achieved. In later years, when more accurate, objective, and continuous recordings of dilatation were available (see Chapter 4), this principle was verified as sound.

Cervical dilatation and fetal station were determined by frequent digital examinations. Estimations were based on rectal and vaginal examinations. From the beginning, we did not hesitate to resort to vaginal examinations for the purpose of obtaining accurate data, particularly if the rectal route was found to be unsatisfactory. Over the years, less and less intensive preparation of the perineum was done for vaginal examinations. Initially, detailed preparation of the perineum as an aseptic field and sterile draping was ritually performed; more recently, merely a sterile rubber glove and simple soap preparation were found to be almost equally innocuous. Currently, the vaginal route is used almost exclusively.

Parenthetically, determinations were found to be most accurate at the onset and at the termination of dilatation; that is, at less than 3 cm and at more than 7 cm. Fetal station increased in accuracy with progressive descent of the fetal presenting part toward the perineum. A study was carried out to probe the question of the degree of error inherent in digital estimations of cervical dilatation. Examinations by 40 individuals with varying degrees of experience, utilizing models constructed to represent various dilatations, degrees of effacement, and softness, yielded an error rate of 3 percent. There did not seem to be any significant improvement with experience. Similar results were recently found with station determinations. On the basis of these data, therefore, our subsequent studies were deemed to be on relatively firm ground.

Plotting estimates of cervical dilatation against the time that has elapsed in labor, one derives the type of cervical dilatation pattern depicted in Figure 2 in all normal labors. This sigmoid or S-shaped curve is quite characteristic. Study of its normal variants and its aberrations has provided much useful clinical information. Plotting station against time yields the typical hyperbolic curve shown here. It, too, serves a similar role.

A technique has evolved for evaluating the individual patient in labor while her labor is in progress. Groups of labors can also be studied to learn

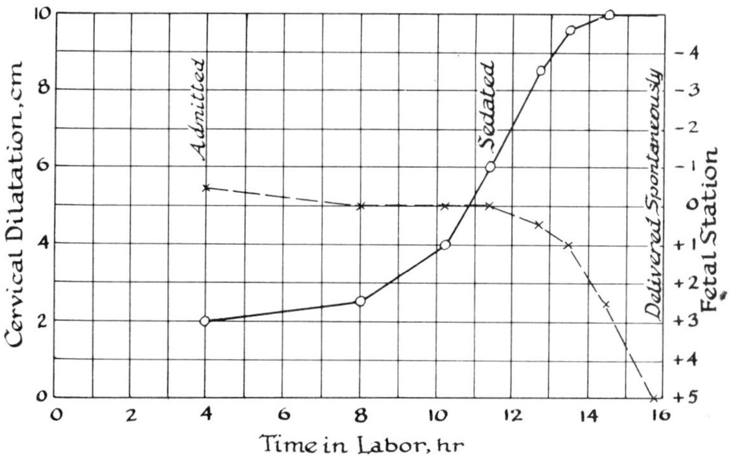


*Fig. 2.* Evolution of normal patterns of cervical dilatation (*solid line*) and fetal descent (*broken line*). Dilatation is plotted in centimeters (left scale) and entered according to the number of hours elapsed in the course of labor to trace the characteristic sigmoid curve shown, typical of all normal labors. Similarly, the hyperbolic curve of descent is traced in all normally progressive labors by plotting estimates of fetal station (right scale) against time in labor.

the effect that various factors may have on labor. The curves obtained in all normal cases were found to be nearly identical. They varied from individual to individual in the length of the various portions and in the inclination of the central part.

Recognizing this, we were eager to proceed to evaluate individual labors in progress and to analyze the course of groups of labors statistically, with particular reference to the effects of exogenous and endogenous factors upon the duration and the slope of the several portions of the curve. Our studies were developed based on the foundation of simplicity and ready adaptability to the clinical problems at hand.

It was hypothesized that labor could be defined in more precise terms than previously available by means of simple graphic representations. The patterns thus obtained were suitable for purposes of statistical breakdown for the study of numerous factors that might affect the course of labor. The proof of this hypothesis rested on the subsequent objective verification of the existence of the sigmoid curve of cervical dilatation and of the hyperbolic curve of descent.

# Objective Verification

## CHAPTER 4

The sigmoid pattern of cervical dilatation has been confirmed by objective means. The range of physiologic instrumentation devised for monitoring dilatation is reviewed. The shortcomings of these experimental tools are dealt with in order to stress their limited applicability to clinical usage in their current state of development.

Confirmation of the characteristic cervical dilatation patterns awaited the development of techniques for continuous and objective measurements of cervical dilatation in labor. The aims of such instrumentation included accuracy, detail, and uninterrupted recording of these changes as they occurred. Prior to the availability of suitable apparatus, the only realistic and practical means for determining the size of the cervical opening were digital examinations by way of the vagina or the rectum or inspection by vaginal speculum. As to descent, attempts to objectify station observations by instrumental measuring devices have to date been largely unsuccessful. Estimations of fetal station are still best obtained by digital examination; a less preferable and somewhat less accurate method involves suprapubic abdominal examination of the cranial prominences with relation to the pelvic inlet.

Palpatory observations of cervical dilatation date back to 1816, when Ebermaier first described the changes in the cervical os that could be palpated by the examining fingers in the vagina (Langreder, 1959). In 1894, independently of each other, Kroenig and Ries first recommended palpation by way of the rectum.

One of the earliest reported attempts to measure the cervix instrumentally was that by Wolf in 1951. He recorded cervical dilatation by applying small induction coils to the external os. No details of this method are available. Transmitting a small electric current through one of the coils should be expected to set up an electromagnetic field that might be detectable in the opposite coil if the current and the coils are large enough and the distance sufficiently small. Changing the distance between the coils (as a result of cervical dilatation, for example) would then be reflected in an altered output from the secondary coil. Attempts to reproduce this technique in recent years have failed.

Smyth, in 1954, measured cervical dilatation employing the principle of linear differential transformers. Movement of a ferromagnetic core (20-gauge iron wire) with respect to the windings altered a measurable electric output. The primary winding of the transformer was excited by a current of 5000 cycles per second. Output was produced in the opposing secondary windings. When the resting position of the core was arranged to provide a readable output, movements of the core about this position caused the output to increase or decrease. A modification of this device with two cores suitable for registering the difference between two movements was used for recording cervical dilatation. Despite its firm theoretical basis, this instrument was of limited use in practice.

The first workable mechanical device was reported by Friedman in 1956a. The apparatus was designed to function on a simple geometric principle: isosceles triangles whose arms and apical angles are equal have equal bases. The earliest form consisted of two thin nonmalleable metal rods of equal length that were attached to the cervix at 3 and 9 o'clock, respectively, by means of sharp hooks. These rods articulated at their midpoints. The linear distance between the distal extravaginal ends was equal to the distance between the proximal cervical ends, thus providing a means for measuring cervical dilatation. Although it was easy to apply the hooks to the cervix, they were too easily dislodged in the course of labor. Several varieties of metal clips and sutures were tried. A small bulldog battery clip, 8-mm wide with spring clamp and serrated jaws, was found to be best with regard to ease of application, ease of removal, tenacity, and lack of trauma.

The levator ani muscles impinged on the lateral excursion of the proximal arms, preventing accurate measurement of dilatation greater than 7 cm. This was overcome in two ways. First, the inner arms were shortened so that the point of articulation became located just inside the introitus. Second, the proximal arms were bent to cross at their midpoints without articulating. This effectively halved the lateral range of motion at the level of the levators, permitting critically accurate readings to well beyond full dilatation. Unfortunately, this modification no longer permitted the instrument to measure cervical dilatation directly because as the intravaginal ends separated, the extravaginal ends approached each other. Accordingly, the instrument required calibration. In its final form, the proximal arms were bent to accommodate the pelvic curve, thereby effectively eliminating almost all distortion.

The instrument consisted of a pair of 25-cm-long uterine dressing forceps, articulating by a removable thumbscrew at the midpoint. The intravaginal extremity incorporated the aforementioned pelvic curve, compensating lateral bend, and bulldog clamps welded to each tip. A hinged centimeter rule at the distal end measured cervical dilatation after calibration. The readings were found to be accurate within 0.5 mm over the entire range of dilatation. This compared rather favorably with the error inherent in digital estimations. The major shortcomings of this instrument were the discontinuity of readings of dilatation and the lack of a means for incorporating the output into a recording device.

At the same time, Siener (1956) described an instrument by means of which the dilatation of the cervix could be continuously recorded. It, too, had two intravaginal arms with built-in, compensating, reversed bends. These articulated at the introitus. Siener's Zervixwehenmesser was attached to the cervix by means of hooks. The extravaginal arms incorporated a pneumatic system: When displaced by cervical dilatation, the movement of the arms could be recorded kymographically. In this way, gross instantaneous changes in the cervix could be recorded.

In 1957, Siener presented a somewhat different type of instrument. Cords attached by hooks to the four quadrants of the cervix (at 3, 6, 9, and 12 o'clock) were led out through a tubular structure and fixed to kymographic recording needles. Motion of the cervix during contraction and dilatation was transmitted to the kymograph. The value of this device was limited because it required absolute fixation and immobility of the patient.

Siener reported an improved modification of his instrument in 1963. He employed two sets of intestinal clamps with detachable handles to secure it to the lateral margins of the cervix. The receptor portion was attached to the outer ends of the clamps protruding from the vagina. This part was equipped with a potentiometer, from which changes in electrical potential could be transmitted to a recorder.

In the same year, Friedman and Von Micsky (1963) presented a similar electromechanical device. This modified Friedman's original instrument by incorporating a potentiometer at the point of articulation. It recorded the angular displacement of the intravaginal arms as the cervix dilated. The original cervimeter had been found to give reasonably accurate determinations of cervical dilatation objectively, but it lacked means for continuous recording. This feature was essential in studies involving the physiology of labor, particularly for confirming the dilatation–time relationship. The tedium of multiple readings and calibrations limited the usefulness of the original device and curtailed its effectiveness. Instantaneous recordings were expected to give information on the more subtle changes of the cervix and perhaps provide data to help elucidate the in vivo function of the cervix in labor. These needs were satisfied by the development of the electronic cervimeter.

The basic design was that of a compact rugged instrument that could be sterilized by autoclave. It weighed 90 g, the intravaginal portion, only 50 g. A pair of lever arms could be secured to the opposing rims of the external os of the cervix by means of a retractable row of needles that held a portion of the cervical lip fixed within a molded socket. The needles were engaged and disengaged from the lateral aspects of the cervix by means of an external cable-release device that terminated directly in the housing in the proximal ends of the lever arms. The arms in turn were attached to a potentiometer, to which a small voltage was applied.

As the cervix dilated, the upper portion of the arms separated while the lower portion closed. As the angle between the arms at the end of the potentiometer decreased, the voltage output of the potentiometer changed. This voltage in turn was applied to an electronic unit whose amplifier system provided current for registration on a graphic recorder. The instrument was also designed with an alarm system that indicated when a preset dilatation had been reached. This could trigger the automatic release of the needle attachments to the cervix.

As cervical dilatation progressed in the course of labor, the aforementioned exaggerating factors were seen to come less and less into play. The instrument then took on greater accuracy. This became apparent when it was appreciated that the separation of the shanks diminished as the cervix opened. Near full cervical dilatation, the shanks were almost juxtaposed.

The readings were not perfectly linear, since the dilatation was translated into angular changes at the potentiometer. Electronic adjustments within the recorder, however, compensated for this nonlinearity to provide a very good approximation of the absolute values. The apparatus gave reproducibly accurate readings after calibration with a mean error of less than 1 percent. The instrument yielded excellent recordings of cervical dilatation of far greater accuracy than could possibly be obtained with the examining finger.

Of interest here were the results obtained when the peaks of the curves were plotted graphically against time. The curves were sigmoid in shape, confirming previously recorded clinical observations. Slight changes in dilatation early in labor but before the upswing of the sigmoid curve were shown in some cases. The existence of the deceleration phase, characterized by a flattening of the curve just before full cervical dilatation, was confirmed in normal nulliparous labors. Deviations due to variations in duration and slope were noted, but all normal uncomplicated labors fell into the same general pattern. The slow, characteristically prolonged sigmoid patterns encountered in some dysfunctional labors were also seen. Major alteration in pattern occurred in arrested labors, with marked flattening of the curve prior to full dilatation. Minor degrees of slowing were also apparent after the administration of large doses of analgesic–sedative medication. These were real changes, but so small that they were undetectable by digital examination.

The normal pattern of cervical dilatation was thus verified by objective cervimetry to be sigmoid in character. Dilatation was seen to occur slowly at first, then to accelerate until a maximum constant slope was attained, and finally to decelerate just prior to full dilatation. The duration of the respective phases was determined not to differ significantly from those values obtained by digital estimations. The mean maximum slope was likewise similar.

Zador et al devised an instrument for measuring cervical dilatation in

1974, using small ceramic piezoelectric crystals as ultrasound transducers. These were mounted on spring clips and thereby attached to the opposite lips of the cervix. A signal generated by the transmitting crystal excited the receiving transducer. The transit time served as a measure of the distance between the crystals and was displayed continuously on a recorder. Use of this device in labor by Sokol et al in 1976 again verified the sigmoid curve of dilatation, but observations suggested displacement of the spring clips during intravaginal examinations or manipulations, a phenomenon encountered by others in the past (Friedman and Von Micsky, 1963). As a consequence, dilatation appeared to decrease transiently during the course of labor. Since it is unclear that the transducers remained attached to the most lateral aspect of the cervical os, these observations need clarification.

Another form of ultrasonic instrument for measuring cervical dilatation has also been described (Kok et al, 1976). The labor pattern it traces compares with the sigmoid curve we have detailed here.

It is apparent that the error associated with rectal and vaginal examinations is relatively small when compared with the wide variations among labors. Any limiting inaccuracy of digital examinations, upon which subsequent data and evaluations of labor are to be based, is rather insignificant. While cervimetric instruments may be considered accurate for purposes of measuring cervical dilatation, it is clear that frequent digital examination is both useful and much more expedient for achieving the same ends. This is perhaps particularly the case because the variations among labors are far greater than the superior accuracy of the objective cervimeter warrants. Although useful, it is seriously doubted that such devices will ever become universal in application other than for experimental purposes. Nevertheless, for academic study they are regarded as valuable adjuncts in the study of parturition.

# Cervical Dilatation Pattern

## CHAPTER 5

The method of tracing the pattern of cervical dilatation in labor is described. Technical details are presented for evolving the typical S-shaped curve of normal labor. The component phases are defined and characterized, together with brief discussion of their probable developmental mechanism and significance.

Search for a method of evaluating labor in progress ultimately focused on an investigation of the relationship between progressive cervical dilatation and the elapsed time in labor. Subsequently, comparable information relating to descent was developed (see Chapter 6). Tens of thousands of labors have now been studied.

With reference to the pattern of cervical dilatation, rectal and vaginal examinations were carefully noted and estimations of dilatation entered on square-ruled graph paper. The paper was printed with two ordinate (vertical) scales: on the left, ascending cervical dilatation in centimeters from 0 to 10 cm; on the right, descending scale of station from −5 to +5. The time abscissa (horizontal) was divided in hours from onset of labor. All medications given and procedures performed were noted. Other clinical features of potential importance were likewise listed, including maternal age, type of pelvis, fetal presentation, and position.

A point entered on this graph could be joined by a straight line to the preceding entry. The sequence of dilatation points evolved the characteristic sigmoid curve of dilatation; the station entries yielded the hyperbolic curve of descent. Relative uniformity of the interpretation of cervical dilatation and station was maintained wherever possible by insisting that one individual perform all the examinations during any given labor; this was not feasible, of course, in all instances.

The patients who presented themselves for study were those arriving sufficiently early in labor to permit adequate numbers of observations for our purposes. Analysis was confined to those who provided dilatation patterns that could be considered adequate in terms of detail, accuracy, and completeness. Those who arrived at the hospital in advanced labor were of necessity eliminated from consideration because their dilatation and descent curve could not be reconstructed with any degree of certainty.

This method of sampling might appear to weight the series somewhat in favor of prolonged labor, because many rapidly evolving labors would not be taken into consideration. Moreover, it was reasonable to assume that other biases of this kind had been introduced and could not be ignored. It was found, however, that the extremes of labor patterns tended to cancel each other out. Patients with inadequately graphed, rapid labors equilibrated with patients who were delivered electively by cesarean section prior to or early in their labors. Similarly, the bias introduced by the patient whose poorly progressive labor was terminated by early operative intervention was balanced by the patient who delivered shortly before or immediately after arrival in the hospital. Additionally, breech presentations were delivered abdominally when progress in labor was poor or when there was presumptive fetopelvic disproportion. In other patients, graphs could not be constructed because examination was interdicted for vaginal bleeding or other reasons. The actual number of such cases that could not be studied was relatively small.

The frequency of examinations depended on the progress of labor. Half-hourly examinations were sometimes found to be insufficient to depict the slope of a rapidly progressive labor accurately. Usually, however, hourly or bihourly examinations were found to be entirely suitable for this purpose.

In practice, the technique is the essence of simplicity. The graph paper utilized is constructed with ten divisions along the vertical axis to represent cervical dilatation in centimeters, or station in centimeters; each corresponding division along the horizontal axis denotes an hour in labor. The onset of labor is taken according to the classic definition as that time when regular uterine contractions as perceived by the patient were first established. Ten centimeters of cervical dilatation is taken as the arbitrary value of full dilatation and the onset of the second stage. It is recognized, of course, that this figure need not necessarily be realistic in any given patient, since the diameter of the cervical os at full dilatation is probably equal to and never greater than the largest diameters of the fetal presenting part. Thus, full cervical dilatation in a premature birth might be only 7.5 or 8 cm; for a fetus with hydramnios, it might be as much as 12.5 or 13 cm. It is important that this be borne in mind when constructing these curves. As readings are made, they are entered on the graph in appropriate locations and joined to preceding notations by a straight line. To avoid confusion and for convenience, estimates of cervical dilatation are usually indicated by a small circle, and those of station, by an X.

The curves obtained by the simple expediency of plotting cervical dilatation against time are all quite similar in general shape, resembling sigmoid curves. Variations are encountered most frequently in the initial portion from the onset of labor to the upswing of the curve. After this, the main variations appear in the midportion, representing the maximum rate of cervical dilatation. Where this is steeply inclined during rapid cervical change, the total labor tends to be short; where more flattened or associated with slower change, the labor is prolonged. Careful study reveals that the rate of change within the limits of error is specific for each patient during a given labor. Mathematically, we are referring to the slope of the curve and, more specifically, to the increment of cervical dilatation per unit of time.

The pattern of cervical dilatation that is seen in all normal labors is thus characteristically S-shaped. Each patient constructs her own unique dilatation pattern to provide a reliable means for following the course of normal labor and for distinguishing it objectively from dysfunctional labor. The maximum slope of active dilatation can be readily calculated whenever two consecutive observations have been made in the active portion of the dilatation slope. Merely dividing the difference in cervical dilatation (calculated in centimeters) by the intervening time interval (in hours and fractions of an hour) will give the value for the slope in centimeters per hour. This is an important measurement which offers a means of assessing the overall effect of all the forces of labor acting on the cervix to effect dilatation. It is an indirect measure of the efficiency of the complex mechanism with which we are concerned (see Chapter 3). The slope of dilatation undergoes predictable changes during the course of normal labor. Just as the rate of change is adversely or beneficially affected by many factors, so the expected variation in the rate of change is likewise influenced.

The mathematical analysis of this type of curve tends to be quite complex. The curves are similar to those first described by Gompertz in 1825 (Davis, 1943). They are represented by the equation, $y = ab^{c^x}$, and applied as a growth curve in business and population problems. The modified Gompertz equation, $y = \alpha + ab^{c^x}$, is more useful for our purposes in that it takes into account the variability of initial cervical dilatation. The time variable $x$ refers to time from upswing of the curve, ignoring the latent phase components; $y$ is cervical dilatation. A recently published, programmed routine for use with a programmable hand calculator (Collier and Savage, 1975) has made application of this approach practical if sufficient data are given. The equation can be solved now for groups of cases as well as for individual labors in progress.

In order to reduce the mathematical complexity, transformation of this function to linearity may be accomplished by using the method of probit analysis developed by Bliss for the statistical treatment of the sigmoid curve (Finney, 1952). The effect of this transformation from absolute values or percentages to probits is to convert the normal sigmoid curve to a straight line on a linear scale of probits. This effectively stretches the percentage scale of cervical dilatation to straighten the sigmoid curve. In essence, the probit is no more than a convenient mathematical device for solving otherwise intractable equations. Its application here is limited by the asymmetry of the curves obtained in evaluating cervical dilatation against time and by the loss of accuracy at the extremes.

One may further simplify the mathematical analysis of the sigmoid curve by examining the several parts independently. By dissecting the curve into its component segments, the problem becomes soluble. It is this last approach that we have used almost exclusively in deriving the data upon which the material discussed in this book is based. Thus, the sigmoid curve obtained in a given case can be divided into well-defined phases, as shown in Figure 3.

The *latent phase* extends from the onset of labor, timed from the onset of regular uterine contractions, to the beginning of the active phase. The onset of the *active phase* is quite apparent on the graphs as that point in time at which the rate of dilatation begins to change acutely, the curve becoming more steeply inclined. The active phase ends at full cervical dilatation when the cervix is fully retracted and is no longer palpable, having essentially become continuous with the upper vagina. The active phase gives way to the second stage of labor.

The active phase may be further subdivided into three distinctive phases. The middle of these is made up of that portion of the curve undergoing the most rapid change, the *phase of maximum slope*. The essential linearity of this phase is apparent. It is introduced by the *acceleration phase* and followed by the *deceleration phase*. It is important to note that these independent phases are unrelated to each other.

The latent phase tends to be flat or nearly flat. Very little by way of significant dilatation occurs during the latent phase. It appears to be that part of labor which is occupied with orientation, coordination, and polarization of uterine contractions and with preparation of the cervix for later active dila-

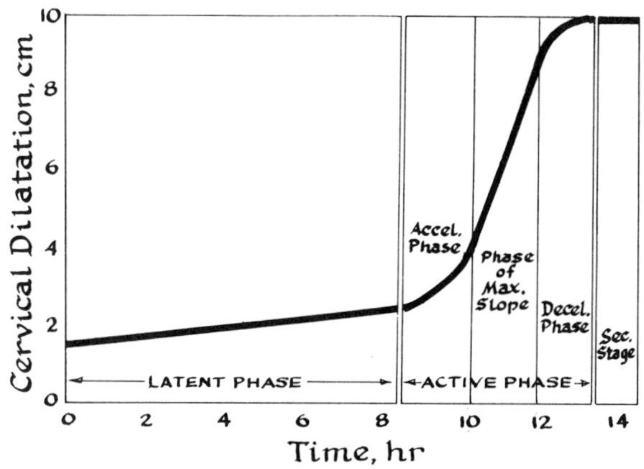


*Fig. 3.* Composite of the average dilatation curve for nulliparous labor based on analysis of the data derived from the patterns traced by a large, nearly consecutive series of gravidas. The first stage is divided into a relatively flat latent phase and a rapidly progressive active phase. The active phase has three identifiable component parts—an acceleration phase, a linear phase of maximum slope, and a deceleration phase.

tation. It has been determined that the duration of the latent phase is very sensitive to outside interference. It is prolonged with heavy sedation and shortened with stimulation. The duration of this prodromal period of labor has no apparent bearing on the future course of labor. Thus, there is no statistical correlation between the length or the slope of the latent phase and the course of the remaining portion of labor.

The acceleration phase is short and variable, but is important in determining the ultimate outcome of the labor in question. It leads from the minimum slope of the latent phase to the maximum slope that follows. A slow acceleration phase generally presages a lower maximum slope and therefore a prolonged total labor. A rapid change in the acceleration phase precedes a short residual labor. From this it might follow that the onset of labor should be measured from the onset of the active phase, since the ensuing changes are interrelated and apparently mutually determinant. However, we would take issue with this. Incorporation of the antecedent elapsed time of the latent phase into the total duration of labor does give an erroneous impression of the uterine work involved and does not permit critical comparisons of labors to be made. It is for this reason that evaluations of total duration of labor lack meaningful significance. Nevertheless, ignoring the early portion of labor may well mean neglecting important evidence of existing or impending problems (see Chapter 9).

The phase of maximum slope is a good measure of the overall efficiency of the "machine" with which we are dealing (see Chapter 3). Its inclination or slope gives one a rather clear idea of how effective the motive force of the uterine contraction is in producing dilatation. The slope of this phase is inversely related to the total duration of the first stage of labor. Since the major portion of cervical change occurs during this interval, it is an apparent and not unexpected relationship. The essential linearity of progressive dilatation reflected in an unchanging slope allows for quick appraisal of any deviations that may occur. During this portion of the first stage of labor, short-term effects of various factors may be observed readily.

The final phase of the first stage of labor, the deceleration phase, reflects fetopelvic relationships. Cervical retraction about the fetal presenting part is essential in obtaining full dilatation. In simultaneous plotting of station on these graphs (see Chapter 6), one can recognize that descent of the fetal presenting part begins in this phase of the first stage and continues uninterruptedly during the second stage of labor under normal circumstances. Descent accompanies the final aspects of full cervical dilatation and retraction and seems to be intimately related. Often this terminal phase of the first stage is short or absent, probably because it is merely not being observed.

As mentioned earlier, deceleration does not closely parallel the rate of acceleration that precedes it. This suggests that these are independent functions. Furthermore, deceleration is probably an artifactual phenomenon. It is not associated with any true deceleration of myometrial function. On the contrary, studies have clearly shown more or less steady progression of uterine work throughout the course of unstimulated labor, apparently quite

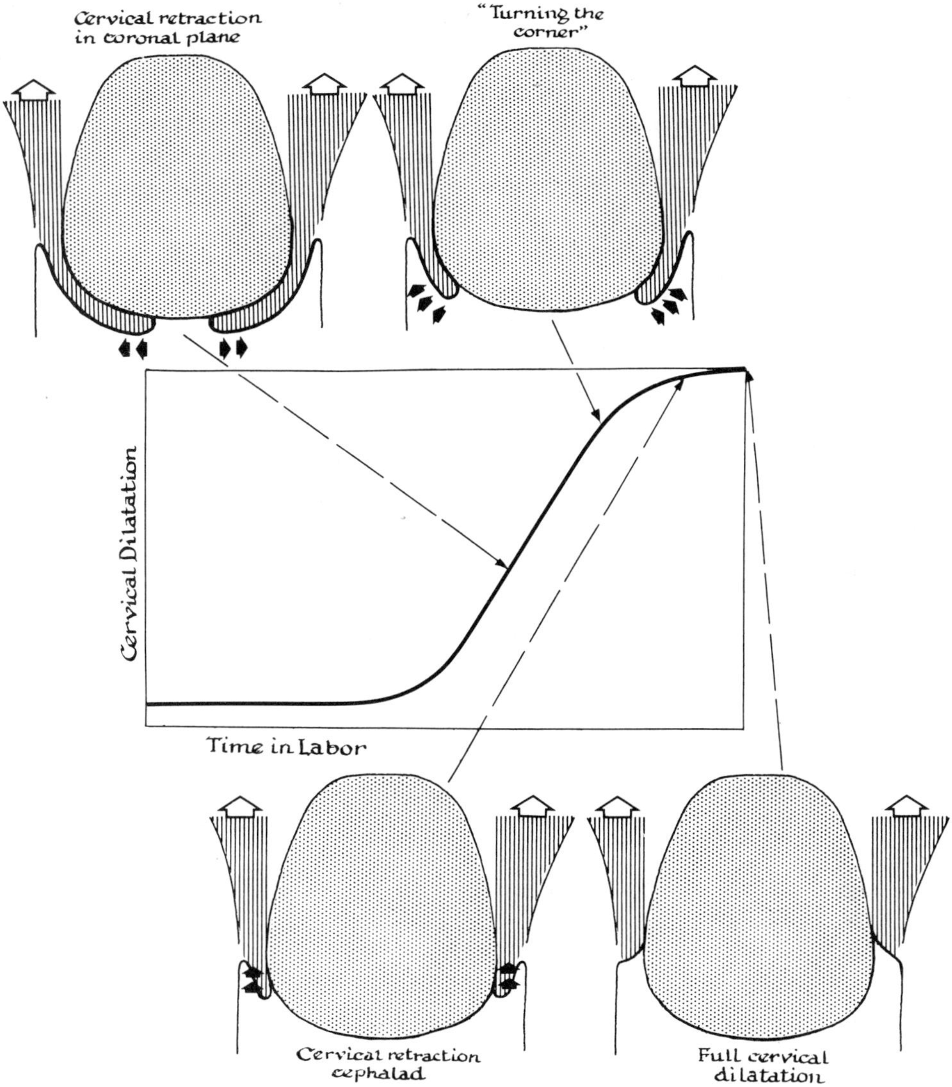


*Fig. 4* Graphic explanation for the development of the deceleration phase, showing *(1)* linear retraction of the cervix along the coronal plane during the phase of maximum slope *(upper left)*, *(2)* turning the corner as the cervix is being retracted around the fetal presenting part at the beginning of the deceleration phase *(upper right)*, *(3)* continued cephalad retraction with little additional increment in cervical dilatation *(lower left)*, until *(4)* second stage is reached when full cervical dilatation and retraction is achieved.

unrelated to progression in the dilatation pattern (Zambrana et al, 1960). The deceleration phase can perhaps best be looked upon as that portion of labor during which the cervix is "turning the corner." During the course of the phase of maximum slope, dilatation involves progressive widening of the cervical os in an essentially flat, horizontal plane. It is responding passively to the active centrifugal traction forces of the upper uterine myometrium. With increasing dilatation, the cervix begins to be retracted around the fetal presenting part, and it is then pulled in a more cephalad direction. As it nears full dilatation, the cervical os no longer increases in its side-to-side or anterior-to-posterior diameter, even though it continues to be retracted at the same rate. Figure 4 illustrates this sequence of events.

Obviously, no further change in the cervix can be detected after it has been completely dilated and retracted. When this occurs and the second stage has been entered, only observations of progressive descent are available for continuing the assessment of labor. The sequence of the descent pattern is treated in the next chapter.

# Descent Pattern

## CHAPTER 6

Progressive change in fetal station is a useful objective approach for assessing descent in labor. Graphic methods for tracing the pattern of descent are shown. The usual hyperbolic pattern of normal labor is illustrated. The relationship between cervical dilatation and descent is noted to be reliably consistent.

The concept of fetal station was first expressed by Müller in 1868 as a means for conveying the idea of the location of the fetal presenting part and its degree of progression in the birth canal. The term has since been popularized and further qualified because of its practical clinical applicability. Station, or degree of engagement or location, is used extensively today in clinical obstetrics both in its absolute form for prognostication, its relative form as a rough measure of progressive descent, and as a guide in evaluation and management of the laboring patient. Early studies of Calkins (1944) related to the duration and number of contractions necessary to complete the descent phase of the second stage. More recent work (Friedman and Sachtleben, 1965c) characterized the relationship of progressive descent with elapsed time in labor as a clinically useful index.

Classically, the first stage of labor is concerned with cervical dilatation; the second stage, with descent and expulsion of the fetus. Engagement of the fetal presenting part followed by descent through the birth canal are primary features of labor mechanisms. These are detailed in arbitrarily discontinuous fashion in all obstetric textbooks. These sequential events must normally occur before vaginal delivery can be accomplished. It has been observed that nulliparas enter labor with the fetus well engaged and frequently do not show further descent until late in labor. By contrast, those not deeply engaged may show some additional slow descent throughout a large segment of the first stage. As a corollary, nulliparas with unengaged fetal head at the onset of labor are viewed with some concern, since this situation may presage inadequate fetopelvic relationships or abnormality of

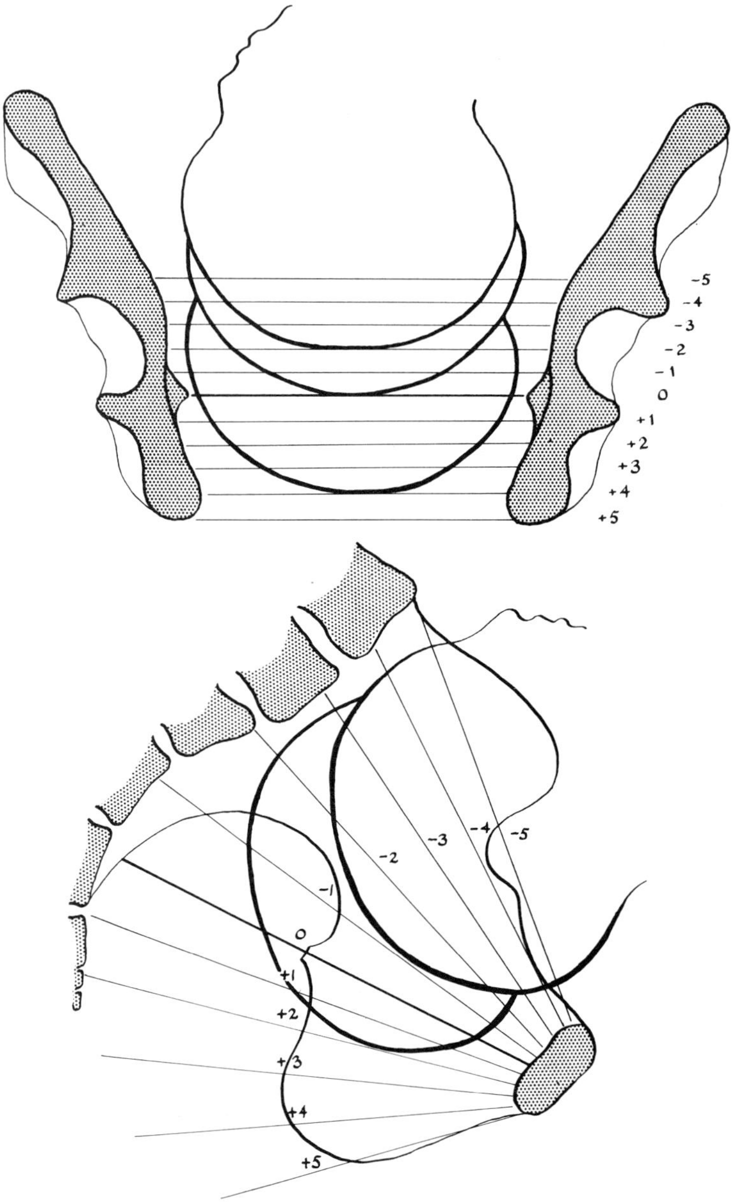


*Fig. 5.* Representation of the designations of fetal station, anteroposterior (top) and lateral (bottom) aspects, as the relation of the forward leading edge of the fetal presenting part to the plane of the ischial spines (*station 0*), in centimeters above (minus values) and below (plus values) this reference plane. While parallel in the anteroposterior view, the planes diverge in the lateral view (wider posteriorly than anteriorly) as they follow the curvilinear pelvic architecture. In the anteroposterior view, fetal heads are shown at station −2 (dipping), 0 (engaged), and +4 (on pelvic floor); in lateral view, −1 and +2.

fetal presentation. Station in multiparas, on the other hand, is generally not considered to be meaningful in the evaluation of the individual patient. In normal labor it is a matter of conjecture whether station of the fetal presenting part might not play a more important role than previously appreciated (see Chapter 25).

On the same graphic form used for the construction of the cervical dilatation pattern, one may readily construct the descent pattern of a given labor in progress. This requires that the obstetric attendant acquire some proficiency in estimating the station of the fetal presenting part with reference to the plane of the ischial spines (Fig. 5).

Some information is obtainable by means of external abdominal examinations. Suprapubic palpation can usually help to determine whether the presenting part is floating (freely movable above the inlet), dipping (having entered the inlet but still somewhat mobile), or fixed in the inlet. While useful information, it does not delineate the degree of engagement with the kind of accuracy that is attainable through periodic assessment of station by internal examination. Such abdominal observations form the basis for the method of assessing the level of the fetal head by suprapubic palpation widely used abroad (Crichton, 1974; Philpott and Castle, 1972a). This provides a scale (Fig. 6) expressed in terms of fifths of the fetal head still palpable above the pelvic rim: five-fifths is equivalent to a floating head and zero-fifths to one that is deeply engaged.

Determining the level of the fetal head in reference to the pelvic inlet in fifths can be a helpful adjunct in diagnosing engagement under these circumstances. While not as accurate as vaginal examinations in ascertaining the station of the forward leading edge of the fetal presenting part with reference to the plane of the ischial spines, this method will ensure that

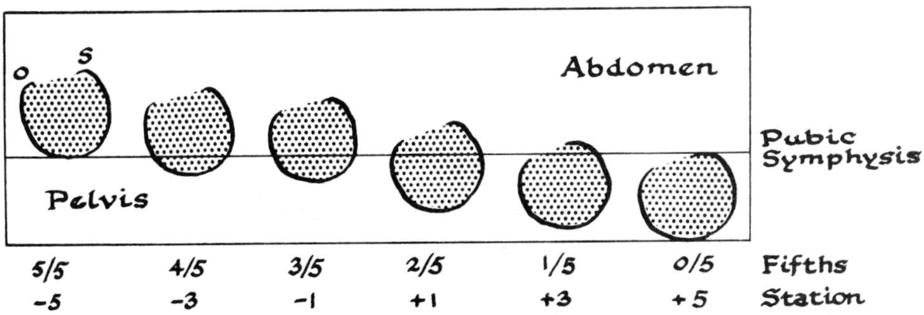


*Fig. 6.* Assessment of the fetal station by abdominal palpation of the relationship of the sinciput (*S*) and the occiput (*O*) above the symphysis pubis, designated in fifths that are each equivalent to about 2 cm of station. The station designations are approximate and vary according to height of symphysis, size of fetal head, degree of extension, and molding. The information provided is especially useful in verifying descent and distinguishing it from progressive molding (From Crichton D: S Afr Med J 48:784, 1974).

perceived descent is true descent and not merely a reflection of molding of the fetal cranium.

This is somewhat analogous to the planes of Hodge, still in use in Europe and recently reintroduced here (Sicuranza et al, 1970). They constitute four parallel planes, the first corresponding to the pelvic inlet, the second drawn from the inferior border of the symphysis pubis to the midportion of the second sacral vertebra, the third through the ischial spines, and the fourth through the apex of the coccyx. The single most serious shortcoming of this latter approach is that it does not take into account the curvature of the pelvis and assumes descent to occur in a straight line from the inlet downward. Neither method quantitates descent in a reproducible manner, using the familiar centimeter scale.

It is essential to delineate the degree of engagement and the progressive descent of the fetal presenting part by means of accurate examinations of station. The engaged head in a vertex presentation is one in which the biparietal diameter has reached or passed the inlet. Usually, the leading edge is at or below the plane of the ischial spines when this is accomplished. One can imagine a coronal plane passing through the ischial spines, which will serve as a reference plane. To determine the relationship of the fetal head (or breech) to this plane, one need only palpate the lowermost aspect of the presenting part during a vaginal or rectal examination, and then pass the fingers across to the ischial spines on the pelvic sidewalls. One should try to visualize the pelvic planes at 1-cm intervals above and below the reference interspinous plane. The inlet is designated at station −5 (5 cm cephalad to the interspinous plane), the perineal floor at station +4 (4 cm caudad), and the introitus at station +5. If the lowermost part of the fetal head has reached the spines and is just engaged, the head is at station 0. If higher, say, 2 cm above the interspinous plane, it is not engaged and can be designated as station −2. If the presenting part has descended below the interspinous plane by 1 cm, for example, engagement has already occurred and the station is designated as +1.

Needless to say, station designations merely refer to the forward leading edge of the fetal presenting part as related to the interspinous plane. They do not actually specify where the biparietal diameter of the fetal head is. Since the planar distance between the forward leading edge and the biparietal diameter is usually 5 cm, one may generally assume that the biparietal diameter is at the inlet plane when the forward leading edge is at station 0. However, this relationship does not always hold, particularly in patients with cephalopelvic disproportion who are allowed to labor for prolonged intervals of time. Here, considerable molding may give the impression that descent is occurring, but the fetal biparietal diameter may still be at or above the inlet. This potentially serious situation must always be considered.

The descent pattern that evolves in normal labors traces a characteristic hyperbolic curve when the station is plotted against elapsed time. Following the descent pattern can be just as useful for uncovering serious labor disorders as tracing the dilatation pattern. Both afford the obstetric attendant considerable insight into the nuances of labor progression. Active descent generally occurs after active cervical dilatation has been in progress for some time. Descent proceeds to its maximum near the end of the first stage of labor. It continues in a constant manner until the perineum is reached by the presenting part. The maximum slope of active descent is calculated in the same way as the slope of active cervical dilatation, by dividing the difference in consecutive station readings (in centimeters) by the intervening time interval (in hours and fractions of an hour) to yield the rate in centimeters per hour.

An extensive analysis was undertaken to determine what part station plays on the course of labor. We utilized a comparable approach to that described in Chapter 5 to evolve patterns for investigation. The constraints imposed are reviewed in detail there. We first directed attention to the problem of characterizing the phenomenon of descent objectively by relating the changes in station to the elapsed time in labor, with special regard to the first stage of labor and to the possible interrelationship of the descent function with the cervical dilatation–time pattern. The curves relating station to time that were constructed from the data obtained were examined, dissected, tabulated, and correlated with the various portions of the corresponding cervical dilatation patterns that had been similarly drawn. These data will be discussed in more detail in Chapter 7.

It is striking to note that, contrary to previously held functional concepts, descent generally appears to begin well before the second stage (Fig. 7). From the onset of regular perceived contractions, little by way of descent takes place for some time. The rate of descent accelerates late in the first stage of labor. The earliest point of acceleration in nulliparas coincides with that portion of labor in which the cervix is dilating at its most rapid rate: namely, the phase of maximum slope. During this interval, the speed of descent increases to a maximum. The maximum is usually reached just at the onset of the deceleration phase of dilatation and then continues in a linear manner into the second stage of labor. Descent normally maintains

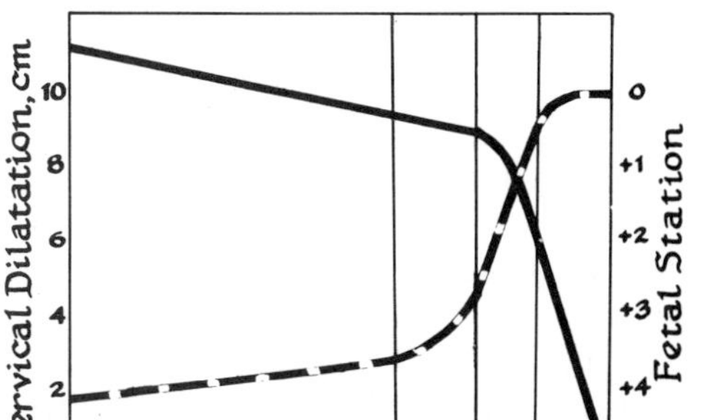


*Fig. 7.* Interrelationship between descent curve (*solid line*) and concurrently developing dilatation pattern (*broken line*), shown in composite form representing the average labor course for nulliparas. Active descent generally begins when the dilatation curve reaches its phase of maximum slope; the rate of descent reaches maximum at the beginning of the deceleration phase of dilatation and continues in a linear manner until the perineum is reached.

this maximum rate until the perineal floor is reached. It is obvious that descent often progresses well beyond the midplane of the pelvis before the second stage of labor begins. In multiparas, active descent may not begin until the dilatation curve reaches the beginning of the deceleration phase. It is most unusual in normal labors for descent not to proceed maximally from the beginning of deceleration onward.

The hyperbolic curve we have described for descent may be said to represent the expected pattern of descent. In nulliparas it can be described in two parts, analogous to the phases of the cervical dilatation curve of the first stage. The *latent period* of descent extends from the onset of labor to that point in time when active descent begins. This latter transition is concurrent with the time that the dilatation curve is entering its phase of maximum slope. The *active period* of descent occupies the remainder of the first and second stages. The initial *acceleration period* of the descent curve coincides almost precisely with the phase of maximum slope which characterizes cervical dilatation in nulliparas. In the remainder of the active period of descent, the rate is normally maintained as a constant. This continues unchanged at the maximum rate that has been established for that patient throughout the deceleration phase of cervical dilatation and during the course of the second stage. A *deceleration period* probably exists for the descent curve, corresponding to a perineal phase during which progressive caudad descent is temporarily slowed immediately prior to delivery. However, this has not yet been objectively demonstrated. It is a clearly recognizable clinical phenomenon, especially when it is abnormal or significantly prolonged. Under normal circumstances, because it is difficult to demonstrate, it must await the development of a more critically objective instrument for continuous, accurate measurement of station than the examiner's finger.

The durations of the various parts of the descent curve indicate the close correspondence of the latent period of descent with the combined latent and acceleration phases of dilatation. Similarly, the acceleration period of descent corresponds to the phase of maximum slope of dilatation in duration. Finally, the phase of maximum slope of descent is concurrent with the combined deceleration phase of dilatation and the second stage.

Similar data show comparable curves for multiparas. The descent curve in multiparas can be subdivided in a manner similar to that done for the nulliparous curve. The latent period of descent for multiparas corresponds almost precisely with the combined latent and acceleration phases of cervical dilatation, but often also includes a part or all of the phase of maximum slope of dilatation as well. The acceleration period of descent may also correspond in time with the phase of maximum slope of dilatation, but often is concurrent only with the deceleration phase of dilatation. Again, the interval of maximum rate of descent may coincide with the combined deceleration phase of dilatation and second stage of labor, as in nulliparas, but often merely involves the second stage. A perineal phase has not been specifically delineated for multiparas. Furthermore, the transition from latent descent to active descent is not as clearly pinpointed at the onset of the phase of maximum slope of the dilatation curve. As stated above, it often occurs later in the deceleration phase, but may also take place within the acceleration phase of dilatation.

The maximum slope of descent is just as good a measure of the overall efficiency of the uterus as the maximum slope of dilatation was. Moreover, it incorporates the resultant effects of both uterine contractility and expulsive efforts as they are reflected in the essential work that must be accomplished, namely, evacuation of the uterus and delivery of the fetus. As with the maximum slope of dilatation, the inclination of the slope of descent gives one an indirect means for quantitating how effective the motive forces are in producing descent. Thus, the slope is inversely related to the total duration of the combined deceleration phase and second stage. The more steeply inclined the descent pattern, the more efficient the progression of labor. The linearity of progressive descent again allows for quick appraisal of any deviations that may occur. It also permits one to observe the short-term effects of factors that are at play.

The relationships between simultaneous observations of station and cervical dilatation have been studied (Fig. 8). Correlation is quite constant for the active portion of dilatation, from 3 to 8 cm. It is of interest to note that the relationship holds almost identically without regard for parity, despite the fact that multiparas so frequently labor with high fetal presenting parts. We note that the multiparous correlative relationship in Figure 8 falls to the left of the nulliparous function, indicating both higher station early in labor and more rapid descent subsequently. In addition, the rapidity of descent in multiparas is enhanced considerably when one takes into account the more expeditious rate of cervical dilatation that usually occurs in them. This latter is not reflected here because the station is related to the factor of cervical dilatation rather than to the factor of time. In relative terms, descent occurs in nulliparas at a rate of 0.25 cm of station per centimeter of dilatation in the active phase; in multiparas, at 0.30 cm of station per centi-

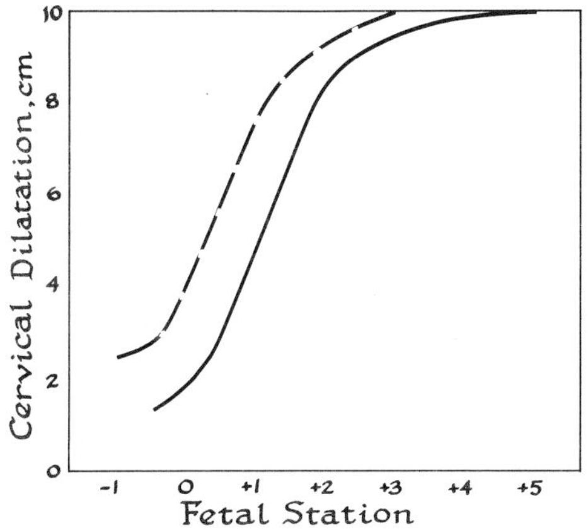


*Fig. 8.* Correlation between cervical dilatation and fetal station for nulliparas (*solid line*) and multiparas (*broken line*), demonstrating the linear correspondence between the two variables for the major portion of dilatation from 3 to 8 cm. During this interval the rate of descent averages 0.25 cm per centimeter of dilatation in nulliparas and 0.30 cm per centimeter in multiparas.

meter of dilatation. The difference in average rates is negligible, verifying that the correlation between descent and dilatation is strong. It follows that they are interdependent variables and should, under normal circumstances, be expected to relate one to the other.

The concept that descent is essentially and almost exclusively limited to the second stage of labor has been rather widely held. Progressive descent in the second stage is assumed to be the norm, but quantitation of expected rate of progression has not been clarified. Clinical impression requires continuous advancement, but the degree and the amount over a given period of time is at best vague. Since in normal cases brisk progression is the rule, this lack of concrete information is of little more than academic interest in the majority of instances. Only in abnormal or potentially abnormal situations does this void in our knowledge become critical.

That all available clinical information must be fully utilized for the evaluation of the laboring patient is clear. We have shown the value of critical analysis of the relationship of cervical dilatation as related to time in labor. Its importance is the demonstration that minimal variations from the expected normal in the active phase of dilatation indicate the approach of serious abnormalities. The shortcomings are readily appreciated by the absence of such well-defined critical measures of normalcy in the latent phase of the first stage in which little if any cervical dilatation takes place; a similar situation prevails in the second stage of labor after full cervical dilatation has occurred and no further observations relating to cervical dilatation can be made.

There is, therefore, real need for expanded study of additional variables such as station in a similar comprehensive manner. Notwithstanding the development of instrumentation for objective physiologic surveillance of mechanical and electrical phenomena of uterine contraction, the readily available clinical measure of station may serve this useful purpose. This holds despite its admittedly limited accuracy, which is of the order of 3 to 5 percent in trained hands. Such data, when related to elapsed time, may help the practicing obstetrician form more meaningful ideas of what constitutes normal labor.

# Normal Labor

## CHAPTER 7

Comprehensive analyses of the graphic patterns of cervical dilatation and fetal descent yield data useful for characterizing the normal range of labor progression. Information based on measurements of the component parts of the labor curves help to define normal limits objectively for unselected gravid populations as well as for those undergoing a natural, unstimulated, and unimpeded labor process. Labor can be divided into three functional divisions according to the demonstration of different and distinctive clinical characteristics. The special features of these functional divisions of labor are detailed.

Recognizing the sigmoid nature of the cervical dilatation pattern of normal labor and the hyperbolic curve of descent were relatively simple matters of objective observation. Although these patterns are interesting, they serve little really useful purpose either for clinical practice or for academic study. They might be made meaningful if it were possible to define their limits in some clear-cut way. Indeed, it was obvious that the limits of normal had to be determined before we could proceed with any study of the phenomenon of labor.

Since definitions of what constitutes normal labor were nebulous at best, we had no guidelines for the determination of these limits. We approached the problem empirically by describing some of the measurable characteristics of the gravid population with regard to patterns of cervical dilatation and descent. In this manner we obtained distribution data to help us determine where normality ends in the wide spectrum of labor variations and where abnormality begins.

## *DATA BASE*

We first succeeded in obtaining sufficiently adequate information on a large series of nulliparas to make the analysis meaningful (Friedman, 1955a). In subsequent years, many more patients have been studied, and the findings have remained essentially unchanged (Friedman and Kroll, 1969, 1971a, b). Our findings have also been verified on the basis of data obtained from diverse populations here and abroad, including such widely separated areas as Thailand (Lekprasert, 1972), Uganda (Glick and Trussell, 1970), and South Africa (Margolis, 1974). A recent report from England showed comparable results and no differences among white, Asian, and black women whose labor patterns were separately studied (Duignan et al, 1975).

The potential distortions by sampling errors in our data have already been mentioned. We also recognized the biases introduced by the need to eliminate those patients who arrived in the hospital too late to permit construction of their dilatation and descent curves, as well as those in whom internal examinations were interdicted because of bleeding or other hazards, those delivered electively by cesarean section, and those whose labors were rapid or unobserved. Such biases have been shown not to affect the reported results to any significant degree.

Our material was carefully examined to assure ourselves that we were dealing with a truly cross-sectional sampling of the nulliparous gravid population. We felt this to be imperative in order that the data subsequently derived might then be usable and applicable in clinical practice and experimental study. The case material was evaluated according to as many variables as could be examined in order to test our sampling techniques and to verify that we were dealing with a representative population. In addition to the usual actuarial items of interest, such as age, parity, gravidity, hospital status, race, height, and weight, we also looked into the factors of fetal position and presentation, gestational age, birth weight, delivery outcome, fetal results, fetopelvic relationships, and the use of sedatives, analgesics, uterotonic agents, and anesthesias. This type of survey clearly indicated that we had obtained an adequate sampling of our hospital population. Since this group presented no significant deviation from the overall nulliparous hospital population, it could be used to provide baseline data for subsequent statistical comparisons.

A similar group of multiparas was subsequently studied (Friedman, 1956b). A much larger series was later evaluated (Friedman and Kroll, 1971b) for verification. The continuity of patient selection in this group was intermittently disturbed by the multipara who arrived at the hospital when delivery was imminent. Deletion of this group of multiparas, which group constituted a sizable number, weighted our data somewhat against more rapid labors. Nonetheless, the material was found to represent an adequate sampling of multiparas. The multiparas presented no significant deviations in frequencies of the many potentially relevant variables that were evaluated.

## *COURSE OF NORMAL LABOR*

On the basis of data derived from such groups of patients, it was possible to determine clear-cut definitions of normality by statistical analysis. Our interest was directed at both the duration and the shape of the dilatation and descent patterns. The curves were subdivided into phases, designated as previously described (see Chapters 5 and 6) in order to simplify this process. The separate phases of all the curves were examined and distribution curves established. From these, the relative merits of each of the different parts of the curves could be ascertained.

It was clear that the total duration of the first stage was not too valuable to us as an index of progression, particularly in view of the broad spread of the data. Similarly, but to a lesser extent, the data for the latent phase duration displayed a large range. By contrast, the distribution curves for the data on active phase duration was sharply peaked, as was that for maximum slope of dilatation, deceleration phase duration, second stage duration, and maximum slope of descent. This observation demonstrated the more precise definition of these variables and provided evidence that small deviations from the average were probably significant. In passing, it was felt that the narrow range of the distribution curve for the second stage duration was probably specious, because labor was commonly terminated as expeditiously as possible after an arbitrary time limit of 2 hours in second stage had elapsed. Since interference occurred so frequently, one could not accept these data as representative of untampered labor progression. Because the distribution curves were asymmetrical, standard statistical techniques for determining limits of normal were felt to be inapplicable. Accordingly, specific 95th-percentile limits were determined in order to define normality.

The mean value for each phase as well as the statistical deviations were obtained. From these, the mean composite dilatation and descent patterns were derived. Of greater importance, the statistical limits were determined based either on a deviation of two standard deviations from the mean or the 5th- or 95th-percentile limit, whichever was more appropriate.

## *PROGRAMMED ANALYSIS*

The critical data derived in this way were subsequently verified by means of an intensive computer analysis of a series of 10,293 gravidas (Friedman and Kroll, 1969). These patients had been preselected to include only singleton pregnancies with infants in excess of 1000 g birth weight. The base population from which the study series was chosen totaled 58,831 women. Demographically, they consisted of a cross-sectional sampling of the gravid population at large (Friedman and Kroll, 1971a). The slope of descent was derived from a similar series (Friedman and Sachtleben, 1970a).

A working solution to the problem of machine case-finding and analysis was developed by which the computer was programmed to accept clinical estimations of cervical dilatation and duration of elapsed time in labor in order to decide whether the data were acceptable, and then to define critical durations and slopes. It is important to review this operation, because its principles can be applied to clinical practice as well.

The computer was instructed to search the available observations for a particular case to determine whether there was sufficient information to permit it to reconstruct the labor pattern. Since the machine had no way of determining the reliability of a given piece of information, it was decided to accept all nonregressive points. By this we mean that we could discard any estimation of cervical dilatation that is followed by a smaller estimate. We can illustrate this essential part of the "cleaning" operation by the temporal sequence of dilatation data:

2.0, *6.0,* 3.0, *5.0,* 4.0, 7.0, *10.0,* 9.0, 10.0

Among these, the points that subsequently regressed are indicated in italics. By eliminating such points, we obtain the usable sequence of nonregressive points:

2.0, 3.0, 4.0, 7.0, 9.0, 10.0

When dilatation values are placed in order of ascending time sequence, any estimate that is followed by a smaller value for dilatation is automatically deleted. Two or more consecutive equal values are not considered regressive. From these nonregressive points a reasonable approximation of the labor pattern can be produced, provided the following minimum criteria are met: (1) known time of onset of labor, (2) known time of delivery, (3) at least one documented nonregressive point between 3.0 and 6.0 cm dilatation, and (4) at least one documented nonregressive point between 6.5 and 9.0 cm dilatation.

The importance of these last two points in permitting total reconstruction of the labor curve is paramount. These two points and others, if available, permit the active phase pattern to be reconstructed and its maximum slope to be calculated with considerable accuracy. Furthermore, these points permit one to extrapolate the active phase slope downward to define the end of the latent phase, and upward to define when the deceleration phase is expected to begin.

Another important, but not essential, piece of information is the first nonregressive 10-cm point, indicating the onset of the second stage. If unavailable, it could be estimated by further upward projection of the slope line to cross 10 cm cervical dilatation.

Selecting cases presenting with the minimum criteria allowed us to reconstruct labor curves by providing the missing data graphically. It became a simple matter thereafter to calculate the several variables that describe the course of labor for each patient; then the material obtained in this way was manipulated to produce important information on frequency distributions.

For each variable, calculations were made of the mean, standard deviation, standard error of the mean, and standard error of the standard deviation. Frequencies (numerical incidence), percents, cumulative frequencies, and cumulative percentage tables were constructed for the entire series as well as for each participating institution. The mean duration of the various phases and stages of labor and relevant slopes are presented in Table 3,

*Table 3. COMPOSITE DATA ON COURSE OF LABOR*

| *Group* | *Latent Phase (hr)* | *Active Phase (hr)* | *Maximum Dilatation (cm/hr)* | *Deceleration Phase (hr)* | *Maximum Descent (cm/hr)* | *Second Stage (hr)* |
|---|---|---|---|---|---|---|
| Nulliparas | | | | | | |
| Mean | 6.4 | 4.6 | 3.0 | 0.84 | 3.3 | 1.1 |
| SD* | 5.1 | 3.6 | 1.9 | 1.0 | 2.3 | 0.8 |
| Limit† | 20.1 | 11.7 | 1.2 | 2.7 | 0.96 | 2.9 |
| Multiparas | | | | | | |
| Mean | 4.8 | 2.4 | 5.7 | 0.36 | 6.6 | 0.39 |
| SD* | 4.9 | 2.2 | 3.6 | 0.3 | 4.0 | 0.3 |
| Limit† | 13.6 | 5.2 | 1.5 | 0.86 | 2.1 | 1.1 |

* Standard deviation.
† 5th or 95th percentile distribution value.

together with the distribution characteristics. In addition, the median (50th percentile point) and modal (point of maximum frequency of occurrence) values were also available. Both the median and modal values are probably more important here in measuring the central tendency than the mean, by virtue of the skewed distribution of these variables. Figure 9 serves to illustrate the degree of skewness, emphasizing the deviation of our data from normal distribution. It presents the histogram (frequency distribution curve) for the maximum slope of dilatation. Similar curves were constructed with all the other dimensions we studied.

The ogive, or cumulative frequency distribution curve, was found to be particularly useful as an adjunct for determining meaningful limits of normal. It has the major advantage of being independent of the variations introduced into the histogram by arbitrary groupings of the continuous variable; that is, the shape of the histogram may change according to the increment of the variable used for purposes of grouping the data. Unfortunately, as can be seen in Figure 9, the ogive for the skewed data was both asymmetric and somewhat imprecise at the critical extremes, where our interest was primarily directed.

Accordingly, we reverted to probit transformation (see Chapter 5) for purposes of adjusting the scalar representation mathematically so as to effect linearity. This was accomplished by the simple expediency of expressing the several durations and slopes as logarithmic functions while simultaneously expressing the cumulative frequency in terms of the normal probability function (probit). The manner in which these scalar alterations affect the

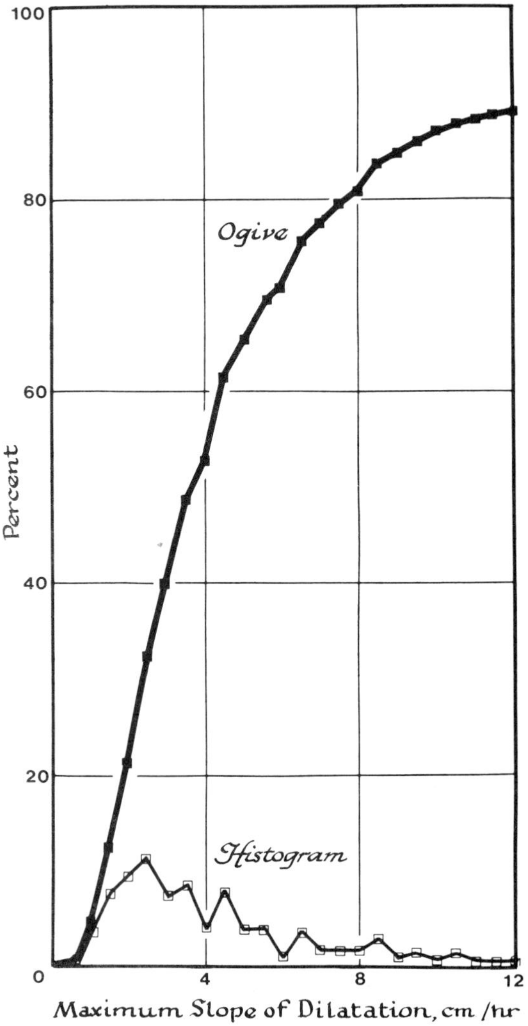


*Fig. 9.* Distribution data for maximum slope of dilatation on linear scale, showing asymmetrically skewed histogram reflecting wide spread at the upper ranges and nonlinear ogive representing the cumulative frequency distribution curve. As depicted, these curves are not sufficiently precise at either extreme to aid in selecting cut-off limits for clinical diagnosis.
(From Friedman EA and Kroll BH: J Reprod Med 6:20, 1971.)

appearance of the histogram and ogive, respectively, is shown in Figure 10 for the maximum slope data. The histogram takes on a regular, symmetric appearance and the ogive becomes essentially linear.

This critical transformation allows us to select appropriate and meaningful limits for the data. Note, for example, that the 5th percentile point for the maximum slope occurs at 1.2 cm per hour. This conforms precisely with the data previously obtained on a strictly clinical basis. Comparable cumulative frequency distribution curves for the other dimensions that are of interest to us provide similar limits at the 5th or 95th percentile points, whichever is more appropriate.

When examined on an institutional basis (among 12 collaborating university hospitals), we found surprisingly good uniformity. Extreme ranges

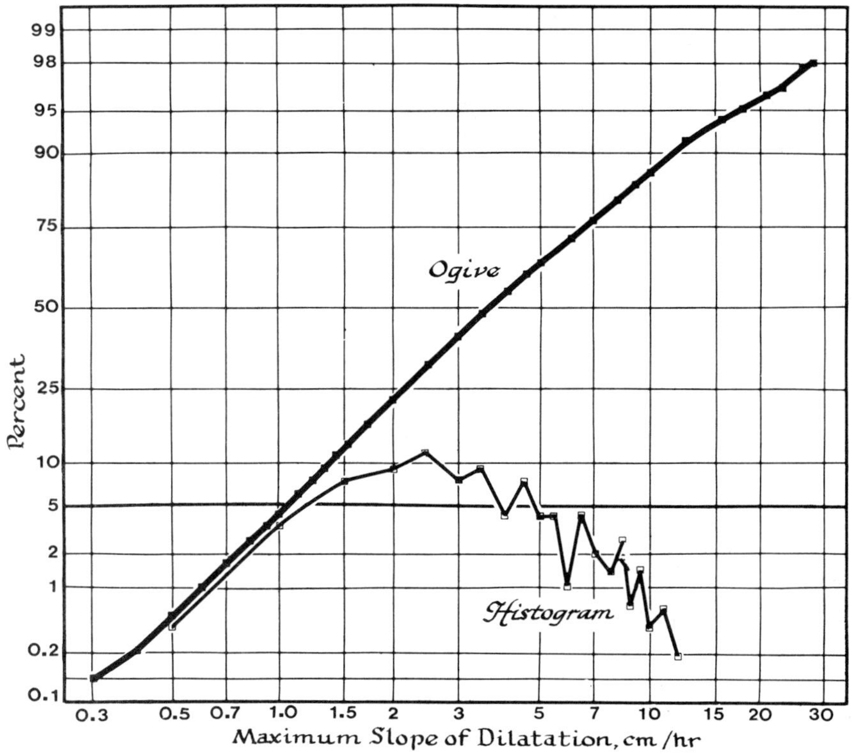


*Fig. 10.* Same data as in Figure 9, with the abscissa adjusted to a logarithmic scale and the ordinate to a probit scale. This achieves normal (Gaussian) distribution of the histogram and linearity of the ogive. Distributions depicted in this transformed way provide means for assessing the limits of normality, shown here as 1.2 cm per hour at the 5th percentile point on the maximum slope distribution.

(From Friedman EA and Kroll BH: J Reprod Med 6:20, 1971.)

closely approximated the mean ogive. At the 5th percentile level for the maximum slope, for example, the entire spectrum of institutional limits around the mean of 1.2 cm per hour extended from 0.7 to 1.5 cm per hour only. Similar verification of the probable significance of the limits for other dimensions was also found.

## *LIMITS OF NORMAL*

The intrinsic importance of this approach is what we may have gained in being able to define the limits of normal objectively. The rationale by which these limits are derived requires some elaboration. Our basic premise concerns the "personalistic concept" of probability that recognizes the usefulness of estimating the degree of confidence or probability that a given event will or will not happen. This concept is rationalized according to the properties of the probability theory. The occurrence of an event (or dimension) within the "tail" of the distribution curve (at an extreme from the mean) can be regarded as one with a minimal likelihood of having taken place purely on a chance basis. Our confidence that such values occur without some outside influence is small.

Based on statistical probability, we may begin to look at the extremes in the distribution curves as if they belonged to a population that was different from the population constituting the remainder of the material. The choice of the 95th percentile value as the limit of normal is admittedly an arbitrary decision, but it is based on a logical and reasonable compromise between hypersensitivity and underselection. To elucidate, hypersensitivity refers to making the limits very broad to avoid excluding any abnormal cases, and at the same time probably including large numbers of normal cases. Underselection, on the other hand, confines the limits too sharply to avoid including normal cases, but simultaneously deletes some cases that are likely to be abnormal. It is not possible in the statistical sense to find a sharp demarcation between observations that are realistically abnormal and those that clearly are not. The point we choose depends on our personal concept of what an improbable or rare occurrence is. In this regard, we are here interested in being able to identify significant labor abnormalities. The limits we have selected are indeed arbitrary, but they have subsequently been demonstrated to be both appropriate and practical.

## *IDEAL LABOR PATTERN*

The composite labor patterns described here were felt to represent average nulliparous and multiparous labors as encountered in our gravid population. However, they do not necessarily reflect the course of the undisturbed parturitional process. There are wide variations in how obstetrics is practiced in different communities. Thus, in one area sedation may be used frequently and heavily, in another conduction anesthesia may be preferred, and in a third natural childbirth may be the standard. In order for our data to be universally applicable, therefore, they must be based on some common frame of reference. Accordingly, it was necessary for us to describe the ideal state of unhampered and unstimulated labor.

This was accomplished by preselecting a large group of gravidas who did not have fetopelvic disproportion, any form of fetal malposition or malpresentation, or multiple pregnancy, and who were not subjected to heavy sedation, conduction anesthesia, uterotonic stimulation, or operative intervention. The group consisted of gravidas at term, all with adequate pelvis, vertex presentation, and well-flexed, occiput anterior position, whose labors progressed normally without interference and who delivered average-sized infants spontaneously or by outlet forceps.

Their labors were studied in great detail to elicit data on the course of

*Table 4.* COMPOSITE IDEAL LABOR COURSE

| *Group* | *Latent Phase (hr)* | *Active Phase (hr)* | *Maximum Dilatation (cm/hr)* | *Deceleration Phase (hr)* | *Maximum Descent (cm/hr)* | *Second Stage (hr)* |
|---|---|---|---|---|---|---|
| Nulliparas | | | | | | |
| Mean | 6.1 | 3.4 | 3.5 | 0.72 | 3.6 | 0.76 |
| SD | 4.0 | 1.5 | 3.0 | 0.7 | 1.9 | 0.5 |
| Multiparas | | | | | | |
| Mean | 4.5 | 2.1 | 5.9 | 0.30 | 7.0 | 0.32 |
| SD | 4.2 | 2.0 | 3.4 | 0.3 | 3.2 | 0.3 |

"ideal" labor (Table 4). Nulliparas yielded data obviously rather different from the composite course described earlier for nulliparas at large. By contrast, the ideal curve based on a series of selected uncomplicated multiparas was determined not to differ in any significant way from the average curve for multiparas in general. This was undoubtedly due to the very low incidence of complicating factors among nulliparas.

These data are particularly important from the academic point of view because they provide the baseline data that can be employed for experimental comparisons between groups of patients. They can help in determining the effects of various exogenous and endogenous factors on the course of labor. Analyses based on such comparisons will be presented in subsequent chapters to illustrate the inherent usefulness of this approach.

## *FUNCTIONAL DIVISIONS OF LABOR*

As this and other material evolved, it became more and more obvious that the labor phenomenon lent itself to division into three parts. Each of these parts was clearly different and functionally special. Each could be easily recognized; each was affected by different factors; each responded in a singular manner to various influences; each was subject to its own set of aberrations (Friedman, 1971). Recognizing and understanding these differences is essential for the practitioner in this field. For the sake of convenience, we can refer to these functional divisions of labor in terms of their physiologic objectives (speaking teleologically), namely, preparatory, dilatational, and pelvic divisions, respectively. These are illustrated in Figure 11.

In order to understand these functional divisions and their distinctive clinical characteristics, the terminology we use must distinguish them from the classical stages of labor in which labor is divided into a first stage, from onset to full cervical dilatation, and a second stage, from full dilatation to delivery of the fetus. This arbitrary division of labor is used universally. It is based on the convention that recognizes a period of dilatation followed by another of descent. The so-called mechanisms of labor (the cardinal movements of the fetus), referring to the accommodations of the fetal presenting

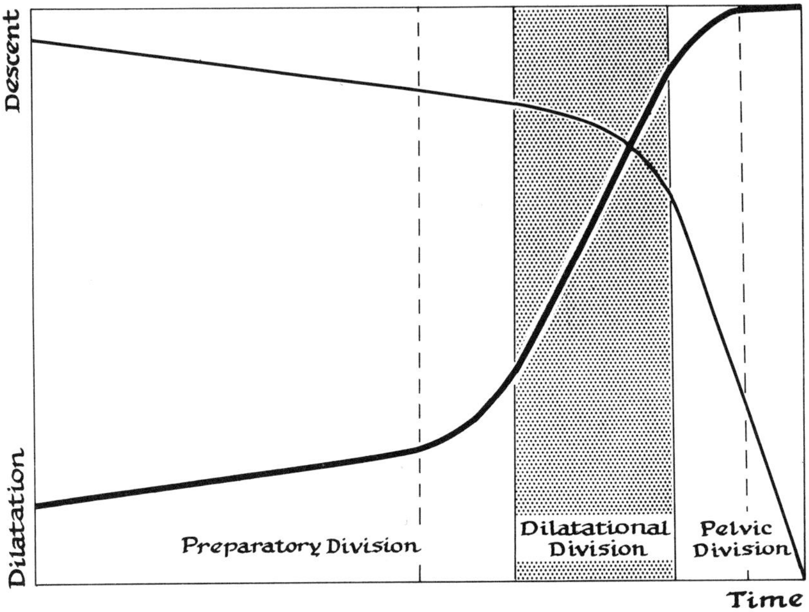


*Fig. 11.* Labor course divided functionally on the basis of expected evolution of the dilatation and descent curves into *(1)* a preparatory division, including latent and acceleration phases, *(2)* a dilatational division, occupying the phase of maximum slope of dilatation, and *(3)* a pelvic division, encompassing both deceleration phase and second stage while concurrent with the phase of maximum slope of descent. Recognizing these distinctive functional divisions proves useful in clinical practice.

part to the pelvis during its descent through the birth canal, are merely superimposed on this scheme without specifically designating where they might fit during the course of time. We now recognize that only a very small portion of the first stage is actually occupied with cervical dilatation, and descent is not exclusively limited to the second stage.

Intuitively, we can examine the dilatation and descent curves to identify three distinctive time periods. First, after contractions begin, little is happening by way of dilatation and descent. It is during this interval that the cervix is being prepared for later active dilatation. Simultaneously, myometrial contractility is undergoing orientation, polarization, and coordination. This is the *preparatory division* of labor. Second, there is the brief interval during which almost all cervical dilatation occurs, constituting the phase of maximum slope of the dilatation curve. This is the *dilatational division.* Third, there follows the remainder of labor, including the deceleration phase of dilatation and the second stage in its entirety. It is during this division of labor that much of descent occurs and all the fetal mechanisms of labor take place. This is the *pelvic division.* The principal characteristics of these functional divisions are listed in Table 5.

*Table 5. PRINCIPAL CLINICAL FEATURES OF THE FUNCTIONAL DIVISIONS OF LABOR*

| *Characteristic* | *Preparatory Division* | *Dilatational Division* | *Pelvic Division* |
|---|---|---|---|
| Functions | Contractions coordinated, polarized, oriented; cervix prepared | Cervix actively dilated | Pelvis negotiated; mechanisms of labor; fetal descent; delivery |
| Interval | Latent and acceleration phases | Phase of maximum slope | Deceleration phase and second stage |
| Measurement | Elapsed duration | Linear rate of dilatation | Linear rate of descent |
| Diagnosable disorders | Prolonged latent phase | Protracted dilatation; protracted descent | Prolonged deceleration; secondary arrest of dilatation; arrest of descent; failure of descent |

## *Preparatory Division*

The preparatory division comprises that portion of labor from the onset of regular, perceived contractions to the end of the acceleration phase of dilatation. It ends when the labor enters that part of the active phase characterized by linear maximum slope of dilatation. During the preparatory division, the descent curve is flat in its own latent period.

We can look at the latent phase and the acceleration phase of dilatation together as a single unit from the functional point of view. This is so because we recognize that both appear to be affected in the same direction and magnitude by the same factors and both manifest related disorders that are correctable by similar management regimens. We have learned, for example, that the preparatory division is particularly sensitive to sedation and anesthesia. It is readily inhibited by these agents. The poorly polarized uterine contractions of this interval are easily disturbed. Myometrial function has not become sufficiently coordinated to withstand the inhibitory aspects of such exogenous influences.

The changes that occur in the cervix during this interval are both overt and subtle. Some apparent transformation is seen with softening, effacement, and the beginning of dilatation. More subtle variations occur in the subcellular alteration of ground substance, collagen, reticulum, and other fibrillar connective tissue components (Danforth et al, 1960).

There is no clear explanation for the acute changes that take place in the functional capacity of the cervix at the end of the preparatory division. Without any noteworthy changes in myometrial contractility, the cervix begins to respond by more rapid dilatation. We might draw an analogy to the phenomenon of stone cutting. Many dozens of strokes with hammer against chisel seem to have no apparent effect, yet one more blow of the same intensity cleaves the stone sharply. The explanation must exist in some change that is yet undetectable, perhaps in molecular orientation, that is produced by subliminal increments of force.

### *Dilatational Division*

The dilatational division, as stated earlier, occupies that time interval during which cervical dilatation is proceeding at its most rapid pace. In addition to the dilatation that has occurred before labor begins (Hendricks et al, 1970) and the negligible additional amount that takes place during the preparatory division (that is, during the latent and acceleration phases combined), all of dilatation except the terminal retraction aspects of the deceleration phase takes place during the relatively short interval of the phase of maximum slope.

It is during this important, although brief, span of time that the results of all the driving forces of uterine contraction become manifest in effecting dilatation. Thus, dilatation of the cervix can be regarded in an engineering sense as the effective end result of these forces. It very specifically reflects the efficiency of the complex machine with which we are dealing (see Chapter 3).

The linearity of the normal dilatation process permits us to determine the degree of effectiveness of a particular contractile pattern in overcoming the specific resistance present in a given patient in labor. To repeat, a steeply inclined slope of dilatation is the result of a favorable combination of factors, regardless of the particular clinical picture of labor in terms of contractility pattern. Contrariwise, slow progress results from disadvantageous combinations. This is an important concept that must be understood in order to make optimal use in practice of the measurements of dilatation and descent.

The deceleration phase of dilatation is not included in the dilatational division because of its functional differences. Despite the fact that the retractional aspects of dilatation are continuing without interruption during this interval as the cervix "turns the corner" (see Chapter 5), the descent phenomenon, then in full progress, takes on much greater significance. Since we are concerned primarily with means for determining normal progression and uncovering abnormalities, this distinction between dilatation and descent has practical significance. For our purposes of functional considerations, therefore, the dilatational division should comprise only the phase of maximum slope of dilatation.

In contrast to the preparatory division, the dilatational division of labor is essentially unaffected by sedation or anesthesia administered for analgesic purposes. Myometrial function tends to be well established, as illustrated by its ability to effect active dilatation. The inhibitory pharmacologic effects of various exogenous agents, so readily demonstrated in the latent phase, are rarely seen here. It is only in the presence of a preexisting disordered state of myometrial function or with some major intrinsic impedance or obstruction that any potentially deleterious influences of extraneous factors become manifest. In general, it is difficult to disturb the rapidly progressing dilatation curve. However, when the phase of maximum slope is progressing slowly or abnormally, the effects of inhibitory factors become more apparent. Under such circumstances, excessive sedation or anesthesia can readily diminish or even stop further progress.

### *Pelvic Division*

As the cervix nears full dilatation, it opens sufficiently to permit the fetal presenting part to descend in a linear manner (see Chapter 5). Descent generally begins earlier during the dilatational division of labor. The rate of descent reaches its maximum rate at the beginning of the deceleration phase of dilatation; descent proceeds thereafter without interruption until the perineum is reached.

In this context, the deceleration phase of dilatation marks the onset of the pelvic division of labor. Its significance may be more readily understood if one considers all of cervical dilatation to be a retraction phenomenon. At the beginning of active dilatation, the passive cervix responds to the centrifugal myometrial forces by retracting in a horizontal plane. Nearing full dilatation, the retraction of the cervix progresses in a more cephalad direction around the fetal presenting part. Now the increments in the lateral dimension of the cervical os diminish, resulting in an apparent deceleration of dilatation. The deceleration phase, therefore, is an artifact because neither myometrial activity nor passive cervical retraction is actually diminishing. If one accepts the hypothesis explaining the deceleration phase in terms of retraction around the fetal presenting part, then one should expect to encounter maximum rates of descent at this time.

The essential feature of the rest of labor is the negotiation of the pelvis by the fetus. The classic mechanisms of labor, describing the cardinal movements of the fetus as it adjusts to the various pelvic dimensions during its descent, take place almost exclusively during this interval.

The linear descent pattern constitutes a fine measure of the overall efficiency of the labor process, analogous in value to that of the linear active dilatation curve. Its inclination provides a measure of the effectiveness of the motive force in producing the work required of it, namely, descent of the fetus through the birth canal.

We can justify this type of classification of the functional divisions of labor because of the clear-cut distinctions between them as to function, technique of assessment, manifestations of disorders (see Chapter 8), management regimens, and prognosis. These essential characteristics must be recognized so that appropriate diagnostic, evaluative, and therapeutic approaches will be available in the armamentarium of the practitioner. This simple view provides a meaningful and practical framework for understanding the complex process of labor and its abnormalities.

To this point we have dealt with normal labor and with attempts to define the limits of normal based on statistical deviations from the average dilatation and descent patterns. Having accomplished this, we are now ready to embark on the detailed study of aberrations of labor. As an aid to comprehension, the functional divisions of labor should be kept in mind at all times. They will serve as a useful skeleton of information on which to build.

# Dysfunctional Labor

# PART II

# Abnormal Labor Patterns

## CHAPTER 8

A series of easily defined labor aberrations is discussed. Each of them is readily diagnosed by specific graphic manifestations. Diagnostic criteria are presented for differentiation. Frequencies of occurrence are shown for nulliparas and multiparas. The relative inaccuracy of diagnostic acumen in clinical assessment of labor is contrasted with the greater objectivity of the graphic approach.

It is essential to clarify the beclouded issues that surround the subject of disordered labor. By having established the limits of normal of the various phases of the dilatation and descent patterns objectively, we felt we were in a position to examine closely those cases in which abnormalities were found. A series of intensive studies was undertaken to elucidate the component features of labor as defined by the dilatation and descent patterns. Most studies of abnormal labor that had been published in the past preselected cases on the basis of clinical impressions of abnormality or, alternatively, on the basis of the duration of labor having exceeded an arbitrary length. The resulting case studies were unevenly weighted with both normal and false labors, as well as admixtures of various types of disordered labors. These several conditions are not generally distinguishable from one another because of the basic lack of reliable criteria for differentiation. By contrast, abnormal labor is now defined in an understandable and objective way.

### *NOMENCLATURE*

The term *inertia* should be avoided because its meaning is so unclear. It means completely different things to different individuals or institutions and its meaning seems to vary from time to time. Instead, we have adopted Eastman's phrase *"dysfunctional labor,"* a descriptive, all-encompassing term that skirts the issues of definition. It is to be emphasized that we are not concerned here with direct evaluation of uterine activity, as this term might indicate, but rather upon the effect of all the forces of labor acting against the resistive maternal soft tissues. The end results, cervical dilatation and descent, are the summation of the interplay between the various factors that influence the efficiency of uterine activity and those contributing to the production of bony, positional, or soft-part dystocia.

The term *inertia* as applied to labor belies its dictionary definition of a condition manifested by indisposition to action, in which the object is indolent and inherently powerless to produce an expected effect. Only in its limited reference to intrinsic uterine activity does this term approach a realistic interpretation. Conceptually, it does not encompass the numerous other factors that are associated with dyfunctional labor. It implies that all labor disorders are the result of insufficient uterine contractile drive. Clearly, this is not the case. Many disturbed labor courses occur with perfectly adequate contractile patterns. Based on our observations of progressive changes in cervical dilatation and fetal station, it has been possible to redefine the limits of normal progress in labor, and thereby provide a means for quantitative assessment of abnormal states.

## *DEFINING DISORDERS*

An empiric method of study was developed. It entailed grouping patients according to the specific aberration that was encountered. This approach lent itself to objective statistical investigation with a minimum of difficulty. It was found to be sound in indicating probabilities of fact, particularly with reference to the effects brought about by the factors under observation. A massive amount of data has been accumulated in this regard. We have been able to define nine identifiable types of labor disorder (Table 6), seven associated with inherently slow or arrested labor and two at the opposite end of the spectrum characterized by excessively rapid progression. As we shall see, these nine disorders can be considered representative of four major classes of aberrant labor.

The techniques that have been evolved for purposes of study include graphing individual labors in progress, dissecting the patterns that are obtained, and analyzing the data thus collected. We will hereafter refer to this sequence as graphicostatistical analysis or, more simply, as graphic analysis. This approach has made possible the study of these aberrations so as to define causative or contributory factors, diagnostic criteria, and the relative efficacy of treatment for the several major disorders that constitute dysfunctional labors.

Thus, the catch-basket of uterine inertia has been replaced by a series of very specific, distinctively different, and diagnostically homogeneous disorders of progress. Having defined the several major disorders, we proceeded to study each of them separately in turn. Through the intermediary of the simplistic device that allowed us to relate progressive changes in cervical

*Table 6.* *THE PATTERNS OF ABNORMAL LABOR*

| *Pattern* | *Diagnostic Criterion* |
|---|---|
| I. *Disorder of Preparatory Division of Labor* | |
| Prolonged latent phase | |
| Nulliparas | Latent phase duration of 20 hr or more |
| Multiparas | Latent phase duration of 14 hr or more |
| II. *Disorders of Dilatational Division of Labor* | |
| Protracted active-phase dilatation | |
| Nulliparas | Maximum slope of dilatation of 1.2 cm/hr or less |
| Multiparas | Maximum slope of dilatation of 1.5 cm/hr or less |
| Protracted descent | |
| Nulliparas | Maximum slope of descent of 1.0 cm/hr or less |
| Multiparas | Maximum slope of descent of 2.0 cm/hr or less |
| III. *Disorders of Pelvic Division of Labor* | |
| Prolonged deceleration phase | |
| Nulliparas | Deceleration phase duration of 3 hr or more |
| Multiparas | Deceleration phase duration of 1 hr or more |
| Secondary arrest of dilatation | Cessation of active-phase progression for 2 hr or more |
| Arrest of descent | Cessation of descent progression for 1 hr or more |
| Failure of descent | Lack of expected descent during deceleration phase and second stage |
| IV. *Precipitate Labor Disorders* | |
| Precipitate dilatation | |
| Nulliparas | Maximum slope of dilatation of 5 cm/hr or more |
| Multiparas | Maximum slope of dilatation of 10 cm/hr or more |
| Precipitate descent | |
| Nulliparas | Maximum slope of descent of 5 cm/hr or more |
| Multiparas | Maximum slope of descent of 10 cm/hr or more |

dilatation and in station of the fetal presenting part to elapsed time in labor, we were offered a means for assessing progress in labor in a dependable and reliably accurate way. This tool helps us to accomplish critical appraisal of labors in progress, replacing much of the subjective art of obstetric evaluation with the objectivity it provides.

## *TYPES OF ABERRATIONS*

Quantitative assessment of the distribution of the dilatation and descent patterns yields information for purposes of defining abnormalities. We have seen that the normal latent phase in nulliparas should not exceed 20 hours in duration, and in multiparas, 14 hours. Labors with latent phases greater than these limits may be considered abnormal. They demonstrate a disorder that we can descriptively call *prolonged latent phase.*

Similarly, in the active phase of dilatation, a maximum rate of dilatation of less than 1.2 cm per hour in nulliparas, or 1.5 cm per hour in multiparas, should be considered evidence of another variety of dysfunctional labor, which we can call *protracted active-phase dilatation.* In the past, we used the less specific phrase "primary dysfunctional labor," but found it much too confusing for continued use.

The pattern of *protracted descent* is characterized by comparably slow rates of descent of less than 1.0 cm per hour in nulliparas or 2.0 cm per hour in multiparas. A fourth major labor aberration is *prolonged deceleration phase.* It is recognized by abnormal lengthening of the deceleration phase duration beyond 3 hours in nulliparas or 1 hour in multiparas.

These four abnormalities are qualitatively indistinguishable from normal labor in that they follow the general shape of the dilatation or descent patterns. They differ from normal only in a strict quantitative sense, falling outside the normal range of some specific phase duration or slope. Thus, although they trace a sigmoid curve of dilatation and a hyperbolic curve of descent, they can be distinguished from normal objectively.

*Secondary arrest of dilatation* involves a pattern change from the expected S-shaped curve of cervical dilatation. Progressive dilatation in the active phase stops before full cervical dilatation is reached. Generally, a minimum of 2 hours of arrest is needed before the diagnosis can be considered to be confirmed. We have retained the modifier *secondary* in order to emphasize that this pattern must be differentiated from the lack of progress often seen (indeed, usually expected) during the latent phase. This disorder requires that the labor enter the active phase of dilatation and then be secondarily arrested in the course of the phase of maximum slope.

*Arrest of descent* also involves a pattern change, with cessation of progressive linear descent occurring most often in the second stage of labor. Usually, one hour of arrest of descent is sufficient to make the diagnosis of this disorder. Logically, we should argue that this abnormality should also be labeled *secondary*. However, as we shall see, there is relatively little difference prognostically between true arrest of descent (which occurs after active descent has begun) and *failure of descent*. This last is diagnosed in the deceleration phase of dilatation or during the second stage, when active descent is expected to be in full progress.

These seven disorders are dysfunctional as a consequence of their being too slow or too prolonged in certain aspects. They represent the several component disorders that fall under the outdated term *"uterine inertia,"* or similar ill-defined expressions (see Chapter 1).

At the other extreme of labor progression are the patterns of labor which describe progress that is too rapid in the sense of being abnormally fast or tumultuous. They can be grouped under the general term *precipitate labor,* but deserve separate identities as *precipitate dilatation* and *precipitate de-*

*scent,* respectively. These terms do not, of course, refer to the pejorative term *"precipitate delivery,"* which refers instead to rapid delivery usually over an unsterile field and without adequate control or preparation.

Objectively, precipitate dilatation is characterized by a rate of cervical dilatation in the active phase in excess of 5 cm per hour in nulliparas or 10 cm per hour in multiparas. It usually occurs in conjunction with comparable rates of excessively rapid descent. In more realistic terms, rapid changes in dilatation and descent can be recognized more easily as 1 cm every 12 minutes or less for nulliparas and 1 cm every 6 minutes or less for multiparas.

These definitions are summarized in Table 6 and are illustrated graphically in Figures 12 to 15. As can be seen, they fall naturally into groups

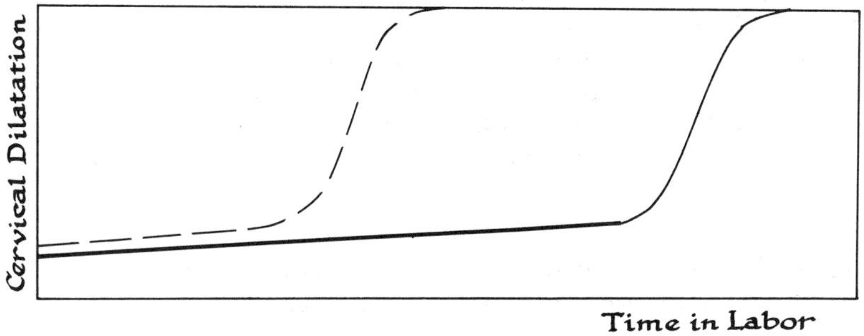


*Fig. 12.* Prolonged latent phase pattern (*solid line*) is the only disorder thus far objectively diagnosable in the preparatory division of labor. It is an abnormality characterized by latent phase duration exceeding established critical limits, shown with typical elongation of the lower initial arm of the sigmoid curve of cervical dilatation. It is followed by a normal active phase here, as is usually the case. The average dilatation curve for nulliparas (*broken line*) is shown for comparison.

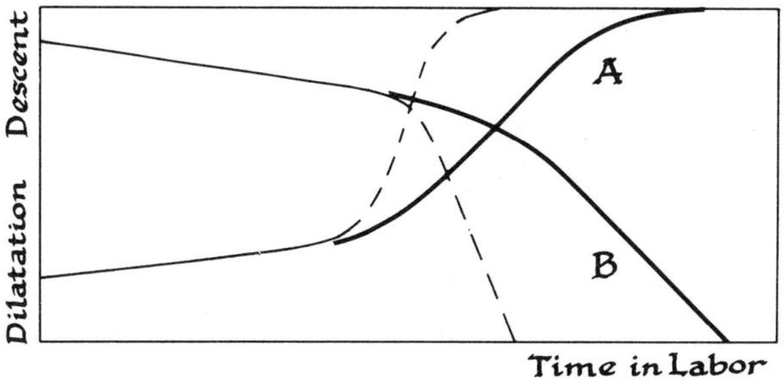


*Fig. 13.* Protraction disorders of labor, depicting (*A*) protracted active phase dilatation pattern with abnormally slow maximum slope of dilatation, and (*B*) protracted descent pattern with maximum slope of descent less than prescribed critical limits of normal. These labor aberrations are similar to each other in many ways and frequently occur together in the same patient. They are clearly different from the average normal dilatation and descent patterns (*broken lines*).

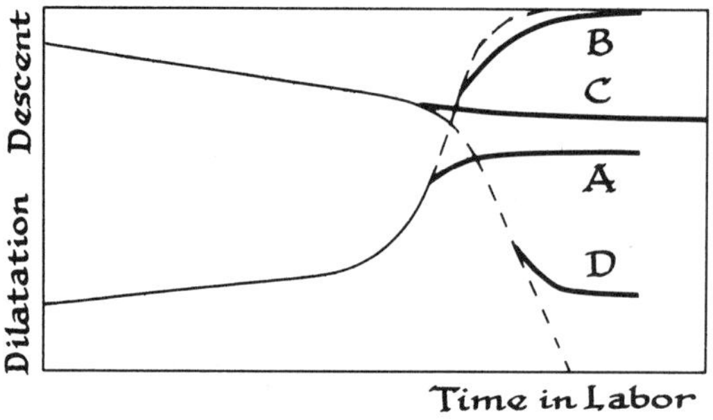


*Fig. 14.* Arrest disorders of labor, illustrating (*A*) secondary arrest of dilatation pattern with documented cessation of progression in the active phase, (*B*) prolonged deceleration phase pattern with deceleration phase duration greater than normal limits, (*C*) failure of descent in the deceleration phase and second stage, and (*D*) arrest of descent characterized by halted advancement of fetal station in the second stage. These four abnormalities are similar in etiology, response to treatment, and prognosis, being readily differentiated from the normal dilatation and descent curves (*broken lines*).

according to the functional division (see Chapter 7) to which they apply. Thus, the disorder of prolonged latent phase can be considered alone as a representative disorder of the preparatory division; the two protraction disorders (protracted active-phase dilatation and protracted descent) can be discussed together under disorders of the dilatational division; the remaining four "arrest" disorders (prolonged deceleration phase, secondary arrest of dilatation, arrest of descent, and failure of descent) belong together under the pelvic division. The precipitate disorders, of course, are in a class by themselves. The next four chapters will deal with these groups seriatim.

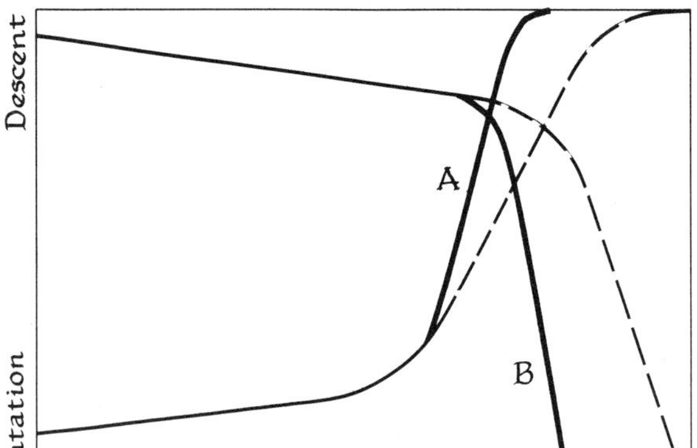


*Fig. 15.* Precipitate labor patterns, represented by (*A*) precipitate dilatation and (*B*) precipitate descent, as defined by their excessively rapid rates of progressive cervical dilatation and fetal descent, respectively, which distinguish them from the course of normal labor (*broken lines*).

## *DIAGNOSTIC CRITERIA*

Clinically, it is of utmost importance in approaching the management of the laboring patient to recognize the particular aberration that she has. This can be done readily by the simple expediency of plotting estimates of cervical dilatation and of fetal station on square-ruled graph paper against the elapsed time in labor. If examinations are done often enough in a given case and if they are done with accuracy, the characteristic S-shaped pattern will evolve and abnormalities will become apparent as they arise.

The diagnosis will be made readily and the physician will then be able to proceed to evaluate the patient for etiologic factors. On this basis, he or she will be able to administer the necessary specific therapy called for by the particular problem situation existing in that patient at that time. The immediate results and the ultimate outcome will depend on the correctness and speed of diagnosis and on the applicability of the treatment that has been chosen for that particular case. Details of diagnosis and differential diagnosis are presented in Chapters 20 and 21.

Investigations along these lines have attempted to make prospective management meaningful by analyzing dysfunctional labors with due regard to diagnosis, etiology, and treatment. Attention has been directed to finding the features that will help to define the type of aberration, the potential causative factors, and the prognostic implications according to the type of therapy that has been utilized.

Difficulties that are encountered in making the correct diagnosis may be reduced by an intelligent and enlightened approach to the problem. It will be apparent, for example, that it is difficult, if not impossible, to distinguish prospectively between prodromal or false labor and the early portion of the latent phase of true labor. If contractions continue uninterruptedly, this distinction is perhaps an unnecessary refinement. If contractions are interrupted in time, it becomes a relatively simple matter in retrospect to ascribe all the foregoing to false labor. This assumes, of course, that some iatrogenic factor, such as heavy sedation or anesthesia, has not been invoked to cause the contractions to stop. As will be seen (Chapter 9), about one-tenth of patients with prolonged latent phase will later be discovered to have been in false labor. Any realistic and practical program of management must necessarily take this possibility into account because obviously there are no methods for making the differential diagnosis correctly on a prospective basis.

The configuration of the abnormally slow active-phase dilatation pattern is not nearly so readily evident as that of secondary arrest of dilatation, in which progress halts prior to full cervical dilatation. Similarly, protracted active-phase dilatation pattern is more difficult to recognize than the entity of abnormally prolonged latent phase, which merely entails recognizing the unduly long duration of expended time in labor without substantive progress in dilatation. Protraction disorders (that is, protracted active-phase dilatation and protracted descent) can be diagnosed with certainty only if the slope of dilatation and the slope of descent are actually measured and calculated for the specific labor in progress. The single criterion of an abnormally low slope of the curve of dilatation or of descent suffices for purposes of diagnosing these serious labor aberrations.

Secondary arrest of dilatation exists in a given labor when previously advancing cervical dilatation stops in the active phase. The arrest of progress is manifested graphically by horizontal flattening of the inclined curve of dilatation. Two hours of arrest documented by sequential vaginal examinations performed by the same individual have been used throughout as a practical minimum criterion for diagnosis. Arrest of descent is similarly manifested by cessation of progressive descent, usually recognized in the second stage of labor, for a period of one hour or more.

A common differential diagnostic quandary encountered by clinicians is associated with precedent undetected (or unrecognized) prelabor cervical dilatation. A patient may arrive for observation in labor with advanced cervical dilatation and several hours later be found not to have progressed further. Here the observer may mistakenly surmise that secondary arrest exists when in fact the patient may still be in her latent phase, even though the cervix is already somewhat dilated. Since not much further dilatation is generally expected during the latent phase, the lack of progression may be normal but can be misinterpreted to represent secondary arrest.

An important diagnostic feature of secondary arrest of dilatation, therefore, is recognition that prearrest active phase dilatation has occurred. Unless one can document that the patient has entered the active phase, one cannot be certain that the interval under observation during which there was no progress actually represents secondary arrest. This documentation can be accomplished easily (if the patient is available for periodic examinations) by plotting estimates of cervical dilatation on a time basis so that the pattern of active phase progression and subsequent arrest can be readily visualized in a graphic manner. The same applies, of course, for arrest of descent. Failure of descent is different in that it can be identified by the observation that the descent expected to take place during the deceleration phase and second stage does not occur.

Unless stringent search is carried out for the detection and the diagnosis of these abnormalities, some may escape notice. It is probable that abnormal labors are sometimes unrecognized, particularly those with prolonged latent phase. This is especially so if subsequent events in a given labor indicate normal progression of dilatation, descent, and delivery. The abnormal latent phase might readily be overlooked or ignored. It might even be imaginatively eliminated. It is surprising how much "interpretation" occurs with reference to the dispassionate computation of the duration of the latent phase or of the total length of labor.

Individual methods for calculating the duration of labor offer an interesting sidelight on the psychology of obstetric attendants. Some will subtract all or a large portion of the latent phase, acting on the retrospective assumption that the patient was probably not yet in true labor because dilatation of the cervix was not occurring. It has been clearly shown that no dilatation or at best very little dilatation has to take place during the latent phase. This is an interval during which the cervix is being prepared by softening and effacement for later rapid dilatation. At the other extreme is the obstetrician who will include in his or her calculations the sometimes obvious duration of false labor, perhaps to support a tenuous contention that intervention was necessary on the basis of excessively prolonged labor.

In a similar way, short intervals of arrest of dilatation or of descent may be ignored retrospectively when the outcome has been good. The whole picture is clouded, moreover, by labeling as abnormal many cases in which progress is deemed to be dilatory (without clear criteria as to what that means) or in which contractions are considered to be ineffectual. The bases for such clinical impressions of abnormal labor are at best vague. Having decided on a nebulous basis that the patient is experiencing an abnormal labor, the physician may then follow through with an arbitrary decision to terminate labor by operative intervention, when in actuality uninterrupted progress was really occurring. It is doubly important, therefore, that diagnoses be made by objective means on clear-cut criteria so that such inappropriate action may not be undertaken.

## *INCIDENCE*

It will be recalled that the criteria for diagnosing labor disorders were derived from the distribution curves for several measurable aspects of the dilatation and descent curves, stipulated as the 5th or 95th percentile values. As a consequence, it should follow that the incidence of each of these disorders ought to be about 5 percent of comparable gravid populations. That such is not the case is attributable to differences among various population samples. In an early series of nearly 29,000 viable births, the overall incidence of occurrence was 3.3 percent, or 1 in 30 deliveries. In our most recent review encompassing nearly 17,000 patients, the rate was nearly 8 percent. Undoubtedly, the frequency in any given community reflects not only the inherent make-up of the gravidas, but also the prevailing obstetric practices. Some of the disordered labor patterns may result from excessive use of analgesic or anesthetic agents in labor, for example.

There is a greater propensity for dysfunctional labors to occur among nulliparas. The probability of a labor problem arising in nulliparas is between six and nine times greater than in multiparas.

The relative frequencies of the major dysfunctional labor aberrations are illustrated in Figures 16 and 17 for nulliparas and multiparas separately. We note that arrest and protraction disorders are relatively more common among nulliparas than among multiparas; they are, of course, more common in absolute terms as well. Prolonged latent phase is the most common disorder encountered among multiparas with abnormal labor. Only about one-third of the dysfunctional labor patterns in nulliparas are char-

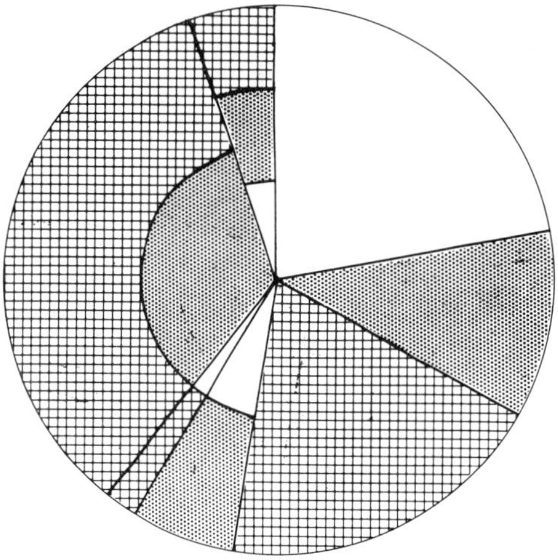

*Fig. 16.* Relative incidence of disordered labors in nulliparas. Prolonged latent phase (*unshaded*) makes up about one-third of abnormal patterns; protraction disorders (*stippled*) are next in order; arrest patterns (*cross-hatched*) occur most often. Combinations of abnormal patterns are frequently encountered in the same labor, especially protraction and arrest.

acterized by a prolonged latent phase, whereas more than one-half of those seen in multiparas have this disorder.

Combinations of labor aberrations occur in the same labors frequently. Such sequential or concurrent combinations are encountered much more often in nulliparas than in multiparas. Nearly one-half of the nulliparas with abnormal labor, for example, have more than one disorder diagnosed during the course of their labor, as contrasted with less than one-third of the multiparas.

## *ACCURACY*

The diagnosis of dysfunctional labor, uterine inertia, uterine dysfunction, and other nebulous conditions by clinical means alone is now recognized to be unsatisfactory. Clinical criteria that utilize subjective impressions are

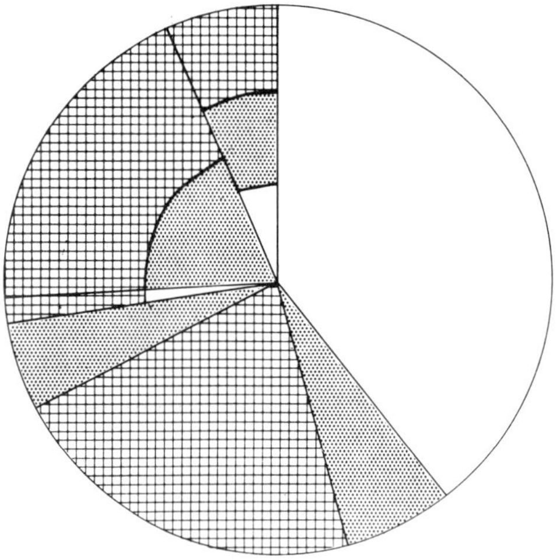

*Fig. 17.* Relative incidence of abnormal labor patterns in multiparas. By far the most common aberration encountered is prolonged latent phase (*unshaded*), which occurs in more than one-half of those with diagnosed dysfunctional labor; arrest disorders (*cross-hatched*) follow closely in frequency; protraction disorders (*stippled*) are rather unusual in multiparas. Combinations, while fewer than in multiparas, do occur rather often and tend to be similar in that arrest patterns are likely to follow protraction patterns.

highly inaccurate. This was demonstrated by examining a large group of patients who were deemed to have entirely normal labors on the basis of clinical evaluation, except that the labors were longer than 20 hours in duration (Friedman et al, 1969a). Dilatation and descent curves were constructed for these patients in retrospect, and it was discovered that only one-quarter (26.3 percent) of their labors were actually normal in all respects. Nearly one-half had a prolonged latent phase, and the remaining abnormal labors were protraction or arrest disorders or both, sequentially. Among labors deemed to be normal but lasting less than 20 hours in duration, the incidence of correct clinical diagnoses was 90.1 percent. Together, the overall frequency of correct diagnoses in labors considered to be normal on clinical grounds was only 51.7 percent.

A comparable study of the relative inaccuracy of clinical diagnostic acumen showed that about one-half (53.9 percent) of a group of patients that had been diagnosed as having uterine dysfunction or maternal dystocia actually were normal with regard to dilatation and descent patterns. The rest of the group comprised patients with a heterogeneous variety of graphic disorders.

This demonstrated that the criteria that had been utilized for clinical diagnosis were not sufficiently adequate or accurate for diagnosing disordered labors where they exist. At the same time, such criteria may actually yield a diagnosis of an abnormality where none is present. Moreover, nongraphic impressions do not appear to be capable of distinguishing between the various specific labor disorders that are readily differentiated by graphic means.

## *CHARACTERIZING SPECIFIC DISORDERS*

In the chapters that follow, results of several studies are presented in which patients were collected and grouped according to the presence of specific aberrations. First, the incidence of various pertinent factors was investigated. In this way, we attempted to determine their possible significance as contributory or determinant factors in producing the disorder itself. Statistical verification was used to confirm or refute potential interrelationships. We felt we could elucidate valid associations between the labor disorders and possible etiologic agents. With this in mind, statistical analyses were carried out to define the significance of the frequencies of occurrence of factors in operation.

In addition, evaluations were undertaken of various treatment modalities. Prognostic implications were sought where the material indicated probable associations. Patients were studied to determine where they might differ from a normal cross-sectional sampling of the corresponding gravid population. This was felt necessary in order to uncover those factors that might potentially have caused or contributed to the development of the labor disorder. Along these lines, factors or agents found in excessive numbers within the several subpopulations were felt to be worthy of study in detail. Special attention was paid to those factors that are widely assumed to act in a deleterious manner in labor. Among others, these included such factors as fetopelvic disproportion, malposition, malpresentation, and excessive sedation and anesthesia. We encountered multiplicities of concurrent etiologic factors. Despite this, analyses did ultimately yield interesting and important information.

Therapeutic regimens were studied at great length, including expectancy, support, rest, uterine stimulation, and amniotomy. Criteria for successful therapy had to be established. In general it was felt that mere correction of the abnormality within a given period of time after initiation of the therapy sufficed for this purpose. This meant termination of the prolonged latent phase by the initiation of active dilatation, additional active cervical dilatation following secondary arrest of dilatation, additional descent following arrest of descent, acceleration of the rate of dilatation in protracted active-phase dilatation, and acceleration of the rate of descent in protracted descent.

As to the evaluation of prognosis, particular emphasis was placed first on the subsequent course of labor after the aberration had been corrected; second, on the ultimate outcome of the labor and delivery; third, on the outcome with regard to fetal morbidity and mortality. A fourth aspect recently pursued was that of long-term outcome with regard to growth and development of the surviving infant.

Failure to make clear distinctions in many prior studies of clinical inertia has confused the differences between the several varieties of dysfunctional labor that may fall into this widely inclusive designation of abnormal labor. Even in our studies, concepts of dysfunctional labor include at least two major extremes, namely, those in which the intrinsic driving uterine forces become insufficient for whatever reason to continue the dilatational and descent process adequately, and those in which dilatation or descent ceases because of local factors, despite apparently adequate driving forces. No provision has been made for this type of differentiation by the graphic analytic technique we have utilized. By our approach, we have examined the course of the resultant summation of the propulsive forces acting on the resistive soft parts. Thus, causative factors are not distinguishable; indeed, they cannot be distinguished.

Despite this limitation, attempts have been made to seek out the mechanisms of the subtle variants that are manifested uniformly by the presence of one or another form of aberration. These have been examined in detail. Graphic portrayal of the progressive changes in cervical dilatation and in descent serves the fundamental purpose of allowing critical identification and appraisal of normal and abnormal parturition. Used in this way, the technique has proved to be invaluable as a clinical and academic tool for the study of labor phenomena.

# Prolonged Latent Phase Disorder

## CHAPTER 9

The common but innocuous disorder of prolonged latent phase is investigated. Its clinical characteristics are detailed. Diagnostic criteria and pitfalls are discussed. Gravidas with prolonged latent phase are shown to differ from those with normal labors in significant ways. These differences aid in providing information concerning the probable etiology of this condition. The usual course of labor among these gravidas yields data on the good prognosis for vaginal delivery and for the delivery of an unaffected infant. Response to various treatments, notably therapeutic rest or uterotonic stimulation, serves as the foundation upon which a meaningful program of management can be built.

In the foregoing chapters, we have provided practical limits of normal labor. By this means we undertook to define the several major varieties of abnormal labor. Prolongation of the latent phase beyond 20 hours exceeds the upper 95th percentile limit of the distribution of latent phase durations in the nulliparous population. This limit is based on the mean plus twice the standard deviation. It should be considered a reference point for defining an important labor aberration. This limit for the latent phase in nulliparas has been incorporated into an expression of normality. The labor with a longer latent phase may be said to be dysfunctional and to demonstrate the specific and readily identifiable pattern of prolonged latent phase. Corresponding limits were evolved for multiparas. The latent phase in the normal multipara was found to be 14 hours at the maximum, based on the 95th percentile point of distribution. Thus, a latent phase longer than 14 hours was arbitrarily (but logically) chosen as the upper limit of normal for the purpose of defining the abnormality of prolonged latent phase in the multipara.

In measuring the latent phase, one must determine the duration of labor from the onset of regular uterine contractions to the beginning of the active phase of cervical dilatation. The latter is represented by the upswing of the dilatation curve. Accurate determination of both onset and end of the latent phase is obviously most important. Unfortunately, neither end is always clearly discernible. At its beginning, the onset of true labor is not necessarily clear-cut. Hendricks et al (1970) have demonstrated that many of the changes which characteristically are expected to take place early in labor, particularly with reference to effacement and beginning dilatation of the cervix, may actually occur well before the onset of perceived labor.

Thus, in many instances, determination of when labor begins may be the source of considerable perplexity and produce errors of variable magnitude. We have preferred to lean toward the conservative side, eliminating doubtful cases, so as to avoid vitiating our material excessively. The transition from false or prodromal labor to the latent phase of true labor, especially where it is smooth and uninterrupted in time, is seldom well defined. It may, however, be pinpointed historically and retrospectively by the astute patient who becomes aware of the rhythmical regularity of the contractions or of a significant and persistent change in her subjective appreciation of the contractions.

At the far end of the latent phase, the transition into the active phase cannot usually be distinguished clinically except by close attention to the plotted curve of cervical dilatation against elapsed time in labor. Only in this way is the end of the latent phase clearly marked by the onset of active cervical dilatation. It should be pointed out, parenthetically, that the transition from the latent phase to the active phase is not necessarily (nor even usually) associated with any abrupt change in contractility pattern or pain perception. Without the information gained from observations of the dilatation pattern, there is generally no reliable way to tell that the active phase of dilatation has begun. From the foot of the patient's bed, so to speak, the early part of the active phase is entirely indistinguishable from the latent phase; neither the patient's subjective appreciation of the contractions of her uterus nor the objective evaluation of the contractility pattern by tocodynamometer or internal strain gauge (see Chapter 2) aid in this regard. The transition from latent to active phase is generally imperceptible insofar as changes in contractility are concerned.

Thus, the requirement that the dilatation–time curve be plotted on an ongoing basis becomes essential. It is a relatively simple matter to delineate the several phases of the curve either while the labor is in progress (assuredly a more preferable practice), or by hindsight if sufficient observations of cervical dilatation are available to help reconstruct the labor curve. This permits one to characterize the individual labor according to its dilatation pattern and to recognize possible deviations from the previously established norm. It also allows for the study of factors that might influence the phases of labor and the relative efficacy of various forms of therapy that might be applied.

## *CHARACTERISTICS OF NULLIPARAS WITH PROLONGED LATENT PHASE*

In order to study the prolonged latent phase, a large series of such cases was collected (Friedman and Sachtleben 1961a). This group plus a more recent series of similar patients was studied in detail. Among nulliparas with abnormal labors, those with prolonged latent phase represented 30.2 percent; among abnormal multiparous labors, 52.8 percent (see Chapter 8 for relative frequencies of abnormal labors). In absolute terms, these cases totaled 2.3 percent of the entire nulliparous population from which they were obtained and 0.44 percent of multiparas.

The relative importance of abnormal prolongation of the latent phase as a clinically identifiable disorder of labor is demonstrated by the statistics: These cases represented 1 in every 43 nulliparas and 1 in every 227 multiparas. To reemphasize this point: Nearly one third of the abnormal labors in nulliparas and more than one half of the abnormal labors in multiparas constitute prolonged latent phase patterns.

The material that follows summarizes the extensive analyses of the data derived from these patients for purposes of determining etiologic factors, responses to therapy, and outcome. The program of management that has been recommended (Chapter 24) was evolved on the basis of this type of analysis. It must be stressed that management principles are based on objective findings rather than on any intuitive, arbitrary, or capricious impressions.

### *Age*

Comparing nulliparas with prolonged latent phase against normal nulliparas delivered during the same interval, we found relatively little difference in various actuarial factors. For example, the average age of those with abnormal labor pattern was 27.3 years, essentially the same as that of normal subjects (26.2 years). On closer scrutiny, however, higher age levels were seen within this group among those subjected to cesarean section without further labor (29.9 years). This may well have reflected the more aggressive attitude on the part of the obstetric attendant in managing gravidas of advanced years. Of greater importance, those who developed an arrest pattern later in the active phase or second stage were generally much older (30.6 years, average age). On the other hand, patients with protraction disorders following their prolonged latent phase were normally distributed with reference to age (25.5 years, average age).

As just stated, it appeared likely that the concentration of older women in the cesarean section group was based on the more liberal indications for abdominal delivery in the so-called elderly nullipara. Explanation for the preponderance of older gravidas in association with arrest patterns may or may not reflect an age influence on labor. However, this latter finding has never been demonstrated objectively, despite prevailing clinical thoughts on the subject. More will be said about the maternal age factor and labor (see Chapter 14).

### Birth Weight and Gestational Age

Birth weights among infants delivered of women with prolonged latent phase were normally distributed, 89.6 percent weighing between 2500 and 4000 g; the comparable frequency among normal nulliparas was 84.5 percent. Similarly, duration of pregnancy was about as expected, 7.7 percent of gravidas delivering in fewer than 39 weeks of gestational age (timed from the first day of the last menstrual period), as compared with 7.8 percent for the normal nulliparous population. Multiple births occurred in 0.9 percent, the same incidence as among normal women.

### Fetal Position

The relative frequencies of fetal positions were of interest by virtue of the high incidence of both transverse and posterior occiput mechanisms in labor. Together, these comprised 78.6 percent of the study population, as compared with 47.4 percent among normal subjects. This represented a sizable increase over the expected frequency of occurrence. There were no face presentations and only one brow presentation. There was a slight increase in the frequency of breech presentations over expected rates (5.4 versus 3.6 percent), but this was not a significant difference. The high incidence of minor degrees of malposition, particularly transverse and occiput posterior fetal positions, should be noted at this point. They will be dealt with in greater detail later (see Chapter 15). Similarly, breech presentation as it might affect the course of labor will be discussed at length (see Chapter 15).

### Pelvic Relationship

Fetopelvic disproportion was documented in 14.3 percent of nulliparas with prolonged latent phase; the comparable incidence in normal nulliparas was 7.8 percent. It should be pointed out in passing, however, that many more of these patients (an additional 6.0 percent) were thought (without documentation) to have disproportion, and were summarily subjected to cesarean section without further labor during the course of the latent phase. The incidence of disproportion remaining after these cases were discounted left an incidence that was still almost twice the expected frequency.

There has been a long recognized association between cephalopelvic disproportion and dysfunctional labor. Among women with prolonged latent phase who went on to develop a protraction disorder during the course of their labor, for example, 25.8 percent had disproportion; those who later developed arrest patterns had documented disproportion in 46.5 percent. More critically, cases of prolonged latent phase without other labor pattern abnormalities had disproportion in 4.7 percent only. On this basis, it was doubtful that the factor of disproportion contributed as such directly to the development of the abnormality of prolonged latent phase.

*Delivery*

As to delivery frequencies, there was an increased incidence of cesarean sections (23.7 percent overall versus 4.6 percent for the normal nulliparous population). Among those in whom the labor process was allowed to evolve, the cesarean section rate was 10.6 percent. Abdominal deliveries were concentrated almost exclusively among those subjected to cesarean section without adequate further trial of labor (62.3 percent of the sections that were done) and among those who subsequently developed an arrest pattern of labor (34.0 percent). There were no abdominal deliveries among those nulliparas with prolonged latent phase whose labors were allowed to proceed normally. This was a critical observation.

Midforceps operations were done in 14.6 percent of nulliparas with prolonged latent phase, as contrasted with 3.8 percent for nulliparas with normal labor. However, they were again concentrated primarily among those who went on in labor to develop either a protraction disorder (20.5 percent) or an arrest problem (23.1 percent). There was a small residual increase in the midforceps rate among nulliparas with pure prolonged latent phase (8.5 percent). This may have reflected the anxiety of the attendant physician in effecting delivery after what may have appeared to him or her to have been a very long and difficult labor.

There was a total incidence of 24.6 percent spontaneous deliveries and 37.1 percent low forceps procedures (comparable hospital rates were 40.4 and 51.2 percent, respectively). It would appear from these data that nulliparas with prolonged latent phase are not at any significantly increased risk for operative delivery unless a subsequent major labor aberration should develop.

*Membrane Status*

The time of rupture of the membranes was classified according to the phase of labor in which it occurred. When compared with corresponding frequencies of our normal nulliparous population, there was a preponderance of rupture of the membranes during the latent phase. The incidence totalled 34.3 percent, or three times the expected frequency of 11.0 percent. Among these, 60.9 percent constituted surgical amniotomies apparently done in an attempt to stimulate progress. These latter accounted for 47.7 percent of all amniotomies among this group of patients. Another concentration of amniotomies here was in the phase of maximum slope of dilatation, totaling 29.6 percent. As might be expected, most of these took place in patients progressing poorly or already arrested at that point (59.3 percent). Spontaneous rupture of the membranes occurred in increased numbers prior to labor

(14.1 percent) as well as at the onset of labor (17.2 percent). This latter phenomenon remains unexplained but will be dealt with in more detail in Chapter 17.

### *Perinatal Outcome*

The overall uncorrected perinatal mortality for this series was about the same as that for the comparable normal nulliparous population. No fetal or infant death was directly attributable to the prolonged latent phase problem. Those cases in which the fetus did not survive had associated protraction disorders, with and without the further complication of arrested labor. Most pertinently, there were no neonatal deaths in cases with prolonged latent phase only.

There is a well-documented direct relationship of increasing perinatal mortality associated with increasing duration of labor (Eastman, 1966). This was not confirmed here. The prolonged latent phase is undoubtedly a major contributing factor toward producing many of these worrisome cases of prolonged labor. However, from our data it does not appear that latent phase prolongation of itself adds significantly to perinatal mortality. This is not meant to imply that other varieties of labor prolongation may not adversely affect the fetus (see Chapter 23), but rather that those prolonged merely on the basis of an unduly long latent phase are apparently not at any substantively increased risk.

### *Labor Course*

As to subsequent labor disorders, nearly two-thirds (62.6 percent) were unassociated with any other aberrations. Those permitted to proceed in labor generally progressed well. Discounting those delivered by cesarean section during the latent phase for various reasons, patients allowed to labor tended to progress well with neither protraction nor arrest disorders during the course of their subsequent labor. The optimistic implications of these data with regard to the ultimate good prognosis for patients with prolonged latent phase are evident. Indeed, while our early series showed a somewhat increased propensity to develop other major aberrations, this has not proved to be the case in recent years.

Thus, patients with prolonged latent phase are no more prone to develop subsequent labor aberrations than those with normal latent phases; at the same time, they are not immune from other problems either, of course. Recent data show that the incidence of subsequent protraction and arrest disorders among such patients are about as frequent as among gravidas with normal latent phases. Moreover, among women who develop either protraction or arrest patterns, the incidence of prolonged latent phase tends to be rather low. This indicates that the abnormality in the latent phase is neither an essential feature in the production of other major labor aberrations nor a critical prognostic element (see Chapters 10 and 11).

*Table 7. LABOR DATA FOR PATIENTS WITH PROLONGED LATENT PHASE (PLP)*

| *Group* | *Latent Phase (hr)* | *Active Phase (hr)* | *Maximum Dilatation (cm/hr)* | *Deceleration Phase (hr)* | *Maximum Descent (cm/hr)* | *Second Stage (hr)* |
|---|---|---|---|---|---|---|
| Nulliparas | | | | | | |
| Mean labor | 6.4±0.25 | 4.6±0.14 | 3.0±0.08 | 0.84±0.04 | 3.3±0.07 | 1.10±0.04 |
| Total PLP series | 27.6±0.71* | 8.0±0.46* | 1.9±0.11* | 1.32±0.14* | 2.0±0.12* | 1.04±0.24 |
| Uncomplicated PLP | 26.7±0.89* | 4.0±0.17 | 2.7±0.15 | 0.63±0.04 | 2.9±0.17 | 0.82±0.06 |
| PLP sectioned | 28.1±2.91* | — | — | — | — | — |
| PLP + protraction | 30.7±1.55* | 10.0±0.60* | 0.8±0.03* | 1.57±0.14* | 0.8±0.04* | 1.25±0.14 |
| PLP + arrest | 28.7±3.02* | 11.0±1.42* | 2.2±0.99 | 3.63±1.18* | 2.4±1.01 | 1.81±0.51 |
| PLP + protraction and arrest | 25.9±0.91* | 18.1±1.15* | 0.6±0.04* | 3.21±0.68* | 0.7±0.05* | 1.69±0.40 |
| Multiparas | | | | | | |
| Mean labor | 4.8±0.18 | 2.4±0.06 | 5.7±0.16 | 0.36±0.02 | 6.6±0.17 | 0.39±0.02 |
| Total PLP | 21.6±0.83* | 4.4±0.53* | 4.2±0.38* | 0.47±0.07* | 4.6±0.40* | 0.29±0.04 |
| Uncomplicated PLP | 21.7±0.96* | 2.2±0.14 | 5.3±0.42 | 0.25±0.02 | 5.8±0.41 | 0.26±0.04 |

* Statistical significance, $p < 0.01$, when compared with corresponding mean labor data expressed in mean ± standard error.

To illustrate the potential effect of prolonged latent phase pattern on the subsequent course of labor, data were amassed for purposes of analysis from the several phases of each labor curve. The composite material is presented in Table 7, which contrasts the mean durations and slopes (and their standard errors) with corresponding data of the normal nulliparous series. Data from various subgroupings are shown as well, most pertinently from those women with prolonged latent phase unassociated with subsequent labor disorder.

We see among these latter patients that the course of the active phase and second stage is entirely normal. There is not even a suggestion that the course of labor following the termination of an abnormally prolonged latent phase is in any way different from normal. By the same token, those patients who later develop either protraction or arrest disorders do not demonstrate that their latent phase prolongations were necessarily any greater on average than other women with uncomplicated prolonged latent phase. We can surmise, therefore, that we need not expect the subsequent course of labor to be abnormal after a prolonged latent phase.

Among gravidas with prolonged latent phase who subsequently developed an arrest pattern, the mean maximum slopes of dilatation and of descent prior to arrest were well within normal limits. This observation suggested a probable dissociation between the two kinds of aberrations (that is, latent phase prolongations versus arrest disorders) because a finite period of normal progressive dilatation intervened between them. We may note in addition that the average duration of the latent phase in patients subjected to cesarean section without further labor was not different from that of any other subgroup. This implied that the trial of labor in these cases was probably not excessive; indeed, it was not necessarily adequate.

## *ETIOLOGIC FACTORS*

We now recognize that the latent phase is remarkably sensitive to narcotic–analgesic–sedative medications administered to the gravida. This applies especially to the inhibitory effect of heavy sedation (see Chapter 19). We investigated the degree of sedation among patients with prolonged latent phase and confirmed this relationship. It should be noted in passing that we were concerned not with specific dosages of given agents, but rather with their effect on the patient in terms of her ability to respond to the discomforts of contractions. In a sense, we were attempting to estimate the effects on her sensorium in a semiquantitative manner.

The incidence of oversedation among women with normal labor patterns in our population was 8.6 percent; among those with prolonged latent phase it was found to total 38.7 percent. More than one-half of these (58.1 percent) occurred in women with prolonged latent phase only, unassociated with other forms of labor aberration. It is pertinent that no other factors seem to be acting in most of these patients. After the effects of the medication had been allowed to abate, subsequent labor patterns were essentially normal in almost every one of these individuals.

Both general inhalation and conduction anesthesia, when administered to women in the latent phase of labor, seemed to present comparable problems. Peridural anesthesia was especially inhibitory in that none of the 5.9 percent of gravidas to whom it was given in the latent phase progressed in labor until the level of the anesthesia had been allowed to subside or until the labor had been stimulated with oxytocin infusion. The sensitivity of early labor to major regional-conduction anesthesia was thus confirmed in this series (see also Chapter 19). Those few patients given transitory general inhalation anesthesia in the latent phase (usually administered in the erroneous assumption that the patient was ready to deliver) invariable prolonged the latent phase until some time after the anesthesia had been allowed to wear off and active labor could be reestablished spontaneously.

A rather common finding in this group was the so-called unripe cervix at the onset of labor. This is variously characterized as tough, rigid, or thick and uneffaced. This condition has been clearly associated with prolonged labors by the work of Calkins (1958). Among normal nulliparous patients, it is encountered in 2.8 percent; by contrast, it is found in 18.0 percent of women with prolonged latent phase. Therefore, it is strongly implicated as probably causative in most of these labors. In a parallel series studied prospectively, we found that patients who entered labor with an unfavorable cervix developed prolonged latent phase precisely one-half of the time.

In this series of women with prolonged latent phase, 10.4 percent were determined in retrospect to have been in false labor. This emphasizes the real difficulties of distinguishing true from false labor clinically. We examined this series of patients with prolonged latent phase in order to ascertain whether or not various conditions commonly believed to be associated with abnormal labor were actually present in meaningful numbers. Our search failed to reveal any but a paltry number of cases with hydramnios, leiomyomata uteri, and multiple pregnancy. On this basis, we felt that these several factors were probably irrelevant as causative or contributory factors in the production of prolonged latent phase abnormalities.

As to causation, the factors of excessive sedation, anesthesia, unripe cervix, and false labor accounted for nearly three-quarters of these cases (73.9 percent). There remained a residual group of gravidas to whom no specific cause for the latent phase prolongation could be assigned. It was noteworthy that 9 percent of them went on to develop some form of protraction disorder. By hindsight, this could serve to imply that an underlying disorder of uterine contractility may have produced or contributed to the development of the prolonged latent phase in some or all of these patients. For some time we conjectured that there may have been some intrinsic myometrial problem of a neurologic or biochemical nature among this group; however, this hypothesis was discarded when it was learned that nulliparas with protraction disorders do not necessarily repeat this special disorder in subsequent pregnancies. Indeed, it is a very rare problem among multiparas.

No likely cause was discovered in 17.1 percent of women with prolonged latent phase. All of these patients in the idiopathic subgroup evolved normal labor patterns if labor was allowed to proceed. It is conceivable that many of these gravidas were merely unrecognized cases of prodromal or false labor who imperceptibly entered true labor; others may have had some form of uterine dysfunction that was later spontaneously corrected; still others may merely have had unripe cervix at the onset of labor that had not been documented or recognized.

These data are summarized in Figure 18, which presents the relative incidence of various factors that are likely to be etiologic for this condition. It should be noted that causal relationships seem clear-cut when these factors occur alone. In many cases, however, various combinations of factors were encountered, and only the ones considered as major contributory items on clinical grounds were included for analysis.

When one contrasts the frequency of occurrence of these factors in nulliparas with prolonged latent phase against the expected incidence based on cross-sectional sampling of normal nulliparas, one finds statistically significant differences only for excessive sedation, unripe cervix, and uterine dysfunction. These factors, therefore, ought to be considered to represent major etiologic influences that act to prolong the latent phase either directly or

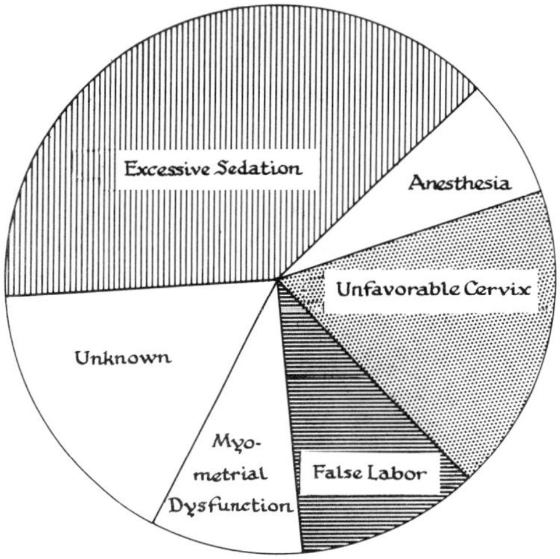


*Fig. 18.* Etiologic factors that appear to be responsible for the development of prolonged latent phase disorders in nulliparas, including most often excessive sedation administered during the course of the latent phase and and poor prelabor soft-tissue preparation; in addition, false labor and myometrial dysfunction are found, but they can be diagnosed only retrospectively. Factors commonly appear conjointly in a given patient, making assignment of proximal responsibility difficult.

indirectly. False labor is obviously another important consideration, based on our inability to distinguish it prospectively from true labor. Moreover, we also ought to include general inhalation and regional-conduction anesthesia for its obvious effects, although the numbers are relatively small and therefore without statistical significance. It is certainly clear that if sedation can inhibit progression in the latent phase, anesthesia will do likewise. Insofar as irrelevant factors are concerned, it is important to recognize that the factor of cephalopelvic disproportion does not influence the course of the latent phase; this holds for other miscellaneous conditions as well.

## *TREATMENT*

In our endeavor to evaluate the effectiveness of treatment modalities used to correct prolonged latent phase disorders, the most immediate problem encountered was the frequent intermixing of techniques. In view of this, criteria of success were necessarily made very stringent. For all modalities of active treatment, a successful effect was considered to be the termination of the latent phase, as demonstrated by the upswing of the dilatation curve within an arbitrary limit of 3 hours. Any effect beyond 3 hours was considered fortuitous and probably unrelated to the treatment administered, except where such treatment was still actively in progress, as during oxytocin infusion. The critical time for effectiveness after therapeutic rest was arbitrarily set at 10 hours.

We were concerned that we might attribute a fortuitous "cure" to a given mode of treatment. Our concern was well founded and confirmed by our observation that some patients who received no treatment whatsoever did progress promptly into the active phase of dilatation; such patients comprised 39.2 percent of the series, and spontaneous cure occurred in 88.5

percent of them. The rest had been delivered abdominally without further attempts to effect correction. We hasten to point out that this apparent rate of effectiveness should not be misconstrued as a realistic estimate of the actual success rate that will be obtained from watchful expectancy. The problem in this regard stems from our inability to judge critically which cases were actually subjected to this form of nonaggressive management. The only relevant cases that were easily identified were those in which prompt progression occurred or, alternatively, those in which cesarean section was done without the interposition of other treatment modalities. The effect among such patients was clearly weighted toward the beneficial side. Unidentified patients in whom expectancy yielded nothing by way of effective results undoubtedly included some who showed no effect and were therefore given other forms of active therapy. It was rarely determinable whether this was always actually required in any given case.

Treatment modalities were administered rather haphazardly, so that objective analysis was not always possible to determine the advantage of one over the other. Those therapeutic regimens administered earlier as a rule would perforce be at a distinct disadvantage when contrasted with those more likely to be held in reserve. This seemed to be especially true with reference to the technique of resting patients with the use of narcotic agents. Moreover, there were obvious preferences among physicians, as illustrated by the relative frequencies of use. Oxytocin infusion, for example, was used for the treatment of prolonged latent phase in 38.7 percent; amniotomy was performed during the latent phase in an effort to enhance the labor in progress in 23.4 percent; 14.0 percent were vigorously and effectively rested with large doses of narcotics; other forms of uterotonic stimulation were given in 8.6 percent. In all, 24.3 percent received two or more forms of treatment management. Evaluation of treatment combinations could not be accomplished because of the paucity of numbers of similar combinations.

Oxytocin infusion was administered to these patients in the form of dilute intravenous solution of 10 international units of synthetic oxytocin diluted in 1000 ml of 5 percent aqueous dextrose. This was given by slow and carefully controlled intravenous drip or by infusion pump, increasing the dosage at approximately 20-minute intervals until effective uterine contractions were produced. Therapeutic rest consisted of the administration of morphine sulphate in an initial dose of 15 mg subcutaneously. This first dose might be increased to 20 mg for a large patient. If contractions were still appreciated by palpation after 20 minutes and no further cervical dilatation had yet occurred, an additional 10 mg morphine (or 15 mg for an obese gravida) would be given, provided of course there had been no inhibition of respiratory function.

As to results, 83.9 percent of patients who were actively rested terminated the latent phase within 10 hours after therapy was initiated. Aware that excessive medication tends to produce prolongation of the latent phase, we may note this paradoxical action. The very same factor that prolongs the latent phase may frequently be followed by a normal labor pattern in the active phase. Whether this came about as a direct result of beneficial uterine rest in the patient with an abnormal labor or the consequence of withdrawal of deleterious sedation in an otherwise normal labor cannot always be determined in retrospect.

Among patients whose membranes were artificially ruptured in the latent phase for purposes of stimulating the labor, only 26.9 percent evolved promptly into the active phase. It should be noted that this figure is actually too high, because many such amniotomies were done during the acceleration phase. In other words, the active phase had already begun when the membranes were ruptured. We included such cases, however, because we could not clearly distinguish those in which acceleration was the immediate result of the amniotomy from those in which it was merely a fortuitous coincidence. Since only this small number progressed into the active phase within the arbitrary three-hour limit after amniotomy, we considered that amniotomy was of rather dubious value in the treatment of the abnormally prolonged latent phase.

As to oxytocin infusion, it was found to be effective in terminating the prolonged latent phase in 85.0 percent overall; prompt effect within three hours occurred in 65.6 per cent. The average interval from initiation of the infusion to the beginning of an identifiable active phase was 3.4 hours among gravidas who ultimately did respond. No other form of pharmacologic uterotonic stimulation was found to be regularly effective, including sparteine sulphate and, more recently, prostaglandin.

A more critical technique was sought for purposes of making the evaluation of treatment modalities more meaningful. This was found in the qualitative approach relating the distribution of cases to the time interval from the initiation of a form of treatment to the point of effectiveness. Effectiveness in these cases meant the onset of the active phase. Distribution curves were constructed and yielded much useful information. They pointed out whether or not a peak of activity existed. Such a peak indicated a direct post hoc relationship between the treatment and its overt effects in terminating the prolonged latent phase. Moreover, when such peaks occurred, the point in time of their appearance was well defined.

Some of these distribution curves for treatment effect are shown in Figure 19. Oxytocin infusion produced a sharply peaked hyperbolic curve. This indicated its prompt and significant efficacy in terminating the prolonged latent phase, whenever such an effect took place (as it did in 85 percent of the cases in which it was used). The flat nondescript amniotomy curve reflected its haphazard distribution of effect (or noneffect). The time at which amniotomy was done appeared to have no bearing on the subsequent results. This supported the contention that artificial rupture of the membranes contributes little or nothing to the treatment of the abnormal latent phase.

The results with aggressive therapeutic rest were impressive. Patients who were given large doses of narcotic analgesics for purposes of inhibiting uterine activity entered the active phase most frequently between 6 and 10

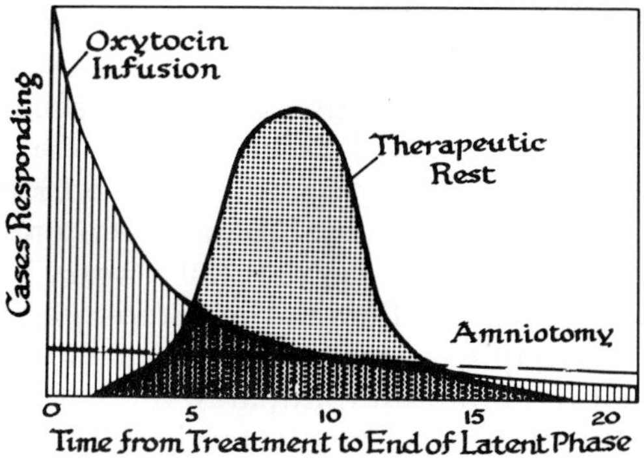


*Fig. 19.* Distribution curves for demonstrating relative effectiveness of therapeutic regimens used to terminate prolonged latent phase. Oxytocin infusion and therapeutic rest are equally efficacious, although their peaks of response appear at distinctively different times. Amniotomy provides a flat distribution of response, failing to demonstrate reliably consistent effect in this disorder.

hours later. This is shown by the peaked distribution curve for successful termination of the latent phase among those women who were sedated and responded (as nearly 85 percent did). While it is clear that oxytocin and therapeutic rest are equally effective, the distribution curves do not reflect this phenomenon precisely because the curve for rest has a wider spread over the course of time.

## *PROGNOSIS*

The material was also analyzed to ascertain the prognostic outlook for mother and fetus. With regard to the possibility of anticipating the subsequent formation of a dysfunctional labor pattern, our data show that these patients are no more prone to develop problems than gravidas with normal latent phase. Thus, the patient who has a latent phase longer than 20 hours in duration should be expected to evolve a normal subsequent dilatation and descent curve, if permitted to do so.

It cannot be too strongly stated that patients who are delivered by cesarean section during the latent phase for no other reason than their lack of progress are being subjected to this operation unnecessarily most of the time. Needless to say, there are indeed some legitimate reasons for undertaking cesarean section during the latent phase, but prolonged latent phase per se should not be one of them. Among those allowed to labor, very few ultimately require abdominal delivery. In fact, if the subsequent labor pattern is normal, nearly all should deliver vaginally and uneventfully (barring other kinds of fetal or maternal problems).

Therefore, the ultimate method of delivery will depend on the situation prevailing later in the course of the labor. Again, if the ensuing dilatation and descent pattern is normal, cesarean section will be unlikely. If a protraction or arrest disorder follows, much higher cesarean section rates will be anticipated; however, these rates are no higher than those occurring among patients with like labor disorders who did not have prolonged latent phase.

## *PROLONGED LATENT PHASE IN MULTIPARAS*

The data for multiparas with this disorder were essentially the same as those for nulliparas, with minor exceptions (Friedman and Sachtleben, 1963b). We will not dwell on the similarities, but only detail the differences where they are relevant. For example, the average age of multiparas with prolonged latent phase was consistently higher than expected (30.8 years as compared with 28.6 years for normal multiparas). This was not statistically significant except in association with subsequent arrest patterns of labor. Not unlike the fetal positional abnormalities found in nulliparas, there were increased frequencies of transverse and posterior occiput mechanisms in multiparas as well (60.0 percent versus 33.1 percent expected). Excess of breech presentations was also encountered (6.7 versus 2.8 percent). Data for perinatal mortality paralleled that of nulliparas.

Material obtained by analysis of the several components of the dilatation and descent curves from these patients revealed findings that were very similar to those in nulliparas. Those who did not subsequently develop a protraction or an arrest disorder, for example, were well within normal limits insofar as their cervimetric data were concerned, except for the expected prolongation of the latent phase. These findings reconfirmed that latent phase prolongation is an abnormality quite distinct unto itself. It appears not to have any pertinent influence on the subsequent course of labor. The dissociation of prolonged latent phase pattern from all other labor aberrations merits our attention.

Attempts were made to define potential causative factors. Those uncovered in large numbers were deemed to be suspicious. Special attention was paid to those factors known to have been acting deleteriously in nulliparous labors. A multiplicity of concurrent etiologic factors was seen frequently, although not as often as in nulliparas. Two-thirds had two or more concomitant factors acting simultaneously. The relative incidence of probable etiologic factors is presented in Figure 20.

The factors of greatest significance included false labor most often (54.0 percent), excessive sedation (28.6 percent as contrasted with 4.0 percent for normal multiparas), and the presence of an unripe cervix at the onset of labor (14.3 percent versus 2.4 percent expected). In addition, there were 22.6 percent who subsequently developed a protraction disorder in the course of the active phase. Again, retrospectively, this suggested that the disordered uterine function may have caused the prolongation of the latent phase. There was a small residual group (8.8 percent) in which no etiologic factor could be assigned.

Corresponding data in nulliparas indicated that neither false labor nor uterine dysfunction was as frequent. On the other hand, the incidence of excessive sedation was much greater, as was the number with unripe cervix and in whom no etiologic factors could be assigned. The critical influence of prelabor cervical preparation on the course of labor was reconfirmed here (see Chapter 16). Conduction anesthesia had been found to be associated

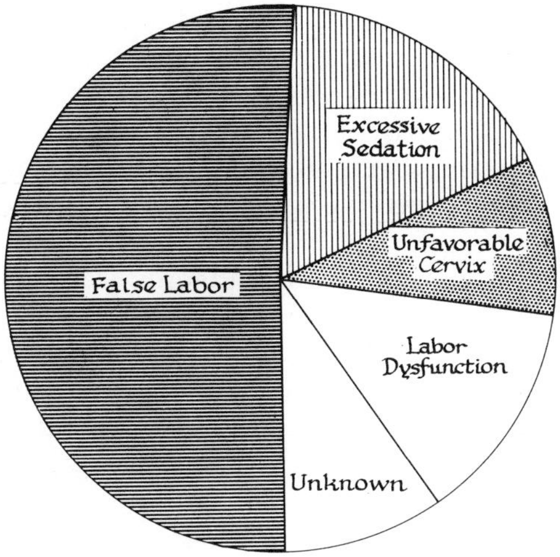


*Fig. 20.* Relative incidence in etiologic factors for prolonged latent phase in multiparas. While the factors responsible are the same as in nulliparas (compare with Fig. 18), false labor leads the list here as a much more common cause. Excessive sedation and myometrial dysfunction are still important, but are encountered less often. Factors commonly occur concurrently.

with prolonged latent phase in nulliparas if administered during the latent phase. It was encountered in 4.8 percent of multiparas with prolonged latent phase as well. It appeared, therefore, that the etiologic factors contributing to the development of prolongation of the latent phase were the same in both multiparas and nulliparas. However, the order of frequency was different. Excessive sedation took the lead in nulliparas; false labor and uterine dysfunction were more common in multiparas.

Evaluation of treatment modalities was carried out in a manner analogous to that in nulliparas. The frequent intermingling of techniques made the task equally difficult. As before, the categories of therapy included observation, support and rest, and uterotonic stimulation. The criterion for successful and efficient therapy was the documentation that the abnormality had been corrected within a suitable period. This was arbitrarily set, as previously stated, at 3 hours after the initiation of active therapy (stimulation) or 10 hours for inactive therapy (observation and rest).

Among those patients rested therapeutically by narcosis, further prolongation of the latent phase occurred as expected; there often followed prompt response without further therapy, usually within 5 hours. Other patients who had been sedated inadvertently during the latent phase, thereby prolonging the interval abnormally, responded well within the requisite time, with documented upswing of the dilatation curve when such sedation had been allowed to abate. The peak response for successful termination of the latent phase after heavy sedation in multiparas occurred between 5 and 9 hours after treatment. This is similar to the peak of response seen after therapeutic rest in nulliparas. In our series, resting the multipara with prolonged latent phase pattern was effective in 92.3 percent within 10 hours. This was only slightly higher than the success rate in nulliparas.

Negligible response was seen with amniotomy as a mode of treatment for prolonged latent phase. Oxytocin infusion, on the other hand, was effective in 85.0 percent overall. Exactly one-half responded within 3 hours of the initiation of the drug. The average interval from the beginning of the infusion until the effect was seen was 3.6 hours—nearly identical with nulliparas. Other uterotonic agents were less effective in general, although decidedly better than in nulliparas. Overall, our data showed that prolonged latent phase in the multipara was much more easily correctable than in the nullipara.

The end results among these patients, as far as delivery outcome was concerned, reflected the subsequent course of labor. If a normal pattern of dilatation and descent followed, no unusual difficulties were encountered. On the other hand, protraction or arrest disorders or both were ominous. The outcome for such patients, however, was no different from that of other multiparas who developed such disorders without precedent abnormal latent phase.

As with nulliparas, certain clear principles evolved. One obvious truism was that cesarean section in the latent phase has no place as a method of treatment for the prolonged latent phase (without other clear indication). Those patients who were subjected to abdominal delivery stand as grievous testimonials to this contention. With a possible exception of those with documented cephalopelvic disproportion of major order and those with objective evidence of fetal distress, one would be hard-pressed to justify the aggressive approach that was employed. There is no way during the course of the latent phase to predict what the subsequent evolution of the dilatation and descent pattern will be. One cannot foresee which of the several patterns will be described in any particular patient while she is still in the latent phase. Termination of labor by cesarean section, therefore, is clearly unwarranted without other more concrete reasons.

# Protraction Disorders

## CHAPTER 10

The related disorders of protracted active-phase dilatation and protracted descent patterns are examined in detail. The special characteristics of patients with these labor abnormalities suggest common factors for the development of the disorders, but etiology remains undefined. The lack of consistent response to any form of known treatment is recognized. These labors are adversely affected rather easily by various inhibitory factors. Prognostic outlook for mother and fetus is considered briefly.

Diagnosis and management of the nebulous disorder called uterine inertia are unclear. It undoubtedly encompasses a conglomerate of conditions and constitutes a major clinical problem that requires careful clarification. Graphic evaluation of both cervical change and progressive descent provide data that have proved useful in this regard (Chapter 8). To review, when estimates of cervical dilatation are plotted against time on a system of coordinates, the maximum rate of dilatation in the active phase should normally exceed 1.2 cm per hour in nulliparas. Correspondingly in multiparas, the lower statistical limit of the mean maximum slope of dilatation is 1.5 cm per hour.

The active phase, briefly outlined again, has been defined as that portion of the first stage of labor that begins with the accelerative change in dilatation at the end of the latent phase—seen on cervical dilatation–time curves as a distinctive upswing—and terminates with full cervical dilatation and retraction. Thus, in the active phase a maximum rate of dilatation or slope of less than 1.2 cm per hour in the nullipara or 1.5 cm per hour in the multipara is clear evidence of the presence of one specific variety of dysfunctional labor: namely, protracted active-phase dilatation.

Similar limits have been evolved from graphic analysis of the patterns of progressive descent with elapsed time in labor. The limits of normal for the maximum slope of descent in the nullipara is 1.0 cm per hour; for the multipara, 2.0 cm per hour. Patients with descent patterns demonstrating a maximum rate of descent of less than these critical limits provide objective evidence that another related variety of disordered labor exists; specifically, protracted descent.

Progressive and uninterrupted advancement of the fetal presenting part is a prerequisite of normal labor, most particularly during the deceleration phase of dilatation and throughout the second stage of labor. Recognizing the limits of the rate of progression to be expected in descent under normal circumstances (Friedman and Sachtleben, 1970a) has permitted us to define, detect, and investigate recognizable aberrations of a specific nature. Our ability to identify such specific abnormalities of labor allows us to sequester homogeneous groups of patients with like problems, in order to derive information that will be utilized to help provide objective bases for establishing meaningful programs of management for these important disorders.

Many published studies on clinical inertia in labor have employed various criteria to help define the abnormality. Some of these are quite uncritical, such as the common practice of assigning an arbitrary limit to the total duration of labor. The normal sigmoid curve of dilatation is readily apparent, as is the hyperbolic curve of descent. The configuration of the abnormally slow active phase of dilatation or of the abnormally dilatory descent pattern, however, are not so obvious to the clinician unless the slope is actually being measured or calculated. The single criterion of an abnormally low slope of the curve of dilatation or of descent suffices to delineate these serious labor aberrations. It has been used as a means of classification for purposes of study and diagnosis. This has greatly aided us in our attempts to elucidate the mechanisms, etiology, therapy, and prognosis of these serious disorders of labor.

## *PROTRACTED ACTIVE-PHASE DILATATION PATTERN*

We have been fortunate in having been able to study a large group of patients with clearly documented protraction of the maximum slope of dilatation (Friedman and Sachtleben, 1961b). Recent review of a comparable series demonstrates no substantive changes in our original findings. The details of these series reflect only those gravidas who did not later develop an arrest disorder; those who did will be discussed separately in Chapter 11.

### *Age*

Actuarial and obstetric data from such patients were compared with like data derived from the normal gravid population of similar parity. Patients with this problem averaged 26.2 years of age; this is precisely the same as the average age of comparable normal patients. There was no evidence of weighting here toward the older groups, contrary to what had been seen among patients with prolonged latent phase who subsequently developed an arrest pattern. Indeed, we were able to reaffirm our earlier findings (see Chapter 9) that there were no age differences among patients with protraction of the active phase of dilatation. This added credence to our contention that age per se had no direct influence either in prolonging the latent phase or in slowing active phase dilatation.

### *Birth Weight and Gestational Age*

As to gestational age, 10.3 percent of pregnancies were less than 39 weeks in duration and only 1.9 percent were less than 37 weeks. This is somewhat better than the normal population with regard to incidence of prematurity. However, there was an essentially normal distribution of birthweights as compared with the normal population (86.2 percent weighed between 2500 and 4000 g versus 84.5 percent expected). The incidence of multiple gestations was somewhat higher than observed normally (1.9 percent versus 0.9 percent).

### *Fetal Position*

Frequent transverse and posterior occiput fetal mechanisms were encountered in this group of patients, totaling 70.6 percent overall (47.4 percent expected). The major difference was concentrated among those with occiput posterior positions (36.7 percent versus 17.2 percent). Just as in the prolonged latent phase series where similar excesses were found, these minor positional abnormalities were implicated here as potentially contributory to the production of protracted active-phase dilatation. Earlier investigation (Friedman, 1955a) had demonstrated a similar relationship between malpositions and the retardation of the deceleration phase and the second stage, but not of active-phase dilatation itself. It is more likely that the high incidence of minor malpositions was the result of poor driving forces associated with this abnormal labor pattern rather than the cause of the pattern.

No face, brow, or transverse presentations were encountered here. A total of 7.5 percent of infants presented by the breech. This represented more than twice the expected incidence (3.6 percent). The question of a possible association between breech presentation and the development of protracted active-phase dilatation was thereby raised (see Chapter 15 for a further consideration of this issue).

### *Pelvic Relationship*

Disproportion was documented by radiographic studies in 28.1 percent of nulliparas with this disorder of labor. This contrasted sharply with that of essentially normal nulliparas (7.8 percent). The correlation between cephalopelvic disproportion and protraction disorders verified the findings of an earlier study (Friedman, 1957a), in which bony disproportion was demonstrated to be a major factor in the production of both protraction and arrest disorders (see Chapter 16).

### *Delivery*

There were high cesarean section (10.2 percent) and midforceps (24.1 percent) rates, both significantly increased over that of the normal nulliparous population. These data played an important role in our subsequent analyses with regard to prognostic outlook (see below).

### *Membrane Status*

Patients were grouped according to the time the membranes ruptured, with particular regard to the phase of labor in which this event occurred. There was an unusual concentration at or before the onset of labor (16 and 22 percent versus 12 and 10 percent, respectively). Most of them were spontaneous rupture of membranes. Membranes ruptured in the latent phase in 15 percent; by contrast, 60 percent of these were surgical amniotomies. The large incidence in the active phase was essentially normal (47 percent), but these were predominantly performed as surgical procedures ostensibly to stimulate labor. Without exception, they were without effect. More will be said about amniotomy as a stimulatory device (see Chapter 17).

### *Perinatal Outcome*

The perinatal mortality among infants born of women with this specific disorder was unexpectedly high. Correcting for anomalies incompatible with life, we obtained an overall perinatal death rate of 38.8 per 1000 births, equally divided between neonatal deaths and stillbirths. The comparable corrected combined rate for infants delivered of normal mothers was 11.8 per 1000 for the same interval. These data suggest that a real increase over expected mortality rates existed in this series.

The possibility that there was a positive correlation between this protraction disorder and perinatal mortality could not be denied. It was perhaps due to increased risks of amnionitis in prolonged labor, to conditions leading to anoxia, and of greatest importance, to traumatic attempts at delivery. All three of these hypothetical possibilities were exemplified in our data. This relationship had not been seen in the prolonged latent phase series. Thus, protracted active-phase dilatation is undoubtedly a far more serious disorder. It was conjectured to be a prominent factor in the documented association between increasing perinatal mortality and increasing duration of labor. Prognosis for the fetus will be discussed in detail subsequently (see Chapter 23).

*Table 8. LABOR DATA FOR PATIENTS WITH PROTRACTION DISORDERS*

| *Group* | *Latent Phase (hr)* | *Active Phase (hr)* | *Maximum Dilatation (cm/hr)* | *Deceleration Phase (hr)* | *Maximum Descent (cm/hr)* | *Second Stage (hr)* |
|---|---|---|---|---|---|---|
| Nulliparas | | | | | | |
| Mean labor | 6.4±0.25 | 4.6±0.14 | 3.0 ±0.08 | 0.84±0.04 | 3.3 ±0.07 | 1.1 ±0.04 |
| Protracted dilatation | 18.6±1.11* | 11.2±0.46* | 0.71±0.02 | 1.8 ±0.10* | 1.1 ±0.04* | 1.4 ±0.11* |
| Protracted descent | 16.2±1.06* | 10.0±0.52* | 1.2 ±0.12* | 2.1 ±0.14* | 0.76±0.06* | 2.1 ±0.09* |
| Multiparas | | | | | | |
| Mean labor | 4.8±0.18 | 2.4±0.06 | 5.7 ±0.16 | 0.36±0.02 | 6.6 ±0.17 | 0.39±0.02 |
| Protracted dilatation | 15.1±2.84* | 8.1±1.13* | 1.1 ±0.07* | 1.35±0.20* | 1.4 ±0.12* | 0.59±0.13 |
| Protracted descent | 14.6±1.90* | 7.1±1.02* | 1.4 ±0.08* | 1.51±0.18* | 0.82±0.10* | 0.96±0.14* |

* Statistically significant, $p < 0.01$.

## *Labor Course*

All patients in this series were examined critically with reference to their overall patterns of dilatation and descent. Mean data for constructing composite curves were obtained by subdividing the pattern of each gravida into its component phases. These are compiled in Table 8 along with similar data for comparison obtained from normal nulliparas. It is apparent from this material that protracted active-phase dilatation does not occur in isolation. Significant prolongations of latent, active, and deceleration phases are found together with comparable prolongation of second-stage duration. These observations emphasize that protraction of the rate of dilatation in the active phase is a sufficient criterion to delineate an intrinsic condition of labor that appears to carry through from the onset of labor to delivery.

It is of considerable interest that the latent phase was so frequently prolonged in this series. It is tempting to deduce from this that underlying etiologic factors in the production of the disorder of protracted active-phase dilatation were in effect long before the active phase began and that these may have also been responsible for prolonging the latent phase. This mechanism was implied to be important in some cases in the prolonged latent phase series (see Chapter 9) .

## *Etiologic Factors*

It was found to be especially difficult to assign etiologic importance to various factors in this series of cases because it is likely that the disorder did not actually begin in the active phase, but instead was merely first identified there. Agents occurring with unusual frequency in the active phase, therefore, although perhaps contributing to the further retardation of cervical dilatation, need not necessarily have been directly causative of the underlying protraction disorder.

Nevertheless, there were certain very suggestive cause-and-effect relationships based on unusually large numbers of patients with specific factors. Included among these were cephalopelvic disproportion, the minor malpositions of occiput posterior and occiput transverse, and amniotomy before or at the onset of labor. Each of these factors, alone or in combination, was in effect throughout both the latent and active phases of dilatation in 84.1 percent of these patients. Therefore, it is certainly possible that they might have been instrumental in producing the abnormal pattern of dilatation. How this might have been brought about is unknown, of course.

The association between this protraction disorder and bony disproportion has been fairly well documented (Friedman, 1957a). Therefore, it was not unexpected here. The high incidence of minor fetal malpositions was somewhat surprising, since they had not previously been implicated as potentially causative except in the related series involving prolonged latent phase labors. We might conjecture whether it was truly etiologic or merely a fortuitous discovery based on early detection of fetal position made possible because such patients were under observation for long intervals of time as a consequence of their prolonged labors. The high incidence of premature and early rupture (35.5 percent) could not be explained.

We searched for other less obvious etiologic factors. The degree of sedation was examined, for example. We saw (Chapter 19) that the latent phase and, to a lesser degree, the active phase of dilatation are sensitive to the inhibitory influence of sedation administered to the mother. In this group of gravidas with protracted active-phase dilatation pattern, 16.8 percent were heavily sedated in the latent phase and 42.1 percent in the active phase (8.6 and 30.8 percent, respectively, in the normal nulliparous population). Heavy sedation here refers, of course, to the effect of such sedation on the patient's sensorium, not on the dosage administered or the type of agent used. This observation of increased use of narcotic analgesics confirmed earlier contentions of a possible cause–effect relationship. It reasserted the likelihood that excessive sedation is indeed contributory toward the slowing of progress in labor.

Similarly, 14 percent of this group had been given peridural anesthesia in the latent phase or during the early active phase of dilatation. We have previously demonstrated that such conduction anesthesia is potentially inhibitory, particularly if administered before the active phase is well under way (Friedman and Sachtleben, 1959). The finding in this series that so many peridural anesthesias had been given early in labor lends support to the probability that conduction anesthesia may cause protracted active-phase dilatation when given so early.

Other possible etiologic factors were sought as well. The paucity of numbers suggested that none were relevant, including breech presentation, multiple pregnancy, prematurity, uterine anomalies, leiomyomata uteri, and hydramnios.

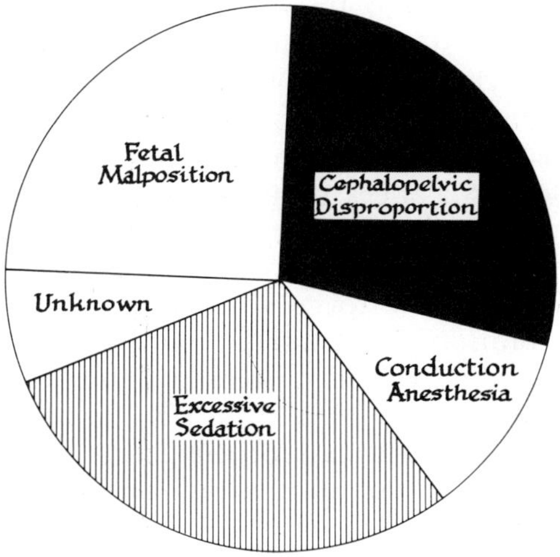


*Fig. 21.* Factors contributory to the development of protraction disorders, emphasizing the importance of cephalopelvic disproportion, excessive sedation, and minor fetal malpositions. It should be stressed that the etiology of these disorders is actually unknown at this time.

The relative incidence of factors deemed likely to be causative or strongly contributory is shown in Figure 21. Actually, more than one factor coexisted in most cases (67 percent). The primary ones, including disproportion, malposition, and early amniotomy, were encountered in 84 percent of cases. Adding the major secondary contributory factors increased this total to 97 percent.

### *Treatment*

Treatment regimens invoked for managing patients with protracted active-phase dilatation pattern included expectant observation, support and rest, and uterotonic stimulation. As to expectancy, an intensive case-by-case search failed to reveal a single instance of spontaneous increase in the rate of cervical dilatation in the active phase. The use of sedation to effect a period of rest for therapeutic purposes could not, of course, be distinguished from its use for relief of discomfort.

The inhibitory action of sedation was recognized. While particularly inhibitory in the latent phase, narcotic analgesics have been shown to be less effective in delaying progress in the normal active phase (see Chapter 19). However, there was little doubt that it did act in a deleterious manner when the active phase was already protracted.

As to potential therapeutic benefit, we attempted to ascertain whether or not there were subsequent changes in the slope of the dilatation curve during the course of the active phase. A total of 36.4 percent had received large doses of narcotics during the active phase and were thereby effectively rested. The dilatation patterns in many showed slight additional retardation for a variable period. As the effect of the medication wore off, there was a return to precisely the same slope as had existed prior to the treatment. In others, no change in the linearity of this portion of the curve could be detected.

The overall effect was to achieve a period of well-needed rest, following which the labor pattern resumed its earlier slow and dilatory course. There was not a single example encountered in which the slope became steeper.

The same approach was used to examine the effect of oxytocin infusion. We sought a criterion of success by examining the linear maximum slope of the active phase of cervical dilatation for changes brought about by such uterotonic agents. We felt that any positive increment in the slope during the course of stimulation would reflect its effectiveness. Oxytocin was administered to 74.7 percent of these patients in the form of modulated intravenous infusions of dilute aqueous solution. It is worth noting that the pattern of protracted active-phase dilatation evolved in some patients while they were receiving their oxytocin stimulation.

Among those receiving oxytocin during the course of the active phase, many were found to undergo changes in the nature of their uterine contractions. This change was characterized by varying degrees of increase in frequency, intensity, and/or duration. However, no effect was seen insofar as the dilatation pattern was concerned. This was another example of the dissociation between contractility and the effect of the contractions.

Amniotomy was used as a stimulatory device in 32.7 percent during the active phase. The linearity of the dilatation curves in these patients was completely unaltered by this procedure. It must be stressed here, however, that this finding is probably subject to misinterpretation, because this group did not include those that subsequently went on to develop an arrest pattern. As will be seen in Chapter 11, when one takes into account those patients with protraction disorders who subsequently developed arrest patterns, the results are quite different. Indeed, amniotomy under those circumstances tends to yield rather untoward effects. Nonetheless, we may see here that amniotomy is clearly not beneficial in accelerating the protracted dilatation pattern. In view of the potential risk of intrauterine infection that may follow amniotomy, especially in such prolonged labors, it may actually serve as a source of harm to both mother and baby.

Our findings with reference to treatment regimens for this disorder may be summarized briefly. The linearity of the curve of dilatation in the active phase, once established, is difficult to alter. Progressive dilatation, even though occurring at abnormally slow rates, does not seem to be amenable to being changed beneficially by any currently available means. On the other hand, protracted dilatation may readily be inhibited to yield an arrest pattern (see Chapter 11).

### *Prognosis*

For purposes of analyzing our data for prognosis, it was necessary to combine this group with those who subsequently developed an arrest pattern. When combined in this way, we found that 69 percent arrested secondarily. The circumstances leading to the later cessation of progress in these cases will be discussed in Chapter 11. The remaining patients continued to advance at their preset, constant, and abnormally slow rate of dilatation. They were not influenced by either deleterious or stimulatory agents.

The increased fetal hazards occurring with such labor patterns (see Chapter 23) were felt to be largely associated with the trauma of the delivery procedures that followed. There were (and continue to be) an unacceptably high frequency of operative vaginal deliveries, particularly midforceps procedures, among these patients. This will be treated in greater detail during our discussion of the management of such patients (see Chapter 24).

## *CHARACTERISTICS OF MULTIPARAS WITH PROTRACTED DILATATION*

Multiparas with this relatively rare labor abnormality were also studied in detail (Friedman and Sachtleben, 1963b). They were found to differ somewhat from comparable nulliparas. Maternal age and parity were normally distributed. Contrary to the finding among nulliparas, there were no fetal losses. This confirmed our contention that this abnormal labor pattern per se did not contribute directly to perinatal mortality, but that the increased losses encountered among nulliparas were more likely due to the delivery procedures instead.

The labor data analysis showed a very low maximum slope, as expected, together with markedly prolonged active and deceleration phase durations as well as significant lengthening of the latent phase. These findings parallel those of nulliparas with this disorder, reasserting the intrinsic nature of the problem that appears to exert its influence at the onset of labor and continues to act throughout the course of labor.

As to factors possibly contributing to the development of this pattern in multiparas, again it was clear that combinations of factors were common (56 percent). Prominently among these was excessive sedation (61 percent), fetal malpositions (67 percent), and conduction anesthesia (28 percent), all of which were found in significantly increased numbers. Contrary to the findings in nulliparas, neither early amniotomy nor disproportion occurred in meaningful frequencies.

The major etiologic factors of malposition, excessive sedation, and conduction anesthesia were thus shared by both nulliparas and multiparas. The relative frequencies of these factors were in the same order of occurrence in the two parallel groups.

As in nulliparas, specific therapeutic agents were generally ineffectual among multiparas. Of those who received no discernible therapy, slow dilatation in the active phase continued without interruption, ultimately terminating in vaginal delivery. Active uterotonic stimulation with oxytocin infusion also had no influence on the course of dilatation. Similarly, amniotomy was ineffectual.

These findings verify the persistently progressive nature of this disorder; they confirm the contention that abnormally slow rates of dilatation such as are encountered in this disorder apparently cannot be speeded. Of course, these rates may be slowed considerably. Indeed, complete arrest occurred commonly (see Chapter 11). Labor was ultimately arrested in 70 percent of multiparas with protracted active-phase dilatation patterns. This is about the same rate as was seen among nulliparas. Those who continue to progress with unimpeded dilatation and descent were generally delivered atraumatically without the difficult operative procedures that probably accounted for the poor fetal results among nulliparas with this disorder. When there was a subsequent arrest pattern in this group, the results were not so favorable, however. The prognostic outlook changed considerably (see Chapter 11).

## PROTRACTED DESCENT PATTERN

A large series of patients with clearly defined protracted descent was recently studied (Friedman and Sachtleben, 1970b). They constituted 4.7 percent of the gravid population. Maternal age was found to be the same as that of the normal obstetric population. Gestational age was also normally distributed, except for a paucity of premature births. Indeed, there was a general shift upward in the distribution of birth weights. There were very few infants weighing less than 2500 g and an increased incidence of large infants weighing more than 4000 g. This was seen especially among nulliparas (9.0 percent, 4.2 percent expected).

### *Fetopelvic Relationship*

The observation suggested that fetopelvic relationships might be important. It was confirmed by the finding of documented disproportion in large numbers among both nulliparas and multiparas with this disorder (26.1 and 9.9 percent, respectively). Furthermore, minor fetal malpositions were encountered frequently in this group, including persistent occiput posterior and transverse positions (82.9 percent overall in nulliparas and 70.4 percent in multiparas). No trends were encountered with reference to any other major abnormal presentation or position.

### *Membrane Status*

The status of the membranes, with specific reference to the time in labor when they ruptured, was distributed in the same unusual manner that had been seen in protracted active-phase dilatation pattern. The incidence of premature rupture of the membranes exceeded expectations significantly in nulliparas (20.5 percent) and to a lesser degree in multiparas (14.1 percent). Similarly, the frequency of rupture of the membranes during the active phase of dilatation was very high. However, here most (84 percent in nulliparas and 90 percent in multiparas) were ruptured surgically for purposes of ostensibly stimulating the labor in progress.

It seemed in retrospect that perhaps the membranes had been ruptured under these circumstances because of the associated protracted active-phase dilatation pattern that so commonly preceded the protracted descent pattern. Indeed, patients with abnormal descent patterns had precedent dilatation abnormalities totaling 75 percent in nulliparas and 58 percent in multiparas. Both of these frequencies are statistically significant, indicating a real association between these two disorders. It is for this reason that they are considered together here and will be dealt with together in our discussions of management (see Chapter 24).

### *Delivery*

Operative deliveries were quite common. Midforceps procedures were performed in nearly one-half of the nulliparas (44 percent) and nearly one-third of the multiparas (28 percent). Cesarean sections were done in 11 percent of nulliparas and 3 percent of multiparas. The high incidence of operative deliveries here is comparable to that seen with protracted active-phase dilatation patterns.

### *Labor Course*

We have already seen that a significant proportion of patients with protracted descent presented dilatation disorders as well. Only 25 percent of nulliparas and 42 percent of multiparas were shown to have completely normal dilatation patterns preceding the descent disorder. The mean durations and slopes of the several phases of the dilatation curve fell outside the normal range. All phases of labor appeared to have been affected.

The association of protracted descent with precedent dilatation disorders was common. Most impressively, there were high frequencies of foregoing patterns of secondary arrest of dilatation and protracted active-phase dilatation. These were especially prominent among nulliparas. We see evidence here that the disorder of protracted active-phase dilatation is not only frequently (more than two-thirds) followed by secondary arrest of dilatation or other arrest patterns, but is frequently followed by protracted descent as well.

### *Etiologic Factors*

Agents, factors, and conditions that occurred with unusual frequency in these patients were felt to be of potential etiologic significance. We were struck by the presence of abnormally large numbers of patients with cephalopelvic disproportion, minor fetal malpositions, excessive sedation, and peridural anesthesia. The association of active-phase aberrations with all of these factors has been well documented (see relevant chapters). We were not surprised, therefore, to find them acting here as well.

Factors that might be causative or contributory were studied. Heavy sedative-analgesic medication had been used frequently (70 percent in nulliparas and 54 percent in multiparas). Similarly, peridural anesthesia had been invoked quite often as well (21 and 27 percent, respectively). Thus, this group of patients was found to be rather similar to gravidas with protracted dilatation.

The role of the commonly encountered pattern of protracted dilatation in the development of this descent aberration cannot be determined at this point. We may infer from the frequent association of protracted dilatation and descent aberration in the same labor that these have some common underlying etiologic factor. Both may arise from common causes. This is a more attractive concept than the assumption that the preceding abnormality caused the subsequent one to occur. Although some of the descent pattern disorders arose near the termination of the active-phase dilatation-pattern aberrations or may even actually have followed them, many began concurrently. The overlap in time between descent pattern and active dilatation pattern under normal circumstances has been well documented (Friedman and Sachtleben, 1965c). Both patterns commonly arise together. Indeed, among patients who developed both disorders, they occurred simultaneously in 52 percent.

## *Treatment*

We investigated the efficacy of treatment modalities employed for correcting protracted descent patterns. Oxytocin infusion was used in 65.0 percent of nulliparas and 39.4 percent of multiparas. In 40.6 percent, the disorder arose while the patient was receiving oxytocin; continuing the infusion appeared to have had no influence on the course of descent. Those who were actively stimulated during the course of protracted descent showed no documentable alteration in the abnormally slow rate of descent.

Those patients with protracted descent who were stimulated with oxytocin could be compared with a group of comparable gravidas whose labors were allowed to evolve without active intervention of this nature. The aggressive approach to management of women who were given oxytocin as treatment was further reflected in a high midforceps rate among them (51 versus 37 percent). At the same time, the relative frequencies of cesarean section were reversed; more followed expectancy than stimulation (15 versus 9 percent). However, significantly more depressed infants and perinatal deaths occurred following uterotonic stimulation, especially when the deliveries were effected by midforceps procedure.

## *Prognosis*

Subdividing the treatment groups according to delivery technique, we encountered interesting trends. Among those treated expectantly and then delivered by midforceps, there were 26 percent depressed infants, as compared with none following cesarean section. By contrast, among patients stimulated with oxytocin, midforceps procedures were associated with frequent neonatal depression (32 percent) and a high perinatal mortality rate (69 per 1000). Cesarean section performed after similar stimulation, on the other hand, produced 25 percent depressed infants and no deaths. This analysis suggested that midforceps operations after protracted descent carry a high fetal risk, especially if uterotonic stimulation had been used as well.

Comparable data were seen in multiparas in whom the incidence of neonatal depression after midforceps delivery was 18 percent overall. This totaled 23 percent if preceded by therapeutic stimulation with oxytocin, and 7 percent in the absence of such foregoing stimulation. Midforceps operations resulted in perinatal mortality of 50 per 1000, paralleling that seen in nulliparas. All deaths were associated with uterotonic stimulation.

As the protracted descent pattern evolved among these patients, 44 percent developed documented arrest of descent. These included 52 percent of nulliparas and 23 percent of multiparas. Almost twice the number of nulliparas with dilatation disorders subsequently developed arrest of descent when compared with those who had normal dilatation patterns before the onset of the protraction disorder. Among multiparas, there was more than a tenfold increment in the incidence of arrest of descent; 37 percent following abnormal dilatation pattern and 3 percent if the dilatation pattern was normal. Although the frequency of midforceps procedures was high in nulliparas regardless of the kind of dilatation pattern that preceded the protracted descent pattern, the number was significantly increased if the dilatation pattern had been abnormal during the first stage.

The incidence of cesarean section reflected the dilatation and descent patterns as well. In both nulliparas and multiparas, abdominal delivery was required much more often after combined dilatation and descent disorders than when the descent pattern occurred alone. The section rates for women with uncomplicated protracted descent (that is, those with a normal dilatation pattern) were essentially the same as for the normal gravid population. Twice as many patients with cephalopelvic disproportion were found in the group with abnormal dilatation patterns. All cesarean sections here were done for insurmountable bony disproportion. In general, those nulliparas with precedent dilatation disorders had larger infants; this was not duplicated among multiparas.

Additional aspects of the prognostic data will be treated in greater detail in Chapter 23. The results of these studies formed the basis upon which the programs of management for these disorders were designed (see Chapter 24).

# Arrest Disorders

## CHAPTER 11

All four related disorders of arrested labor are studied in order to characterize the gravidas afflicted by them. Their common association with cephalopelvic disproportion emphasizes the overriding seriousness of these aberrations. Other apparent causes are reviewed. Relative treatment effectiveness is shown, especially the generally good response to oxytocin stimulation. The significance of post-arrest progression is stressed.

It is a matter of the most serious importance when progressive cervical dilatation stops or progressive fetal descent halts in labor. It is toward a clearer understanding of this group of disorders that this chapter is directed. We recognize four different and interrelated kinds of patterns here: secondary arrest of dilatation, prolonged deceleration, arrest of descent, and failure of descent.

By way of definition, secondary arrest of dilatation occurs when cervical dilatation stops in the active phase. The arrest is manifested by flattening of the dilatation curve. Two hours of arrest are used as the minimum criterion for diagnosis. It can be documented by two or more vaginal examinations spaced at least 2 hours apart. A variant of this abnormality is prolonged deceleration phase, characterized by a deceleration phase duration lasting longer than 3 hours in nulliparas or 1 hour in multiparas.

Arrest of descent is analogous to secondary arrest of dilatation, in that progressive fetal descent stops during the pelvic division of labor (deceleration phase and second stage). The pattern of descent is expected to be progressing at its maximum during this interval; arrest of descent is readily recognized when descent stops abruptly. The minimum criterion for diagnosis is 1 hour of arrest, as documented by sequential vaginal examinations.

The last variant consists of failure of descent, a condition in which the expected descent during the pelvic division does not occur. By the time the cervical dilatation pattern reaches its deceleration phase at 8 or 9 cm of dilatation, descent should have begun. If the deceleration phase of dilatation or the second stage has been entered, the absence of descent is a potentially serious problem.

## SECONDARY ARREST OF DILATATION

About one nullipara in twenty develops secondary arrest of dilatation during the course of her labor; the incidence is somewhat less in multiparas. A large series of patients has been studied (Friedman and Sachtleben, 1962a), and a more recent review of similar patients has confirmed our original findings. The characteristics of these patients, particularly as they differ from gravidas who follow a more normal labor pattern, will be detailed here.

### *Age*

Nulliparas with secondary arrest of dilatation averaged 27.1 years in age; this is only slightly greater than expected (26.2 years). Multiparas with this disorder, on the other hand, were significantly older than normal multiparas (31.8 versus 28.6 years). Closer examination of the age distribution among nulliparas showed that those who developed arrest during the phase of maximum slope tended to be somewhat older (average age, 28.1 years). The age factor among nulliparas approaches statistical significance in those who develop arrest late in the phase of maximum slope; that is, beyond 6 cm of cervical dilatation (28.7 years).

Our attention is drawn toward the concentration of older gravidas in this series. We had previously encountered a comparable trend among gravidas with prolonged latent phase who subsequently developed secondary arrest of dilatation (Chapter 9). However, it will be seen (Chapter 14) that we are unable to demonstrate any real influence of maternal age on the course of labor. It is possible to explain this apparent paradox on the basis of the relative rarity of the phenomenon of secondary arrest of dilatation in the unselected gravid population. If maternal age does actually affect labor, we cannot demonstrate it clearly; on the other hand, it would be difficult to refute that such an influence might exist. If it does, its point of action appears to be narrowly limited to the late active phase.

### *Birth Weight*

The distribution of birth weights among infants born following secondary arrest of dilatation was essentially normal in nulliparas, provided the preceding labor had not been additionally complicated by a protraction disorder. In multiparas, by contrast, the relative frequency of large babies (more than 4000 g) was much greater than expected (13.5 versus 5.8 percent). Actually, this relationship was not unexpected in view of the close correlation of this disorder with fetopelvic disproportion (see below).

### *Fetal Position*

Minor fetal malpositions were common. Occiput transverse and occiput posterior positions were encountered in 73.2 percent of nulliparas and 70.4 percent of multiparas with secondary arrest. These findings confirmed what had been seen consistently before; namely, that minor positional abnormalities could be implicated in the pathogenesis of these dysfunctional labor patterns.

Additionally, the incidence of breech presentations was greater than expected as well (6.9 and 8.1 percent, respectively). The finding of increased numbers of breech presentations had previously been noted in association with protracted active-phase dilatation pattern (Chapter 10). These data now suggest that a similar relationship may exist for secondary arrest of dilatation. We hasten to point out that the association of abnormal labor patterns with breech presentation has not been detected in the general gravid population (see Chapter 15).

It is likely that such a relationship could not be detected because the relative infrequency of dysfunctional labors among gravid patients would preclude it. A prospective study on the order of several tens of thousands of parturients would be required to collect sufficient numbers of abnormal labors in conjunction with breech presentations to uncover any meaningful association. For example, in a gravid population of 10,000 women, 500 should be expected to develop secondary arrest of dilatation; among these, only between 15 and 20 will have breech presentations. This is obviously an insufficient number for definitive study of the possible influences of the presentation on the course of labor or on the production of labor aberrations. The possibility that a positive correlation exists between breech presentation and dysfunctional labor has nevertheless been suggested and will be discussed further (Chapter 15).

### *Pelvic Relationship*

The association between secondary arrest of dilatation and insurmountable degrees of pelvic dystocia has been documented (Friedman, 1957a). It was not surprising, therefore, that large numbers of patients with secondary arrest of dilatation presented radiographic evidence of fetopelvic disproportion. The incidence in nulliparas was 44.6 percent (expected: 7.8 percent); in multiparas, 19.5 percent (expected: 5.8 percent). These findings clearly confirm the probable cause-and-effect relationship between cephalopelvic disproportion and secondary arrest of dilatation. This will be treated in much greater detail later (Chapter 16).

### *Delivery*

As expected, the incidence of cesarean section (29.0 percent) and midforceps (29.8 percent) was significantly increased in nulliparas; the rates were comparably elevated in multiparas as well (5.6 and 11.1 percent, respectively). Most of the cesarean sections were indicated for documented cephalopelvic disproportion. The midforceps were generally indicated for positional dystocia, particularly in relation to persistent occiput posterior and occiput transverse arrests. The remainder consisted of trials of forceps in the presence of mild to moderate degrees of relative disproportion. It is likely that some of these procedures would not have been required had sufficient time been allowed to elapse to permit the second stage to evolve further.

The aggressive intervention that these operative procedures probably represented is further illustrated by the frequent association with other potentially traumatic techniques and resultant injuries. Among these were manual dilatation of the cervix, intense Kristeller expression, multiple forceps applications, difficult extractions, delivery hemorrhage, as well as vaginal sulcus, cervical and rectal lacerations.

### *Membrane Status*

A slight but consistent increase was seen in early rupture of the membranes, either before or at the onset of labor. Whether or not there is a deleterious effect in dysfunctional labors from early or premature rupture of the membranes will be discussed more fully later (see Chapter 17). An increased frequency of membrane rupture during the active phase of dilatation was also encountered (44.6 percent versus 21.5 percent expected).

This exaggerated incidence was thought perhaps to reflect the use of amniotomy as a stimulatory device for therapeutic reasons in a labor that was not progressing well. However, this contention could not be confirmed, because relatively few were done after the arrest of dilatation had occurred. In 32 percent the arrest circumstantially followed the amniotomy.

Thus, there is an increasingly perplexing implication that amniotomy may be a retarding factor in dysfunctional labor. This is contrary to current opinion and widespread clinical impression and practice. It appears to demand that this matter be clarified further (see Chapter 17).

### *Perinatal Outcome*

Perinatal mortality among infants delivered following secondary arrest of dilatation is similar to that encountered in the protraction disorders, and may actually be greater. This had not been immediately apparent in our original studies, but as data have accumulated, it has become increasingly clear that secondary arrest of dilatation carries a significant risk to the fetus.

When appropriate corrections are applied for congenital anomalies that are incompatible with life, the overall perinatal death rate was 40.2 per 1000 births (compared with 11.8 per 1000 for infants delivered after normal labor). As will be seen (Chapter 23), fetal wastage in association with this disorder was largely related to the kind of delivery that was undertaken. The more traumatic the delivery procedure, the greater the perinatal loss.

## *Labor Course*

Dilatation and descent data were obtainable by abstracting the several component parts of the labor pattern from patients who exhibited secondary arrest of dilatation (Table 9). There is the expected overall prolongation of the durations of the active and deceleration phases and the second stage, together with flattening of the maximum slopes of both dilatation and descent. The latent phase was prolonged only when protracted active-phase dilatation pattern coexisted.

Thus, the latent phase is not specifically affected in gravidas with pure secondary arrest of dilatation. This indicates that this latter condition is an entity quite distinct from the protraction disorders and essentially unrelated to them. The protraction disorders have been demonstrated to reflect an intrinsic process in effect from the onset of labor. The underlying mechanisms of secondary arrest, on the other hand, do not appear to become manifest until after the active phase has been entered. This leaves the latent phase of the first stage intact and unaffected.

The significantly prolonged active-phase durations reflect several factors. The most obvious is the time lost from the arrest of progress itself. In addition, the average maximum slope is distinctively less than expected. Although it does not reach the abnormally slow rates that characterize the protracted active-phase dilatation pattern, the effective rate of change is significantly slowed. It should be pointed out that we have here selectively excluded protraction disorders so that these data may be seriously biased.

The basic distribution data, furthermore, demonstrate that protraction

*Table 9. LABOR DATA FOR PATIENTS WITH SECONDARY ARREST OF DILATATION*

| Group | Latent Phase (hr) | Active Phase (hr) | Maximum Dilatation (cm/hr) | Deceleration Phase (hr) | Maximum Descent (cm/hr) | Second Stage (hr) |
|---|---|---|---|---|---|---|
| Nulliparas | | | | | | |
| Mean labor | 6.4±0.25 | 4.6±0.14 | 3.0 ±0.08 | 0.84±0.04 | 3.3 ±0.07 | 1.10±0.04 |
| Secondary arrest | 10.1±0.78* | 10.4±0.47* | 1.86±0.08* | 4.25±0.44* | 1.98±0.09* | 2.54±0.22* |
| Multiparas | | | | | | |
| Mean labor | 4.8±0.18 | 2.4±0.06 | 5.7 ±0.16 | 0.36±0.02 | 6.6 ±0.17 | 0.39±0.02 |
| Secondary arrest | 6.5±0.94 | 6.9±0.49* | 2.5 ±0.21* | 2.25±0.35* | 2.6 ±0.24* | 0.93±0.22* |

* Statistically significant, $p < 0.01$.

and arrest occur together in about half the cases (see Chapter 12). Thus, there is a tendency toward protraction among cases that eventually arrest. Accordingly, protraction and arrest disorders are not always mutually exclusive and may indeed have some common or interrelated mechanisms.

The fact that the subsequent course of labor in many of these patients is normal, however, tends to confirm the contention that the entities are distinctive. Investigation of protracted active-phase dilatation patterns showed the unchangeable and persistently dilatory nature of that pattern despite any form of therapy. The course of dilatation following arrest, on the other hand, generally returned toward normal. Data derived from those portions of the dilatation curves that followed the arrest confirm this observation.

In a series of patients with demonstrable effect from therapy in the form of further cervical dilatation, the average second slope was 3.1 ± 0.27 cm per hour, a significant increment over that of the slope of the curve prior to the arrest. This value is quite comparable with the mean maximum slope for normal nulliparous labors. Including those with associated protracted active-phase dilatation pattern, the rate of dilatation following arrest averaged 2.5 ± 0.13 cm per hour.

Whereas the overall effect from therapy of secondary arrest in nulliparas was a significant increase in the postarrest slope, this was not the case in effectively treated multiparas. The postarrest maximum slope in multiparas averaged 2.5 ± 0.23 cm per hour. This was identical with the average prearrest slope.

## *Etiologic Factors*

Previously in foregoing studies of labor aberrations, there was often considerable difficulty in uncovering potentially causative factors. This was not a problem here. In our efforts to assign proper etiologic roles to those factors that might have been influential in stopping progress, any factor or agent intrinsically present or administered prior to the arrest was suspect. Accordingly, since the onset of arrest was usually rather well defined, the events that occurred in the interval immediately preceding the actual arrest of dilatation were examined carefully.

In addition to the obvious agents encountered, including the administration of excessive sedation or conduction anesthesia and the performance of surgical amniotomy, endogenous conditions that might have contributed to the aberration were noted for study as well. These latter included bony dystocia, malpositions and malpresentations, leiomyomata uteri, multiple pregnancy, prematurity, and hydramnios.

We encountered an unusual number of nulliparas with malpositions, excessive sedation, cephalopelvic disproportion, and conduction anesthesia (Fig. 22). Combinations of possible factors were more in evidence here than in preceding studies. In 99 percent of the patients, at least one of these factors was operative; in 76 percent, two or more were found. In essentially all instances, disproportion, malposition, and/or excessive sedation occurred. In

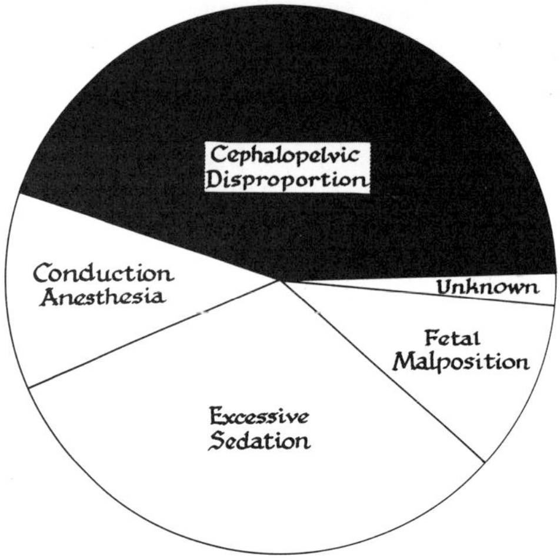


*Fig. 22.* Etiology of arrest disorders. The striking association with cephalopelvic disproportion makes these disorders especially ominous; whenever encountered, arrest patterns should signal the likelihood that a bony impediment exists. Other factors very often occur in combination with each other and with disproportion as well.

those cases in which amniotomy or regional anesthesia was implicated, they generally occurred concomitantly with one or more of the other factors under surveillance here.

Overall, nearly 45 percent of the cases had documented cephalopelvic disproportion. This was significantly greater than the expected frequency in the nulliparous population (almost sixfold). This finding agreed with earlier observations of the concurrence of secondary arrest and bony dystocia.

Excessive narcosis was encountered in 63.1 percent. The expected incidence in nulliparas during the same interval was 30.8 percent. It has been established that the latent phase is considerably more sensitive to sedative-analgesic medication than the active phase. Breakdown of our data by phase of arrest showed a much higher incidence of excessive sedation in gravidas whose labors arrested during the acceleration phase, or phase of maximum slope, than in the deceleration phase. There appears to be a difference in responsiveness to sedation according to how far advanced the active phase is.

Malposition was encountered in 73.1 percent (47.4 percent expected). These cases were more frequently associated with arrest late in the active phase (beyond 6 cm of dilatation) and in the deceleration phase. This trend verified that malpositions may prolong the deceleration phase of the first stage (see Chapter 15).

Conduction anesthesia was implicated because of the increased frequency encountered among these patients (18.5 versus 9.6 percent expected). There was a similar trend toward more frequent occurrence late in labor. The increased incidence of such deleterious factors as disproportion, malposition, and excessive sedation in this series was quite in agreement with the contention that conduction anesthesia would augment the untoward effect of these factors (see Chapter 19).

It did not appear that the anesthesia itself was a common primary factor in producing secondary arrest, but it may indeed have been contributory in many instances. This was particularly so when the level of anesthesia was especially high (above dermatome thoracic–10) and where significant hypotension resulted. The need to avoid such complicating factors has been well documented. The tendency for high anesthetic levels to cause labor to arrest is well known in clinical practice.

Amniotomy preceded arrest within 2 hours in 31.5 percent of the cases. This incidence was not very different from the expected frequency of amniotomies in the active phase. Of course, if we had included those done in this phase as therapeutic measures for the management of arrest of dilatation (see below), we would have brought the total significantly to 44.6 percent.

Unfortunately, meaningful data are not yet available for an evaluation of the potential interrelationship between amniotomy and the subsequent development of secondary arrest of dilatation. Our data suggest that amniotomy may impede progress in dysfunctional labor in some obscure manner, but it is perhaps only a minor contributory factor. This is supported by its very common association with other, better substantiated factors. None of the other factors examined for possible etiologic relationships could be determined to be significant in any way because of the sparsity of numbers involved.

Comparable factors were found to be present among multiparas with secondary arrest of dilatation. These included excessive sedation (47.2 percent), malpositions (58.3 percent), improperly administered conduction anesthesia (33.3 percent), and fetopelvic disproportion (13.9 percent). Comparing these figures with the corresponding frequencies in nulliparas, we determined that the same etiologic factors were acting in both groups. Disproportion was considerably more frequent among nulliparas. In an inordinately large number of multiparas, moreover, none of these factors could be found to be in operation (17.0 percent).

## *Treatment*

The techniques of analysis that we used for the prolonged latent phase series (Chapter 9) were utilized to define the effectiveness of the several treatment modalities in use here. The basic criterion of success was documentation of subsequent progressive cervical dilatation following the period of arrest. This was recognized as a secondary upswing of the dilatation curve.

The regimens employed included no treatment, rest and support, and uterine stimulation. Those stimulated were easily identified. Patients who were rested by narcosis, on the other hand, could not be readily distinguished from those given heavy sedation inadvertently. This was further confused by that group of patients in whom arrest of dilatation was apparently brought about by excessive analgesia. Suitable and effective treatment may have merely entailed permitting the effect of the medication to subside spontaneously. The same held for patients who developed arrest following improperly administered conduction anesthesia.

Among those who received no form of uterotonic stimulation, 52.5 percent showed later spontaneous progress in cervical dilatation and were ultimately delivered vaginally. It is especially noteworthy that so many of these patients subsequently dilated their cervix without the aid of any active stimulation. Among these, one-half had been heavily sedated, and progressive dilatation occurred when the medication wore off; most of the remainder had had conduction anesthesia, and subsequent progress followed abatement of the anesthesia.

Among gravidas to whom oxytocin infusion had been given as specific treatment for arrest of progress in the active phase, only 14.5 percent failed to progress further. The success rate for this form of therapy increased to well over 90 percent when those cases were eliminated in which cesarean section had been undertaken promptly; that is, further labor had not been allowed to evolve.

It is of considerable interest to note that this good result was encountered even in the presence of documented cephalopelvic disproportion. This observation is the source of much consternation and will be discussed at length subsequently (see Chapter 16).

Patients with a secondary arrest who were narcotized for the purpose of providing therapeutic rest responded with later active dilatation in 40.0 percent. The average duration of arrest was 5.3 hours. Among gravidas ostensibly stimulated by amniotomy, subsequent dilatation occurred in 20.0 percent only—a negligible effect.

Evaluation of the relative effectiveness of the several treatment modalities was made difficult by their frequent admixture. In order to quantitate their relative effects, it was necessary to relate the distribution of cases to the time interval from initiation of therapy to a response in the form of subsequent further progressive cervical dilatation. Distribution curves of this type were found to be valuable in demonstrating the presence of a peak of activity, if any, and for indicating potential cause-and-effect relationships.

The graphic representation (Fig. 23) illustrates the rapid, efficient action of oxytocin in correcting the arrest disorder. The absence of a peak of activity following amniotomy is noteworthy and illustrates the relative inefficacy of this form of treatment of secondary arrest. The response following therapeutic rest is diffuse. While there is a peak of activity in patients who are sedated for rest, the distribution curve of that response is spread over an unduly long period of time, indicating that the effect is not one that can be relied upon to any great extent.

In multiparas who were given oxytocin infusion to correct secondary arrest of dilatation, the response was nearly uniform: 89.5 percent dilating the cervix within 3 hours and all delivering normally. These results were somewhat better than those seen in nulliparas after oxytocin.

Expectant treatment consisted of allowing excessive sedation or conduction anesthesia to abate when this was apparently causative; under these circumstances, expectancy proved effective. Amniotomy was not utilized in sufficient numbers to permit meaningful evaluation of its efficacy, but the results were generally disappointing.

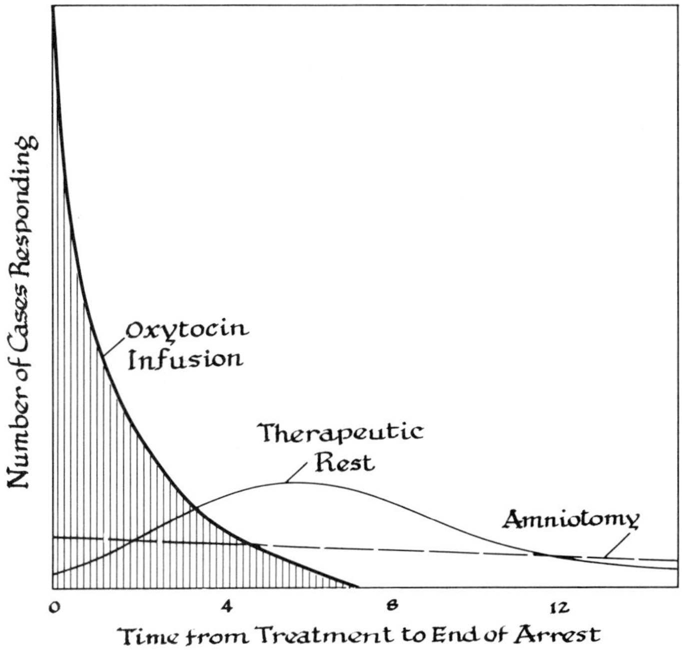


*Fig. 23.* Response to treatment of arrest disorders. Distribution curves based on number of labors responding over a period of time from the beginning of therapy with additional dilatation or descent following uterotonic stimulation, showing the good results generally expected by this means. All those capable of responding (constituting more than 90 percent) have responded by 7 hours, and most by 4 hours. No other form of therapy, including amniotomy, is reliably effective in this regard. A diffuse, poorly peaked response to therapeutic rest suggests that this form of treatment is only of limited usefulness.

## *Prognosis*

Following secondary arrest of dilatation, 69 percent responded with further dilatation. Most of the remaining patients were not given an opportunity to labor; they were either delivered by cesarean section or by a midforceps procedure through the incompletely dilated cervix. Several had unsuccessful trials of forceps and were subsequently delivered abdominally.

The overall response rate of 69 percent to all forms of therapy may actually be a low estimate of the potential rate obtainable in secondary arrest of dilatation with more conservative management. This statement, however, should not be misconstrued to imply that this is the expected magnitude of the cure rate for all secondary arrest problems because we are discussing only cases of pure secondary arrest. Those occurring in conjunction with protracted active-phase dilatation patterns will be discussed later (Chapter 12).

A less favorable response was encountered in labors that arrested early in

*Table 10. DELIVERY OUTCOME IN SECONDARY ARREST BY POSTARREST RESPONSE*

| *Postarrest* | *Cesarean section* (%) | *Midforceps* (%) |
|---|---|---|
| No response | 82.5 | 12.5 |
| Any response | 5.6 | 37.8 |
| Decrement or no change | 11.1 | 55.6 |
| Increment +0.5 or greater | 4.2 | 33.3 |
| Increment +1.5 or greater | 0 | 22.2 |

the active phase (less than 6 cm of cervical dilatation). This observation confirmed similar findings in patients with documented disproportion (see Chapter 16). Among them, there was a tendency toward greater degrees of bony dystocia in association with early secondary arrest. Here the section rate was considerably higher than among those who arrested later (98.8 versus 36.4 percent).

The degree of responsiveness in terms of the rate of dilatation following arrest unquestionably influenced the ultimate outcome (Table 10). For example, among those with no postarrest response, 82.5 percent required cesarean section and 12.5 percent, midforceps operation. Most of the latter were difficult. Among those who did respond with further dilatation, only 5.6 percent came to cesarean section and 37.8 percent, to midforceps delivery. These data are statistically quite significant, supporting the thesis that the degree of responsiveness has prognostic value.

We explored this matter still further. Patients with accurately measurable postarrest slopes were studied. All had arrested prior to the beginning of the deceleration phase. It was determined that the degree of response was greater in patients arresting early than in those arresting late in the active phase (postarrest slope, 4.6 ± 0.77 versus 2.6 ± 0.18 cm per hour). It is pertinent that the response of those who did show subsequent dilatation was quite efficient. It should be noted, however, that early arrests were less often correctable.

It has been shown that the individual patient traces her own characteristic pattern, particularly with regard to the maximum slope of dilatation that she tends to maintain steadily throughout a major part of the active phase. In view of this, it was felt essential to compare the pre- and postarrest slopes. We examined both the magnitude of the slope and the change in the slope (noting the increment or decrement from prearrest to postarrest rate of progression).

Marked differences were seen with regard to the influence of the increment in slope on delivery outcome. Labors with postarrest slopes that were less steep than the prearrest slope (or equally inclined) were terminated by cesarean section in 11 percent and by midforceps in 56 percent. This contrasted significantly with labors characterized by a positive increment in slope of at least +0.5 cm per hour following the arrest; these women required cesarean section in only 4 percent and midforceps in 33 percent. Still more impressive are the data for gravidas with increments of +1.5 cm per hour or more; none required cesarean section, and midforceps were used in 22 percent. The prognostic significance of the occurrence of a postarrest slope was quite evident and the degree of change obviously very important.

Among multiparas with secondary arrest of dilatation, 89 percent responded with further dilatation. All those who did not respond had not been given sufficient opportunity to do so. This overall rate of response is, therefore, a reasonable estimate of the potential outlook in the secondary arrest of dilatation that is not preceded by protraction disorder.

As to delivery, there were no cesarean sections and only 5.6 percent midforceps procedures required among those multiparas in whom treatment resulted in further dilatation. This reflected the similar reduction in cesarean section rates seen above in nulliparas, according to treatment response. However, because the numbers of cases were not adequate, we could not demonstrate a clear-cut correlation between increment in postarrest slope and decreasing frequencies of operative delivery. On the basis of our data, nevertheless, in the presence of any response to therapy in the form of additional progressive cervical dilatation, the likelihood of operative delivery appeared to be reduced to a minimum. When a response to adequate therapy did not occur, the prognostic forecast became rather pessimistic.

## *PROLONGED DECELERATION PHASE*

The duration of the deceleration phase in nulliparas averages 50 minutes; in multiparas, 22 minutes. The 95th percentile limits were determined to be 2.7 hours and 52 minutes, respectively (see Chapter 7). Although the existence of the deceleration phase has been denied by some (Hendricks et al, 1970), it has been verified objectively (Chapter 4). Moreover, it has been found to be very important, particularly when abnormal labor occurs.

Under normal circumstances, the deceleration phase may indeed be difficult to detect since it can be very short, spanning only a matter of minutes. Although it is probably present to some degree in all cases, in the majority of normal multiparas it may be considered to be absent since it is essentially undetectable by currently available, coarse clinical means of estimating cervical dilatation. Obviously, only frequent observations will disclose it in the normal multipara. When it is abnormal, however, it is quite readily detectable by the simple expediency of graphing the changes in cervical dilatation with time.

The mechanism by which the deceleration phase is produced has previously been discussed at length (Chapter 5). We should emphasize again that the rate of cervical dilatation may be decelerating, but myometrial activity and simultaneous passive retraction of the cervix normally continues without interruption and may actually be increasing during this interval.

For the data described here, we chose as our diagnostic criteria specific cut-off intervals beyond which abnormality was considered to be present. In nulliparas, this included all gravidas with deceleration phase greater than 3 hours; in multiparas, 1 hour. The potentially serious nature of complications causing this abnormality or produced by it made it clear that this choice of limits was probably too restrictive. In clinical usage, it has since been found reasonable to accept 2 hours' duration for nulliparas and 30 minutes for multiparas as meaningful upper limits for the normal deceleration phase. Using these more liberal values, the clinician will be alerted earlier and more readily to the impending serious problem.

## *Obstetric Factors*

Previous obstetric history in these patients tended to be similar to that of normal gravidas. Maternal age was normally distributed. The distribution of birth weights was also normal in nulliparas (6.7 percent of neonates weighed more than 4000 g) , but not in multiparas. In this latter group, the frequencies of infants weighing less than 2500 g (10.2 versus 5.2 percent) and more than 4000 g (13.6 versus 5.8 percent) were definitely higher than expected.

The increased incidence of fetal malposition and fetopelvic disproportion will be discussed in more detail below. The time membranes ruptured was rather normally distributed throughout. Multiple pregnancies were encountered in excess numbers among multiparas with prolonged deceleration phase (5.1 versus 1.3 percent expected) , but not among comparable nulliparas.

The incidence of operative deliveries was very high among these patients. In nulliparas, there were 16.7 percent cesarean sections (1.8 percent expected) and 40.0 percent midforceps (3.8 percent expected) . Similarly, in multiparas there were 8.5 percent cesarean sections and 16.9 percent midforceps (0.8 and 1.8 percent expected, respectively) .

All the cesarean sections were indicated for cephalopelvic disproportion, including several that followed failed attempts at vaginal delivery. Most of the midforceps procedures were done for positional dystocia or for midpelvic arrest in progressive descent. About 10 percent of these subjects had been delivered instrumentally through a residual rim of cervix prior to full cervical dilatation and retraction. Some had been subjected to manual dilatation of the cervix as well. The significantly reduced number of uncomplicated vaginal deliveries in this group indicated the serious nature of this disorder.

Dysfunctional labors of other varieties were quite common in association with prolonged deceleration phase. For example, there were 63.3 percent of nulliparas who had a coexisting protraction disorder and 23.3 percent who had another arrest disorder. Among multiparas, 37.3 percent had a dysfunctional pattern concurrent with prolongation of the deceleration phase. This

*Table 11. LABOR DATA FOR PATIENTS WITH PROLONGED DECELERATION PHASE*

| Group | *Latent Phase (hr)* | *Active Phase (hr)* | *Maximum Dilatation (cm/hr)* | *Deceleration Phase (hr)* | *Maximum Descent (cm/hr)* | *Second Stage (hr)* |
|---|---|---|---|---|---|---|
| Nulliparas | | | | | | |
| Mean labor | 6.4±0.25 | 4.6±0.14 | 3.0±0.08 | 0.84±0.04 | 3.3±0.07 | 1.1 ±0.04 |
| Prolonged deceleration phase | 8.8±1.30 | 10.2±0.59* | 1.2±0.10* | 4.6 ±0.22* | 1.4±0.12* | 2.2 ±0.30* |
| Multiparas | | | | | | |
| Mean labor | 4.8±0.18 | 2.4±0.06 | 5.7±0.16 | 0.36±0.02 | 6.6±0.17 | 0.39±0.02 |
| Prolonged deceleration phase | 6.7±0.98 | 5.6±0.34* | 2.9±0.32* | 1.7 ±0.11* | 3.0±0.31* | 1.1 ±0.12* |

* Statistically significant, $p < 0.01$.

most often (35.6 percent) took the form of a protraction disorder. It is of interest to note that concurrent secondary arrest of dilatation was unusual in the multipara with prolonged deceleration phase; however, arrest of descent occurred more commonly among these multiparas.

Analysis of the labor data of gravidas with prolonged deceleration phase (Table 11) demonstrates abnormalities in all phases except the latent phase. We recognize markedly prolonged average active-phase duration. This is not completely explained by the expected prolongation of the deceleration phase. Similarly, the maximum slopes of both dilatation and descent are abnormally depressed and the second-stage duration unusually lengthened.

The essentially normal average latent-phase duration stands conspicuously alone except in multiparas where there is a suggestion of prolongation, albeit not statistically significant. This observation implies that latent-phase dysfunction need not necessarily be reflected in active-phase abnormalities, a phenomenon previously described. Furthermore, dysfunctional labor disorders of the active phase would appear to carry through from the onset of the active phase until delivery, because the manifestation of deceleration-phase prolongation reflects the precedent abnormalities of the acceleration phase and the phase of maximum slope as well as the abnormality of progression in the second stage.

## *Etiology*

Nulliparas with prolonged deceleration phase differ from the normal nullipara in certain specific ways. For example, cephalopelvic disproportion is seen more than twice as often (15.8 percent versus an expected incidence of 7.8 percent). Similarly, 26.3 percent have persistent occiput posterior mechanisms. A total of 75 percent have been heavily sedated with regard to the effect of the medication on the patient's sensorium. There seems little doubt that these factors play a role in producing the prolongation of the deceleration phase.

It has been shown that any factor that tends to impede the retraction of the cervix about the fetal presenting part during the terminal phase of dilatation will prolong that portion of the curve. This was first demonstrated by the radiographic studies of Caldwell et al in 1939. Factors that may bring about this phenomenon include disturbances in fetal position (such as occiput posterior and occiput transverse), in fetopelvic relationships (bony dystocia), and in motive force (myometrial dysfunction, whether idiopathic or due to medication, anesthesia, or exhaustion).

It is pertinent that 13.8 percent of patients had conduction anesthesia administered within a short interval prior to deceleration. This implicates conduction anesthesia as possibly causative in a post hoc relationship. Sedation, excessive as it relates to effect, was administered to 40.0 percent of patients during the deceleration phase, and therefore was felt likely to be an etiologic factor in these instances.

Similar trends were seen in multiparas. There was a 15.3 percent incidence of cephalopelvic disproportion, contrasted with 5.8 percent expected among normal multiparas. Occiput posterior positions occurred in 40.7 percent (15.9 percent expected) and occiput transverse in 25.4 percent (17.2 percent expected).

Caudal anesthesia was administered to 44.1 percent of multiparas at or before the deceleration phase (average rate, 10.6 percent in multiparas), and was improperly administered according to defined standards (see Chapter 19) in 35.6 percent. By the same token, 39.0 percent of patients were heavily sedated prior to prolongation of the deceleration phase, the expected incidence in normal multiparas being 13.6 percent.

Essentially all patients with prolonged deceleration phase had associated excessive sedation, malposition, improperly administered conduction anesthesia, and/or cephalopelvic disproportion. The overwhelming weight of evidence seems to implicate these factors as causative or contributory.

Statistical analysis has thus revealed the significance of such factors as conduction anesthesia, cephalopelvic disproportion, and malposition in the production of prolonged deceleration phase. Similarly, it is likely that excessive sedation plays a contributory role. We see, therefore, that progress in the deceleration phase is influenced by factors giving rise to bony, positional, and inertial dystocia.

## *Treatment and Prognosis*

Excluding uterotonic stimulation for induction of labor, we found that no specific treatment was utilized in just half the nulliparas with prolonged deceleration phase. Most of these included patients in whom heavy sedation had been permitted to abate. In the remaining half, oxytocin stimulation was employed as a method of treating the prolonged deceleration phase.

It is of interest to note that the outcome in both these groups of nulliparas was essentially identical. In reality, the cesarean section rate was somewhat higher, but not significantly so, in the stimulated group. This undoubtedly reflected more impatience on the part of the attendant physicians; it did not necessarily indicate a poorer response from stimulation. It is certainly likely that greater conservatism might have resulted in fewer operative deliveries, particularly among those cases in which disproportion was not a pertinent factor.

The management of multiparas resulted in somewhat different outcomes. Unstimulated labors were delivered by midforceps in 21.6 percent and by cesarean section in 5.4 percent. By contrast, labors stimulated with uterotonic agents showed significant reduction in midforceps procedures to 9.1 percent, but an unexplained increase in cesarean sections to 13.6 percent.

It appears that oxytocin stimulation of the multipara with prolonged deceleration phase is effective in diminishing the incidence of midforceps operations, especially in the absence of cephalopelvic disproportion. However, it does not seem to affect the need for cesarean section. It is clear that the prognosis for uncomplicated vaginal delivery in patients with prolonged deceleration phase is guarded.

## *ARREST OF DESCENT*

In the second stage, the cervix is fully dilated and retracted so that it is no longer available as a means for evaluating continued progress. Here one may profitably use progressive descent of the fetal presenting part for this purpose. The basic assumption is that station progresses continuously, advancing in a linear manner during the second stage. This has been fairly well established and is useful in the practical clinical evaluation of second-stage progress (see Chapter 6).

The diagnosis of the abnormality of arrest of descent is based merely upon the documentation that progress has halted in the movement of the fetus through the birth canal. Such documentation requires two well-spaced vaginal examinations done by the same individual, at least 1 hour apart.

We should be cognizant that there may be instances in which apparent progress is being made, but in which the observer is deluded because he or she misinterprets changes occurring as a consequence of increasing scalp edema or cranial bone molding. Such situations may not be diagnosed promptly or correctly unless the kinds of precautions described in Chapter 6 are taken. These specifically advise the observer to cross-validate observations of fetal station (as obtained by vaginal examination) with suitable suprapubic assessment of the descent of the fetal head.

Interruption of progressive descent of the fetal presenting part late in labor is ominous and should serve to alert the knowledgeable obstetric attendant to the possibility that a serious problem exists. The gravida with arrest of descent has been characterized in some detail (Friedman and Sachtleben, 1976). The condition was found to occur in 6.9 percent or 1:14.5 nulliparas, as contrasted with 1.2 percent or 1:83 multiparas.

### *Obstetric Factors*

Nulliparas with arrest of descent were distinguished from those with normal labor patterns in certain specific respects. Gestational age, for example, was markedly skewed toward term. Essentially all such cases were of advanced gestational age. All infants at birth weighed more than 2500 g. The incidence of large babies weighing more than 4000 g was considerably higher than in the normal population (9.8 percent).

Not unexpectedly, therefore, documentable cephalopelvic disproportion was commonly seen (52.2 percent). This is analogous to the close association of disproportion with secondary arrest of dilatation (see above).

While malpresentations were infrequently encountered among these women, fetal malpositions were rather common. Persistent occiput transverse or occiput posterior positions were encountered in 75.9 percent of this group. The finding of excessive occurrence of minor malpositions is entirely consistent with like relationships seen in association with all other dysfunctional labor patterns.

Coexisting labor disorders were common. These most often consisted of one or both protraction abnormalities (in 65.6 percent). Other arrest variants were also encountered frequently (24.5 percent). Abnormal prolongation of the latent phase was found only slightly more often than expected for comparable normal nulliparas.

More than one-third of the patients with arrest of descent were delivered by midforceps procedures (37.6 percent) and almost as many, by cesarean section (30.4 percent). Both procedures were significantly more frequent than expected. Moreover, there were excessive numbers of forceps rotations (12.7 percent) and failed forceps (5.1 percent). Operative vaginal deliveries resulted in maternal trauma rather commonly, most often following midforceps operations.

### *Labor Course*

When subjected to graphic analysis (Table 12), labors in patients with arrest of descent showed significant deviations from normal, including prolongations of latent, active, and deceleration phases as well as marked slowing of the maximum slopes of dilatation and descent—all in association with increased duration of the second stage. These data reflected the common occurrence of dysfunctional labor patterns in association with arrest of descent. Only 14.2 percent had completely normal dilatation and descent patterns preceding the arrest of descent.

This observation suggests that arrest of descent is rarely an isolated phe-

*Table 12. LABOR DATA FOR PATIENTS WITH ARREST OF DESCENT*

| Group | Latent Phase (hr) | Active Phase (hr) | Maximum Dilatation (cm/hr) | Deceleration Phase (hr) | Maximum Descent (cm/hr) | Second Stage (hr) |
|---|---|---|---|---|---|---|
| Nulliparas | | | | | | |
| Mean labor | 6.4±0.25 | 4.6±0.14 | 3.0±0.08 | 0.84±0.04 | 3.3±0.07 | 1.1 ±0.04 |
| Arrest of descent | 10.0±0.49* | 6.1±0.22* | 2.0±0.08* | 1.20±0.07* | 1.2±0.04* | 2.6 ±0.13* |
| Multiparas | | | | | | |
| Mean labor | 4.8±0.18 | 2.4±0.06 | 5.7±0.16 | 0.36±0.02 | 6.6±0.17 | 0.39±0.02 |
| Arrest of descent | 6.0±0.32* | 3.3±0.18* | 4.2±0.18* | 0.60±0.08* | 4.8±0.20* | 0.98±0.08* |

* Statistically significant, $p < 0.01$.

nomenon. Instead, it is often preceded by other dysfunctional patterns, most particularly a protraction disorder. It is clear that patients with such major aberrations of labor progression are at considerably greater risk of developing arrest of descent than those progressing normally.

Furthermore, labor progression was related to the station of the fetal presenting part that had been reached at the time the arrest of descent took place. The higher the station in the pelvis, the slower and more protracted the labor was likely to have been. A linear trend was encountered in the durations of the several measurable phases, inversely related to the station of arrest. In other words, there were shorter durations with advancing station. Additionally, there were corresponding linear progressions in the slopes of dilatation and of descent; that is, greater slopes occurred with lower stations.

## Etiologic Factors

While the characteristics that distinguish patients with arrest of descent from the general population are not necessarily etiologic or contributory to the development of the labor disorder, they do provide the basis for certain potentially useful inferences. Most noteworthy is the exceptionally high incidence of cephalopelvic disproportion in these cases. Both secondary arrest of dilatation (see above) and protracted descent (see Chapter 10) were similarly correlated with disproportion. Findings in this disorder of sizable numbers of patients presenting with minor fetal malpositions who were given large doses of narcotic-analgesic agents or had peridural anesthesia administered prior to the arrest also paralleled the findings in related dysfunctional labors.

Almost every patient with a malposition in this group had one or more of the other factors operating simultaneously. This relegated the malposition to a minor role at best. Nevertheless, the frequency with which malpositions were found allows one to conjecture that they may be the result of the labor aberration rather than its cause.

### *Treatment and Prognosis*

Mutually exclusive management plans could be categorized into three groups: immediate delivery, expectancy, and uterotonic stimulation. The expectancy group was further subdivided to examine those patients with arrest disorder apparently resulting directly from peridural anesthesia or excessive sedation and who were managed by allowing these inhibitory factors to abate. The several treatment groups were similar in regard to makeup, particularly in the relative frequencies of associated disproportion.

The criterion of successful treatment was the documentation of subsequent progressive descent following the period of arrest. Among nulliparas with arrest of descent, nearly 90 percent failed to progress further, regardless of the form of management that had been tried. No patient managed expectantly progressed other than those treated by allowing the inhibitory sedation or anesthesia to abate. Clear postarrest progress was encountered in 30.8 percent of the abatement group and 30.6 percent of those subjected to therapeutic oxytocin stimulation. Amniotomy was determined to be entirely ineffectual.

It was of considerable interest that no patient who developed arrest of descent during the administration of oxytocin showed any form of postarrest response, even to augmented uterotonic stimulation. Those who responded to oxytocin did so as a consequence of the initiation of such stimulation after arrest had occurred. We should note especially that progression was encountered even in association with clinically evident and radiologically verified fetopelvic disproportion.

Delivery outcome data showed the highest incidence of operative vaginal delivery for patients managed by immediate termination of pregnancy (45.6 percent midforceps). There were few cesarean sections (10.3 percent) and no spontaneous deliveries among this group. A significantly higher relative number of cesarean sections was done in patients treated expectantly, especially among those in whom such an approach extended beyond 4 hours (63.0 percent sectioned). In this latter group, moreover, all of those not delivered abdominally were subjected to midforceps operations (37.0 percent). Little difference was seen among those managed with uterotonic stimulation, except for somewhat fewer abdominal deliveries (36.7 percent) and more spontaneous vaginal deliveries (16.3 percent). Abatement programs yielded still fewer cesarean sections (30.0 percent) and more spontaneous deliveries (20.5 percent).

When postarrest progression was taken into account as a possible index of of prognosis, the situation became clearer. The abatement approach that yielded progress required neither cesarean section nor midforceps for delivery. Similarly, postarrest descent accompanying therapeutic stimulation necessitated few sections and no midforceps. Those who did not respond in either treatment group fared poorly.

Most of the spontaneous deliveries that occurred in this series took place within the group of patients who showed postarrest progression. The others followed vigorous Kristeller expression to effect descent at delivery. Most of the patients with postarrest progression here were delivered by low forceps; the rest came to cesarean section, all for cephalopelvic disproportion.

The prognostic value of the postarrest slope as it relates to prearrest progress will be discussed in detail subsequently (see Chapter 23). At this point it is merely necessary to point out that the absence of postarrest progress made it likely that cesarean section or midforceps operation would be required (44.3 and 36.1 percent, respectively). By contrast, with any postarrest descent, there were very few cesarean sections (11.1 percent) and no midforceps procedures. A response usually signified that vaginal delivery would occur, even in the presence of apparent cephalopelvic disproportion.

## *FAILURE OF DESCENT*

It has become more and more apparent during the past several years that there is a special category of arrest problem characterized by no descent at all. In a sense, it is analogous to prolonged latent phase in that the process never begins. However, in contradistinction to prolonged latent phase, failure of descent is obviously very much more ominous.

We now recognize that descent normally begins in active labor either during the phase of maximum slope of dilatation or, at the very latest, at the onset of the deceleration phase. We have rationalized this relationship in some detail in Chapter 6. If descent has not begun by the time the dilatation curve has reached its deceleration phase, an abnormality must be considered to exist. For the purpose of determining the characteristics of patients who have this labor aberration, the material that follows here deals exclusively with those whose failure to descend extended into the second stage.

### *Obstetric Factors*

The patients who experienced failure of descent constituted 3.6 percent of our gravid population. Their age distribution did not differ from normal in any significant way. In general, their infants weighed more at birth than expected: none weighed less than 2800 g, and 16.7 percent weighed more than 4000 g (including 5.9 percent weighing more than 4500 g), a significant trend.

As a consequence of the tendency toward large babies, the incidence of cephalopelvic disproportion was quite remarkable. Indeed, disproportion was deemed to be present in every instance on clinical grounds. Where radiographic evaluation was undertaken, 54.0 percent of the patients were readily documented as having major degrees of obstructed labor.

Minor malpositions were very common in this group. Only 2 percent had a normal occiput anterior mechanism. The remainder were almost equally divided between persistent occiput transverse and occiput posterior positions. Additionally, there were instances of both parietal and face presenta-

*Table 13. LABOR DATA FOR PATIENTS WITH FAILURE OF DESCENT*

| Group | Latent Phase (hr) | Active Phase (hr) | Maximum Dilatation (cm/hr) | Deceleration Phase (hr) | Maximum Descent (cm/hr) | Second Stage (hr) |
|---|---|---|---|---|---|---|
| Nulliparas | | | | | | |
| Mean labor | 6.4±0.25 | 4.6±0.14 | 3.0±0.08 | 0.84±0.04 | 3.3±0.07 | 1.1 ±0.04 |
| Failure of descent | 8.0±0.79 | 9.1±0.54* | 1.0±0.08* | 2.2 ±0.24* | — | 2.8 ±0.40* |
| Multiparas | | | | | | |
| Mean labor | 4.8±0.18 | 2.4±0.06 | 5.7±0.16 | 0.36±0.02 | 6.6±0.17 | 0.39±0.02 |
| Failure of descent | 5.6±0.70 | 5.0±0.46* | 2.1±0.17* | 0.91±0.14* | — | 1.40±0.29* |

* Statistically significant, $p < 0.01$.

tion. The incidence of breech presentation was not increased over that of the general population. The time of membrane rupture was normally distributed in this series of patients. Similarly, the incidence of conduction anesthesia and excessive sedation was about as expected.

Concurrent labor aberrations were exceedingly frequent. In all, 98.0 percent had some other form of major disorder. Most often this took the form of another arrest variant; 94.1 percent had secondary arrest of dilatation as well. Protraction disorders were also often seen (78.4 percent). It is of interest to note that prolonged latent phase was rather infrequently seen (5.9 percent).

This again verifies that active-phase disorders are distinct from those of the latent phase. More importantly, failure of descent is almost never seen (2.0 percent only) in labors that are progressing normally in the active phase.

The course of labor in these patients (Table 13) differed significantly from the normal gravid population. There was, of course, no maximum slope of descent, no descent having ever occurred. The high frequency of coexisting dysfunctional aberrations was reflected in the markedly prolonged active and deceleration phases and diminished maximum slope of dilatation. The second stage was also prolonged in these cases.

## *Etiologic Factors*

By far the most obvious cause-and-effect relationship appears to exist with regard to cephalopelvic disproportion. As with the other arrest disorders (see above), there is a clear-cut correlation with bony dystocia. The very common association with fetal malpositions is also noteworthy. Here it is again likely that these are the resultant effect of the labor dysfunction rather than the cause.

Since neither conduction anesthesia nor heavy sedation appear to have been administered in excessive numbers, neither need be implicated as necessarily causative. However, there can be little doubt that they can both be contributory, particularly in labors that are not progressing normally. We have already seen (Chapter 10) that progression in labors characterized by a protraction disorder is readily arrested by anesthesia or sedation. This will be discussed further in Chapter 12 in reference to analysis of labors demonstrating both protraction and arrest disorders concurrently.

### *Treatment and Prognosis*

Almost no information is available to aid in evaluating the efficacy of management programs applied specifically for the treatment of failure of descent. The reason for this is obvious. When encountered, this disorder has in the past intuitively implied the presence of disproportion, a relationship now documented. Generally, verification of the fetopelvic relationship is promptly sought. When insurmountable bony dystocia is revealed objectively, cesarean section is then justifiably undertaken without further trial of labor.

In gravidas who were observed to have failure of descent as defined above, oxytocin infusion had been invoked in 35.3 percent. In none of these cases was any descent accomplished as a consequence of the uterotonic stimulation. This is not to imply, of course, that there might not be circumstances under which oxytocin infusion would effect descent.

Indeed, there were rare instances, particularly among multiparas, in which descent did ultimately take place and vaginal delivery occur. These unusual instances involved patients whose fetus remained floating above the pelvic inlet during the entire first stage. In some, the mechanical drive of the uterus was disadvantageous as a consequence of a pendulous abdomen and markedly anteflexed uterus. Correction of these problems (with or without oxytocin augmentation) in the second stage proved effective in permitting descent to occur.

However, these are obviously exceptional circumstances. While they deserve to be recognized as such, they need not detract from the general concept that failure of descent is rarely, if ever, responsive to conservative measures aimed at trying to effect vaginal delivery. Since cesarean section is almost always required in these cases, the prognosis is obviously very guarded.

# Concurrent Protraction and Arrest Disorders

## CHAPTER 12

Gravidas with both protraction and arrest disorders occurring together in the same labor are described in detail to provide data on clinical features, response to treatment, and prognosis for delivery as well as for fetal outcome. In general, they are found in most respects to resemble patients with arrest disorders closely.

When major labor aberrations occur together in a single labor, the clinical problem is compounded. This situation carries an ominous outlook in practice. Its obvious importance makes it imperative that we try to understand why it arises and what its impact might be.

The particular combination with which we are concerned is that of a protraction disorder occurring in association with an arrest disorder. The former includes protracted active-phase dilatation and protracted descent patterns. These have been defined and characterized as isolated entities in Chapter 10. The arrest disorders include secondary arrest of dilatation, prolonged deceleration phase, arrest of descent, and failure of descent—all discussed at length in Chapter 11. Earlier, we alluded to the more serious prognostic outlook to be expected when these aberrations occur together. The basis for this pessimism will now be elaborated.

### *CONCURRENT DISORDERS IN NULLIPARAS*

Protraction disorders coexist with arrest disorders in 1–2 percent of nulliparas (0.84 percent in our original series; 2.04 percent, more recently). These disorders represent about one-quarter of all dysfunctional labors that occur in nulliparas. Among those who develop protraction disorders, 69.3 percent will develop an arrest problem subsequently in the same labor. By the same token, 65.0 percent of gravidas with arrest disorders have concurrent protraction aberrations.

Among these patients, two-thirds arrested in the linear portion of the active phase, including 49.0 percent before 6 cm of cervical dilatation. This is quite unlike the experience encountered in otherwise uncomplicated cases of secondary arrest of dilatation, in which 40.8 percent arrested during the phase of maximum slope, 12.3 percent prior to 6 cm of dilatation. The importance of this observation lies in its apparent support of the contention that the combined disorders are more serious. They have a less favorable outlook because arrest tends to occur relatively early among them. This will be discussed in more detail below.

The incidence of multiple pregnancy was more than twice that expected in our nulliparous population (2.5 versus 1.1 percent). A similar finding was noted in association with protraction disorders occurring in isolation. Both findings point to the possibility that multiple pregnancy may be associated with the development of protraction disorders. However, they do not constitute irrefutable statistical evidence for this contention. This will be further detailed in Chapter 17.

## *Age*

The average maternal age of these patients at delivery was 27.8 years. This was slightly but not significantly greater than that of normal nulliparas (26.2 years). The apparent trend toward concentration of older gravidas that was seen in association with some forms of arrest disorder was not clearly verified here. Nevertheless, there were 9.2 percent of gravidas who were older than 35 years. This is more than twice the expected number in nulliparas (4.1 percent).

It has been demonstrated that age variations do not appear to influence prolongation of the latent phase or protraction of dilatation or descent. Whether or not the factor of advancing age contributes to the development of an arrest disorder could not be determined precisely from these data. As stated before, if there is an age influence on the course of labor, it manifests itself in the arrest disorders (see Chapter 14).

## *Birth Weight*

Infants born after labors characterized by concurrent aberrations were studied to determine their weight distribution. Overall, 84.1 percent weighed between 2500 and 4000 g. This compared favorably with the corresponding hospital incidence of 84.5 percent for normal nulliparas. A total of 6.1 percent weighed less than 2500 g, and 9.8 percent weighed more than 4000 g. These data are essentially the same as expected (7.2 and 8.3 percent, respectively).

Thus, contrary to the findings of large babies in association with isolated arrest problems, birth weight was about normally distributed among these infants. Similarly, gestational age did not seem to play a role in producing these labor disorders.

### Fetal Position

The excessive numbers of occiput transverse and posterior mechanisms that were seen in each of the related dysfunctional labor groups was reduplicated here. Persistent occiput transverse position occurred in 38.6 percent and occiput posterior, in 40.2 percent, both well in excess of expected frequencies (30.2 and 17.2 percent, respectively). The occiput posterior frequency corroborated consistent implications that these ostensibly minor positional abnormalities may play significant roles in the pathogenesis of the dysfunctional labor patterns. Once again, we cannot distinguish cause from effect, however.

There were 5.4 percent breech presentations in this group. This represented a somewhat higher incidence than in the normal nulliparous population (3.6 percent). This is in agreement with findings in both the uncomplicated protraction and arrest series. Although suggesting the possibility of a correlation between breech presentation and both of these major dysfunctional labor patterns, the relationship does not hold up under statistical scrutiny.

### Fetopelvic Relationship

Cephalopelvic disproportion was determined by radiographic survey to exist in 44.8 percent of nulliparas with concurrent disorders. The expected incidence was 7.8 percent. The obviously high frequency of disproportion coincided almost identically with that of gravidas with uncomplicated arrest problems (44.6 percent). This constitutes strong reconfirmation of the rather clear-cut association between bony dystocia and arrest disorders (see Chapter 16).

### Delivery

Nulliparas with concurrent disorders were delivered by cesarean section in 41.5 percent and by midforceps operations in 18.3 percent. The incidence of abdominal deliveries was more than six times the expected rate in normal nulliparas (6.8 percent); the midforceps incidence was almost five times the expected frequency (3.8 percent).

The midforceps rate was not significantly different from that found following protraction disorders (24.1 percent) or after arrest disorders (29.8 percent). The cesarean section rate, on the other hand, was four times greater than the rate in protraction disorders (10.2 percent) and one-half again larger than in arrest disorders (29.0 percent). These latter differences are important from the prognostic point of view and will be discussed more fully below.

Most of the midforceps procedures were done for positional dystocia in association with occiput posterior and transverse arrest. Several were undoubtedly undertaken prematurely (and perhaps ill-advisedly), as evidenced by their having been done through an incompletely dilated cervix or following manual dilatation of the cervix. Further substantiation existed in the rather frequent trauma that occurred and in the traumatic maneuvers that were used, including intensive Kristeller pressure, difficult forceps applications and deliveries, delivery and postpartum hemorrhages, uterine atony, lacerations of the cervix, sulcus, and rectum, as well as an instance of uterine rupture.

More than three-quarters of the cesarean sections in this group were done for cephalopelvic disproportion (77.0 percent). Documentation of the bony relationship by radiographic pelvimetry was confirmatory in one-half of these. Of the remaining, justification took the form of an adequate trial of labor as defined in Chapter 16) in 28.6 percent. Except for instances of persistent fetal distress, in none of the remaining cases was there either sufficient therapy or time allotted after the arrest to determine whether progressive dilatation or descent might have evolved. This left the indication for the cesarean section somewhat in doubt among them. Thus, it is possible that some of these cesarean sections need not have been done. Although it is difficult in retrospect to judge the merits of individual cases, reevaluation suggested that a minimal cesarean section rate of about 17 percent might be anticipated in a comparable series of abnormal labors treated more conservatively.

### *Membrane Status*

There were large numbers of labors in this series that began with ruptured membranes. This is consistent with findings in other studies of dysfunctional labor patterns. A total of 20.6 percent of membranes had ruptured prematurely (11.8 percent expected) and 17.0 percent, at the onset of labor (9.5 percent expected). All had occurred spontaneously. A similar phenomenon had been encountered before in association with other forms of labor aberrations and remains unexplained.

Moreover, 51.0 percent had had the membranes ruptured in the active phase, and of these 79.8 percent were ruptured artificially. This large number of amniotomies in the active phase was believed at first to reflect therapeutic measures aimed at attempting to correct the dysfunctional labor pattern. However, only 3.6 percent (or 7.9 percent of all amniotomies) were actually done during the period of arrest. Indeed, in 22.9 percent of the series—constituting 82 percent of the amniotomies performed during the linear portion of the phase of maximum slope prior to arrest—the arrest pattern followed rather promptly within 2 hours of the amniotomy. This clearly serves to illustrate the general inefficacy of this ostensibly stimulatory device. It may actually provide evidence that amniotomy is deleterious under these circumstances.

### *Labor Course*

The labor curves of dilatation and descent were analyzed for purposes of accurate statistical evaluation of the component phases of labor in these cases (Table 14). As expected, we found significant prolongation of the latent, active, and deceleration phases, as well as of the second-stage duration. In addition, there was marked flattening of the maximum slopes of both dilatation and descent. These were essentially identical with findings encountered in patients with uncomplicated protraction disorders (see Chapter 10).

The quantitative differences could be ascribed in part to the concurrent phenomenon of arrest. The average duration of arrest in these cases was 8.3 hours. This accounted for much of the 11.7 hours of prolongation of the active phase over that of normal nulliparas (4.9 hours), but not for all of that time. The residual difference might be attributable to the especially protracted rate of dilatation characteristic of these labors. This was further illustrated by the 5.4 hours of additional lengthening of the active-phase duration in this series, as compared with that of the pure protraction disorders, including 2.1 additional hours of deceleration phase.

The apparent foreshortening of the latent phase toward normal—although still abnormally prolonged—was an interesting but unexplained finding. The frequent occurrence of prolonged latent-phase duration reconfirmed that the protraction disorder often begins with an abnormally long latent phase. However, it may be unrecognized as such until the active phase has been entered; indeed, it usually cannot be recognized until later in the course of the labor.

Similarly, this observation implied that the underlying problems affecting the efficiency of uterine contractility contribute to the development of both of these kinds of labor disorders (that is, both prolonged latent phase and the protraction disorders). Whether a third major superimposed dysfunction—namely, an arrest disorder—is part of the same process may be ques-

*Table 14. LABOR DATA FOR PATIENTS WITH CONCURRENT PROTRACTION AND ARREST*

| *Group* | *Latent Phase (hr)* | *Active Phase (hr)* | *Maximum Dilatation (cm/hr)* | *Deceleration Phase (hr)* | *Maximum Descent (cm/hr)* | *Second Stage (hr)* |
|---|---|---|---|---|---|---|
| Nulliparas | | | | | | |
| Mean labor | 6.4±0.25 | 4.6±0.14 | 3.0 ±0.08 | 0.84±0.04 | 3.3 ±0.07 | 1.1 ±0.04 |
| Concurrent disorders | 11.3±0.47* | 16.6±0.42* | 0.66±0.02* | 3.9 ±0.30* | 0.72±0.03* | 1.5 ±0.12* |
| Multiparas | | | | | | |
| Mean labor | 4.8±0.18 | 2.4±0.06 | 5.7 ±0.16 | 0.36±0.02 | 6.6 ±0.17 | 0.39±0.02 |
| Concurrent disorders | 9.7±0.99* | 12.2±0.80* | 0.81±0.04* | 2.4 ±0.48* | 0.94±0.06* | 0.56±0.14 |

* Statistically significant, $p < 0.01$.

tioned. It is not likely to be, in view of evidence showing that the latent-phase durations are generally normal in association with pure arrest patterns (see Chapter 11).

The relatively common concurrence of both protraction and arrest disorders, however, preclude their complete independence. This indicates that they may share common etiologic factors. More probably, it suggests that labor may be presensitized by the existence of a protraction state and thereby may more readily be influenced by deleterious conditions that might not ordinarily have had the potential to arrest progress. In other words, it is possible that the protraction disorder synergizes the labor so as to potentiate inhibitory effects of various factors.

## *Etiology*

The methods of assigning etiologic roles to various factors have been reviewed. This approach was applied in our attempt to determine the underlying basis for the development of both the protraction and the arrest disorders in this series. Endogenous conditions acting prior to the beginning of the active phase were noted for their possible contribution to the production of the protraction pattern; factors possibly acting immediately prior to an arrest were examined for their potential effect in causing the arrest.

The most obvious items found in excessive numbers among these patients included cephalopelvic disproportion, fetal malposition, and excessive sedation. There was little doubt as to the part these factors played. They were seen alone or in combination in 95.0 percent of cases.

Comparing the absolute frequency of each of these factors in this series of patients with the occurrence rate among patients with either protraction disorder or arrest problem alone, we found that the incidence of malpositions was about the same. While the frequency of bony disproportion was similar to that seen in association with other arrest problems, it was considerably higher than in isolated protraction disorders. The rate of excessive sedation was much higher than anticipated. This indicated its relatively greater significance as a factor contributing to the development of the combined disorders.

In this regard, 29.9 percent had been heavily narcotized in early labor. The expected incidence of heavy sedation in the general nulliparous population was 8.6 percent; among patients with uncomplicated protraction disorder, 16.8 percent. In the interval just preceding arrest, 81.3 percent of patients with concurrent protraction and arrest had received heavy sedation. This contrasted with a 30.8-percent incidence of heavy sedation in the active phase in nulliparas at large and 63.1 percent in those with arrest alone.

We could verify no trend toward increased frequency of conduction anesthesia as possibly contributing to the development of the protraction disorder here. However, in 18.3 percent of patients, peridural anesthesia had been administered prior to the arrest. This was essentially the same rate that had been seen in patients with isolated arrest problems (see Chapter 11). In nearly every instance the anesthesia had been given to a patient whose labor had already been affected by one or more of the other major factors (that is, disproportion, malposition, or excessive sedation). This indicated the likelihood that the role of this agent is merely a secondary or enhancing one. It corroborates that conduction anesthesia tends to augment the adverse effects of other factors that may impede progression in labor.

In the 2-hour interval prior to the arrest in these cases, membranes ruptured in 32.0 percent. The post hoc occurrence of arrest following amniotomy is suggestive of a possible adverse effect from the procedure. The overall incidence of membrane rupture in the active phase is 32.9 percent in nulliparas, but this information cannot properly serve for comparison. The dilatation-specific incidence to be anticipated under comparable circumstances—based on the number ruptured prior to 6 cm of dilatation when the arrest is likely to occur—is 16 percent. This is a significantly smaller frequency than encountered here.

Additionally, there were 37.7 percent of these patients who began labor with ruptured membranes. The same excess incidence was seen preceding the pattern of protracted active-phase dilatation (see Chapter 10). This leads again to the suggestion that a causal relationship may exist. Against this conclusion is the observation that one or more of the other possible etiologic agents or factors were operating simultaneously in every instance.

### *Treatment*

Effectiveness of the several treatment modalities was evaluated by the analytic methods we described earlier. In this entire group, there was no instance in which the abnormally low slope of dilatation or descent improved regardless of the therapy used. Our analysis, therefore, was limited to evaluating therapy aimed at correcting the arrest problem. The criterion used to indicate effective action of a given regimen was the documentation of subsequent further dilatation or descent following the arrest.

Oxytocin infusion was successful in producing further progress in 72.0 percent. All responses were seen within a 7-hour period of stimulation. This success rate with oxytocin was somewhat less than that seen in the treatment of isolated arrest disorders (see Chapter 11), indicating the more serious outlook in those patients with concurrent protraction disorder. The relative efficacy of oxytocin over any other form of treatment was demonstrated, nevertheless.

The responsiveness to oxytocin was closely related to the presence or absence of bony disproportion. Among nulliparas with disproportion who were given oxytocin, a good response was seen in 47.1 percent. By contrast, those without disproportion who were similarly stimulated responded in 81.3 percent, a statistically significant difference. The prognostic importance of these findings will be discussed further (see below).

Amniotomy was used as a therapeutic means for stimulating labor in some cases, but only a few patients responded without the aid of uterotonic stimulation. The response in these cases, however, usually occurred at about the same time that the heavy sedation, which had apparently produced the arrest, abated. Rest by means of narcotic analgesics was also used occasionally for these patients. About 10 percent responded with subsequent dilatation or descent when they awoke. Most of the remainder were stimulated with oxytocin infusion; 68.2 percent reacted with further dilatation or descent. This rate of success is about the same as had been encountered with oxytocin administration as the primary mode of treatment (72.0 percent; see above).

It was obvious that some of these patients had had their labors arrested following the administration of excessive sedation. These were largely managed expectantly. As the sedative effect abated in those cases in which it was allowed to abate, further progression occurred without the necessity for active treatment. In these cases, the average duration of arrest was 7.3 hours, an interval during which the effect of the narcotizing medication slowly attenuated.

The quantitative approach previously described (see Chapters 9 and 11) was used here to attempt to relate the distribution of cases to the time elapsing between initiation of treatment and its effect. This technique was felt to provide information concerning the relative efficacy of the several management approaches, as indicated both by the amplitude of the peak of activity and by the point in time when it occurred. Among these patients, a peak of activity was seen for oxytocin infusion only (Fig. 24). It is sharply hyperbolic, illustrating the prompt and significant effect that this drug had in terminating the arrest problem. None of the other modalities that were studied showed any peak of activity here. Thus, it appears that this serious combination of major labor abnormalities could not be benefited by treatment other than oxytocin infusion.

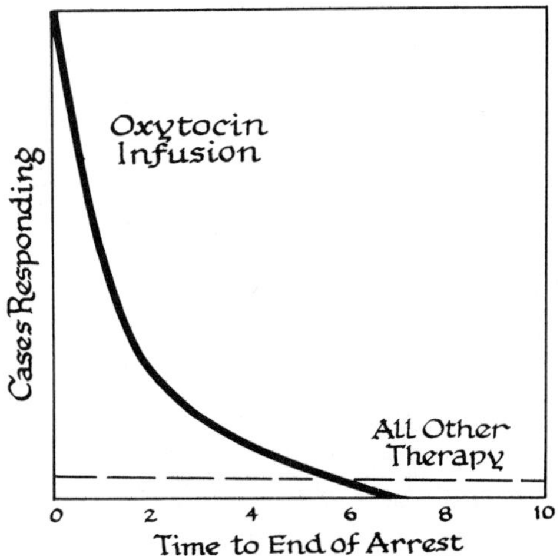


*Fig. 24.* Distribution of treatment response in patients with both protraction and arrest disorders. As with arrest patterns alone (see Fig. 23), all responses occur within 7 hours. Neither amniotomy nor rest yielded identifiable effect in patients with concurrent labor aberrations.

## *Prognosis*

Cesarean sections were undertaken in 41.5 percent of patients with concurrent protraction and arrest disorders. This was much higher than expected for either protraction or arrest aberrations when they occurred alone. The prognostic significance of this observation is obvious.

Differences were observed according to the time in labor when the arrest took place. For example, 54 percent of the sections occurred in labors that had arrested early in the active phase; that is, before dilatation had reached 6 cm. There were 29 percent done late in the active phase, beyond 6 cm of cervical dilatation but before the onset of the deceleration phase; 17 percent were done still later in labor.

These data suggest that arrest before deceleration carries a poor prognosis. It appears to reflect the increased incidence of more serious degrees of cephalopelvic disproportion in labors that arrest early. We found 69.6 percent of gravidas with absolute cephalopelvic disproportion had arrested before 6 cm of cervical dilatation, as contrasted with 17.4 percent later.

Most of the labors that were terminated by cesarean section were done for cephalopelvic disproportion (77 percent). Documentation of cephalopelvic disproportion by digital and radiographic means was reflected in the outcome: not unexpectedly, 71.3 percent were delivered by abdominal section and 20.5 percent, by midforceps. In contrast, among those with normal fetopelvic relationships, cesarean section was ultimately required in 17.3 percent and midforceps was required about as many times. Earlier (Chapter 11) we saw the differences in response to specific therapy according to the presence or absence of bony dystocia. The same relationship obviously applies here.

In 52.3 percent of these patients, some postarrest progression occurred. Many were not given the opportunity to respond by having been delivered promptly, either by cesarean section or operative vaginal delivery. Therefore, the frequency with which postarrest progression was seen is at best a minimal estimate of the rate to be expected in response to conservative nonoperative management of patients with concurrent protraction and arrest disorders.

The outcome was studied with reference to response to therapy directed at correcting the arrest. Among patients who displayed any response in the form of further dilatation or descent, only 7.1 percent required cesarean section and 21.4 percent, midforceps. By contrast, those in whom therapy was ineffectual came to cesarean section in 79.1 percent and midforceps in 14.8 percent. It was clear that the occurrence of any further dilatation or descent after the arrest in these cases immediately improved the prognostic outlook considerably.

The degree of responsiveness provided additional information. The postarrest slope of dilatation or descent was compared with the foregoing prearrest slope in each case. The differences in the relative increments according to the phase of labor in which the arrests occurred were not statistically significant. Nevertheless, there was a tendency toward quantitatively better responses in early arrest. This mirrored the same trend seen in uncomplicated arrest patterns (see Chapter 11). In the latter cases, the earlier the arrest, the less probable the ultimate response to therapy. By contrast, the success rate among gravidas with concurrent protraction and arrest was the same in those arresting early as in those arresting late in labor (52.1 and 52.7 percent, respectively).

The delivery prognosis was influenced to a considerable extent by the degree of response as measured by the critical difference between prearrest slope and postarrest slope. The average increment in labors that were ultimately terminated by cesarean section was +0.60 and by midforceps, +0.79; this contrasted sharply with the increment seen in patients who delivered normally: +1.83 cm per hour.

When the difference between the slopes before and after arrest was small, operative delivery was relatively more common. For example, with increments of less than +0.5 cm per hour, both cesarean section and midforceps rates were 20.0 percent, respectively. Patients with postarrest increments of less than +1.0 cm per hour were delivered abdominally in 11.1 percent and by midforceps in 27.8 percent. Increments between +1.0 and +1.9 cm per hour yielded 7.4 percent cesarean sections and 11.1 percent midforceps. As the increments increased, the outlook became progressively more optimistic. None required cesarean section with increments of +2.0 cm per hour or greater; only 4.5 percent of this subgroup required midforceps for delivery. In fact, neither midforceps nor cesarean section was required with increments greater than +2.5 cm per hour.

## *CONCURRENT DISORDERS IN MULTIPARAS*

### *Obstetric Factors*

Multiparas with both protraction and arrest disorders in labor tended to be older than normal multiparas. This difference in age was statistically significant and appeared to confirm the similar observation encountered in multiparas with arrest patterns alone (see Chapter 11). There were 4.8 percent more than 40 years of age (3.6 percent expected).

Gestational age at delivery was narrowly distributed at or near term. The incidence of small babies was about normal. However, large infants weighing more than 4000 g occurred in greater numbers than expected, but the difference was not statistically significant.

As to cephalopelvic disproportion, the expected increase in incidence was found (30.9 percent), confirming comparable findings in multiparas with uncomplicated arrest patterns. This interrelationship between arrest and fetopelvic disproportion has been well documented. In addition, there were increased frequencies of occiput transverse and occiput posterior positions as well as breech presentations. The incidence of midforceps procedures was 17 percent and of cesarean sections, 24 percent.

Analysis of the labor data (Table 14) in this group showed marked prolongation of the active-phase duration. This reflected both the slow rate of dilatation and the intervals of arrest. The maximum slopes of both dilatation and descent were very low and the deceleration phase was likewise prolonged The second-stage duration was somewhat prolonged, but minimally so. This perhaps reflects the general tendency to expedite delivery in these cases.

## *Etiologic Factors*

As before, a search was carried out to determine which factors might be operating here to produce the protraction and arrest dysfunction. Excessive sedation (78.6 percent), fetal malposition (76.2 percent), and fetopelvic disproportion (23.8 percent) were found in significant numbers. These observations paralleled the nulliparous group of patients with concurrent disorders. The incidence of conduction anesthesia (16.7 percent) was higher than anticipated, although not significantly different from the expected rate of 10.6 percent in this population. In nulliparas, conduction anesthesia had been administered rather often (18.3 percent) just prior to the arrest in such cases.

The incidence of rupture of membranes at or before the onset of labor or just preceding arrest was not excessive here either. This finding was rather different from that seen in nulliparas. The incidence of cephalopelvic disproportion among multiparas, while increased statistically, did not reflect the very marked preponderance in nulliparas.

## *Treatment*

Among multiparas with these disorders who were managed with oxytocin infusion, 83.3 percent responded with further dilation or descent. Almost all who responded successfully did so within 3 hours of the beginning of therapy. Other forms of therapy, including expectancy, rest, and amniotomy, were generally inconsistent in effect.

In some multiparas, of course, it occasionally appeared sufficient to allow sedative effect to wear off when it was clear that the arrest may have resulted from the sedation. Thus, expectant treatment may be worthy of consideration when the circumstances warrant.

## *Prognosis*

The cesarean section rate of 23.8 percent among multiparas with concurrent protraction and arrest was greater than had been encountered for either disorder alone. All the sections were done during a period of arrest and most of them (80 percent) were undertaken without any intervening trial of other form of therapy. In the rest of the cases, the cesarean section was done either after uterotonic stimulation had failed or at the time of a subsequent recurrent arrest. Thus, the section rate among patients who did not progress further after the arrest occurred was 64.3 percent; among those in whom a response to therapy was documentable, it was 3.6 percent.

In all, some progress beyond the arrest was found to occur in 66.7 percent. Obviously, not all patients were given the opportunity to demonstrate whether they could respond with further progress after the arrest was diagnosed. If we were to correct for the cesarean sections done without the benefit of further trial of therapy, we would increase the overall response rate to 77.8 percent. This is one-half again larger than the minimal expected rate of response in nulliparas (52.3 percent) with concurrent disorders.

In nulliparas, it was found that the outlook for patients in whom labor arrested prior to the deceleration phase was especially poor (49.7 percent cesarean sections if arrest occurred early versus 23.0 percent if it occurred subsequently). In multiparas, this was not verified. The section rate remained fairly stable throughout regardless of the phase in which arrest occurred (22.2 percent if early, 26.7 percent if late).

Cephalopelvic disproportion was the most common reason for cesarean section, occurring in all cases. This finding paralleled that seen in nulliparas. The association of disproportion and the potentially serious combination of protraction and arrest disorders is noteworthy. It is not unexpected, therefore, that those patients in this group who had documented disproportion came to cesarean section in 76.9 percent and midforceps delivery in 15.3 percent. In contrast, among those with normal fetopelvic relationships, no cesarean sections were required at all, and there were 17.2 percent midforceps operations.

In nulliparas, we encountered more favorable outcome according to increasing degree of responsiveness in the form of the increment in postarrest slope relative to its prearrest counterpart. This could not be verified here on a statistical basis, but the trends appeared to be comparable in direction if not in magnitude. Nevertheless, in general, the prognosis in multiparas with concurrent protraction and arrest disorders is considerably more favorable than in nulliparas. Among multiparas, it appears that any response in the form of further dilatation or descent should be looked upon as an optimistic sign.

# Precipitate Labor

## CHAPTER 13

Precipitate dilatation and precipitate descent patterns of labor are reviewed. We appear to be unable to characterize patients who are likely to develop these potentially serious disorders, but the abnormalities are important to recognize by graphic means, nevertheless.

Interest in abnormally rapid labor is generated by its clinical importance. There is an appreciable increase in perinatal mortality associated with rapid labor and delivery. Fetal wastage appears to result from diminished intrauterine oxygenation of the fetus and concomitant birth trauma. The trauma may be associated with excessively violent contractions that can damage both mother and baby by direct action. This may bring about rupture of the uterus or, by rapidly changing the intracranial pressure, favor the development of cerebral hemorrhage. Intrauterine hypoxia may result from diminished circulation to the uterus and impeded fetal–placental exchange.

In general, this condition appears to result from overactivity of the myometrium. It is manifest by contractions that occur too frequently and too intensively. It usually occurs in association with negligible resistance from the maternal soft tissues. Additionally, there are frequently concurrent powerful contractions of the abdominal musculature so that labor is further enhanced and delivery quickly effected.

Up to this point, we have limited our survey to those instances in which progress in labor has been abnormally slow or arrested. We can now look at the other extreme of the spectrum; namely, those cases in which progress occurs with excessive rapidity. Based on the limits derived from distribution data obtained earlier (Chapter 7) from gravid patients at large, we are in a position to examine those cases in which the progress in labor is excessively rapid.

Precipitate labor has been variously defined without clear-cut consideration for the physiologic variations known to occur in otherwise normal labors. One generally finds categorical statements claiming that labors lasting less than 2 or 3 hours in duration are precipitate. Such limits are obviously arbitrary.

The problem is further compounded by the confusion in terms. Precipitate delivery—or the misnomer "precipitous," which refers rather to precipices—is a rapid, unsterile, unsupervised, and/or uncontrolled delivery. Although precipitate labor may often terminate in a precipitate delivery, we are not concerned here with this latter phenomenon.

We have examined in detail the maximum slopes of the active phase of dilatation and of descent. From the observations that have been made, average rates of dilatation and of descent have been derived (Chapter 7). From the distribution data, we have been able to determine lower statistical limits based on the 5th and 95th percentile variations from the mean. These have proved rather useful in helping to define disordered labor patterns.

By the same token, it is reasonable to assume that the upper limits will be equally meaningful in defining precipitate labor and in pointing out those cases that exhibit this potentially serious disorder. The 95th-percentile statistical maxima in nulliparas for dilatation were determined to be 6.8 cm per hour, and in multiparas 14.7 cm per hour. For descent, the limits were 6.4 and 14.0 cm per hour, respectively (Friedman and Sachtleben, 1970a).

The rapidity with which changes take place in some patients is so extreme, particularly in multiparas, that it may almost be unmeasurable. These are cases in which significant changes in dilatation occur with each successive contraction. Only with a device such as the continuously recording cervimeter (see Chapter 4) can the slope be measured with any degree of accuracy.

For practical purposes in clinical usage, rates greater than 5 cm per hour (or 1 cm every 12 minutes) in nulliparas, or 10 cm per hour (1 cm every 6 minutes) in multiparas are useful approximations. These serve to help detect and delineate this important abnormality.

## *PRECIPITATE DILATATION*

A series of nulliparas with maximum slope of dilatation of at least 5 cm per hour were studied (Friedman, 1955a), and the results have recently been reconfirmed in a similar series. The labor data derived from this group (Table 15) showed the expected significant increase in the maximum slope of dilatation and a parallel increase in the maximum slope of descent. It will be seen that precipitate dilatation frequently occurs in association with precipitate descent in the same labor. Consistent with this observation is the foreshortening of the durations of active and deceleration phases and second stage.

Interestingly, the latent phase was found not to differ significantly from the average for nulliparas in general. This is of some importance. In this regard, it should be stressed that the latent phase does not seem to be affected by the pathophysiologic mechanism that produces precipitate labor. The

*Table 15. LABOR DATA FOR PATIENTS WITH PRECIPITATE LABOR*

| Group | Latent Phase (hr) | Active Phase (hr) | Maximum Dilatation (cm/hr) | Deceleration Phase (hr) | Maximum Descent (cm/hr) | Second Stage (hr) |
|---|---|---|---|---|---|---|
| Nulliparas | | | | | | |
| Mean labor | 6.4±0.25 | 4.6±0.14 | 3.0±0.08 | 0.84±0.04 | 3.3±0.07 | 1.10±0.04 |
| Precipitate dilatation | 7.7±0.61 | 2.4±0.11* | 6.5±0.19* | 0.55±0.05* | 6.8±0.18* | 0.76±0.06* |
| Precipitate descent | 7.0±0.58 | 2.6±0.13* | 6.0±0.20* | 0.48±0.06* | 7.6±0.18* | 0.60±0.05* |
| Multiparas | | | | | | |
| Mean labor | 4.8±0.18 | 2.4±0.06 | 5.7±0.16 | 0.36±0.02 | 6.6±0.17 | 0.39±0.02 |
| Precipitate dilatation | 5.5±0.57 | 1.0±0.06* | 12.4±0.37* | 0.13±0.02* | 10.7±0.40* | 0.14±0.02* |
| Precipitate descent | 5.1±0.48 | 1.2±0.07* | 11.1±0.36* | 0.12±0.02* | 14.0±0.38* | 0.10±0.02* |

* Statistically significant, $p < 0.01$.

foreshortening of the deceleration phase in association with rapid cervical dilatation in the active phase is expected, as is precipitate descent, since all appear to be functions of an overly efficient driving uterine force coupled with diminished soft-tissue resistance.

Because most precipitate labors were found not to have been enhanced or inhibited by exogenous factors, we felt that it was appropriate to compare their labor data with the ideal labor described in Chapter 7. It will be recalled that this latter group consisted of gravidas at term, all with adequate pelves and vertex presentation, without malposition and with unimpeded labors. When nulliparas with precipitate dilatation patterns were compared with ideal nulliparas, only the mean maximum slopes of dilatation and descent were significantly different.

Almost all deliveries were uncomplicated and spontaneous by the vaginal route. There were 2.8 percent midforceps procedures, a significantly diminished incidence; these were associated with relative cephalopelvic disproportion.

It is of interest to note that 12.5 percent of patients were considered to be heavily sedated on the basis of their suppressed response to painful stimuli. In addition, 43.1 percent were moderately sedated. Nonetheless, there was a diminished frequency of heavily medicated patients in this group. It is of more than passing interest that there were some patients who developed precipitate labor in the presence of what was considered excessive sedation.

A total of 8.3 percent received conduction anesthesia during the course of their labor. All of these anesthesias had been administered according to standard and acceptable practice (see Chapter 19). Thus, none was given too early (in the latent phase), in conjunction with excessive premedication, or to too high an anesthetic level (above dermatome thoracic–10).

Cephalopelvic disproportion was determined to be present by radiographic pelvimetry in 8.3 percent of these cases. Again, it is important to note that precipitate labor can occur in conjunction with bony disproportion. Similarly, persistent occiput posterior positions were seen in 12.5 percent.

Other factors that have been reported to predispose patients to rapid labors were surveyed. None was felt to be relevant here, including youth (average age of these patients, 25.8 years) or prematurity (6.9 percent delivered infants less than 2500 g in weight, and no infant weighed less than 2000 g). This diminished the likelihood that these factors are truly contributory.

Oxytocin infusion was administered in 11.1 percent. Its use was implicated as probably causative in the development of the tumultuous labor that was observed to follow in many of these cases.

Among multiparas, precipitate dilatation was encountered with nearly twice the frequency of that seen in nulliparas. These patients did not differ significantly from the average multipara in age (29.3 years). Contrary to expectations, we did not encounter an unusual number of grand multiparas. Only 4.1 percent had had five or more prior viable pregnancies, compared with 3.8 percent for multiparas in general.

The incidence of fetal malpositions was about as expected (15.1 percent occiput transverse and 16.4 percent occiput posterior). Infant birth weight was likewise normally distributed: 4.2 percent weighed less than 2500 g (5.2 percent expected) and 6.9 percent weighed more than 4000 g (5.8 percent expected). Similarly, the distribution of rupture of membranes was not unusual. For example, 29.6 percent remained intact until delivery (32.2 percent expected).

All multiparas in this series were delivered vaginally, including 12.3 percent by low forceps. There were no midforceps or cesarean sections among this group. Moreover, it was interesting to find no instances of cephalopelvic disproportion in a population in which 5.8 percent were expected to present this problem. In this regard, it should be added that disproportion may have existed, but none was detected in this series. Furthermore, 20.5 percent were unsedated (4.2 percent expected), while 9.6 percent were considered to be heavily sedated (13.6 percent expected). Again, we see that precipitate dilatation is possible in the presence of clinically excessive sedative-analgesic medication.

The labor data in multiparas with precipitate dilatation showed foreshortening of the active and deceleration phases, as well as marked steepening of the maximum slopes of dilatation and descent—all of which were expected and confirmatory of comparable findings in nulliparas. The relatively normal average length of latent phase was also encountered in nulliparas.

It was of some interest to note that there were 4.1 percent prolonged latent-phase patterns in this group. In each of these cases, the abnormally long latent phase spontaneously corrected itself and the subsequent active-phase dilatation was surprisingly rapid, contrary to expectations. All such patients delivered spontaneously and uneventfully. This finding reemphasizes the apparent dissociation between factors influencing the latent phase and those affecting the remaining portion of labor.

Additionally, there were 2.7 percent with prolonged deceleration phase. This abnormality followed the precipitate dilatation and appeared in retrospect to result from the use of heavy sedation in most cases. The medication apparently was effective in slowing the abnormally rapid progression in the active phase. This observation may be useful for purposes of clinical management.

We appear to be justified in concluding that precipitate dilatation is a real clinical entity. It can be detected graphically. Etiologic factors are not clearly defined at all. However, it seems that precipitate dilatation can occur even in the presence of heavy sedation, relative bony disproportion, minor fetal malpositions, and conduction anesthesia.

## *PRECIPITATE DESCENT*

To review in detail the characteristics of gravidas who developed precipitate descent would merely repeat much of the material just presented for the patients with precipitate dilatation. This is so because the conditions so commonly occurred together in the same labor. The constellation of features that make for precipitate dilatation (tumultuous uterine contractions coupled with negligible soft-tissue resistance) also produce precipitate descent. While they do not always go together, they are concurrent in about 91 percent. This figure is likely to be a low estimate, because progression is sometimes so rapid that the diagnosis cannot always be made with certainty on a quantitative basis.

Labor data have been analyzed for groups of patients with precipitate descent, nulliparas and multiparas being considered separately (Table 15). As expected, the composite material is very similar in both direction and magnitude to that derived from gravidas with precipitate dilatation. They differ only in that patients with precipitate descent tend to have greater rates of descent than those with precipitate dilatation, although both are statistically significant when compared with the average maximum slope of descent in normal gravidas. An inverse relationship exists with regard to maximum rates of dilatation: the rates are greater with precipitate dilatation than with precipitate descent, but again both are significantly different from the mean of normal labors.

Other aspects of the course of labor were also foreshortened, except for the latent-phase duration. This is precisely the same as had been seen with precipitate dilatation (see above). Moreover, when compared with the ideal labor course (see Chapter 7) based on data derived from optimal labors, it was found that these labors differed very little, except for the marked increase in maximum slope of descent.

As in the precipitate dilatation series, patients with precipitate descent were sometimes found to have been heavily sedated (9.2 percent). A small number had been given conduction anesthesia (5.1 percent), and some even had cephalopelvic disproportion (6.0 percent). Essentially all deliveries were spontaneous, many having been designated as precipitate delivery (that is, over an unsterile field and without appropriate control). This occurred in nearly two-thirds of the cases and was not unexpected in view of the exceedingly rapid progress that took place in these cases.

In retrospect, precipitate delivery is perhaps understandable and excusable in the multiparas, but it is difficult to justify in the nulliparas in this series, in whom the second-stage duration averaged 36 minutes. In most of the latter cases, there were sufficient numbers of observations to enable the attendant clinicians to foresee the rapid descent and to make the necessary preparations for the impending delivery.

Thus, we see that precipitate descent is just as real a clinical entity as precipitate dilatation. Indeed, both commonly occur together in the same labor. Precipitate descent is readily detected by graphically depicting the course of progressive fetal descent in labor. It can be objectively diagnosed by calculating the slope of descent in a labor in progress. As with precipitate dilatation, etiologic factors are unclear, but we can encounter such cases even in the presence of heavy sedation, cephalopelvic disproportion, and conduction anesthesia.

# Factors Affecting Labor

# PART III

# Maternal Actuarial Factors

## CHAPTER 14

Maternal age appears to have little bearing on the course of labor, except for a small but consistent increase in the length of second stage in older gravidas. The stature of gravidas does seem to affect labor progression. Obese women undergo slower labor courses in general, and their labor patterns are more frequently disordered than gravidas whose weight is more ideal for height. Labors tend to be briefer with advancing parity, largely because of latent-phase foreshortening and, to a lesser extent, speeding of the rates of dilatation and descent.

This section will undertake to study various endogenous factors affecting the course of labor. We will attempt to determine what specific effects they may have, if any. In order to proceed with investigations that are aimed at determining specific effects, it has been satisfactory merely to group patients according to the presence of the factor under surveillance.

The problem of studying maternal age as it might affect labor, for example, was readily solved by classifying patients into broad groups according to chronologic age. Similar stratifications were made for other actuarial factors that were to be studied, including maternal height and weight, parity, and gravidity. Comparisons could then be made among the several groups.

The only statistical provision that required clarification was the need to demonstrate that each subgroup was comparable with others in all features other than that under study. This requirement was not always easily satisfied, nor was it necessarily true that the various subgroups were actually comparable. This complicated our analyses considerably because suitable corrections had to be made frequently for differences in group composition. Such limitations aside, our investigations have yielded important and potentially useful information.

## MATERNAL AGE

The effect that advancing maternal age has on the course of labor is poorly defined. The literature (for extensive references see Friedman and Sachtleben, 1965a) is inconsistent as to the kind of labor to be expected in either the very young or the elderly gravida. Indeed, there are wide differences of opinion as to what the upper and lower age limits should be for optimal performance. Various reports describe labor in adolescents as lengthened, normal, or shortened depending on the makeup of the series being studied. In older women, it may likewise be abnormally long, normal, or shorter than expected.

In our attempt to clarify the relationship between maternal age and labor, a study was undertaken using the graphic techniques that we have described here (see Chapter 7). This approach permitted us to assess the course of labor critically on a quantitative basis by evaluating the functions of cervical dilatation and fetal descent against elapsed time. With these methods, data were obtained from homogeneous groups of patients for purposes of comparison. It has been possible to ascertain the influences of various factors on the course of labor in this way.

### *Age Limits*

We first determined the age distribution of our gravid population. This was necessary in order to find appropriate cut-off limits to describe the extremes in maternal age. A large group of patients was selected for study (Friedman and Sachtleben, 1965a). They consisted of a cross-sectional sampling of more than 3000 consecutive nulliparas. The distribution of this group by age is shown in Figure 25. From this distribution curve, limits were selected: the 5th and 95th percentile limits were determined to be 17.8 and 35.4 years, respectively. Thus, ages 18 through 35 years were assumed to be close approximations of the range of normal.

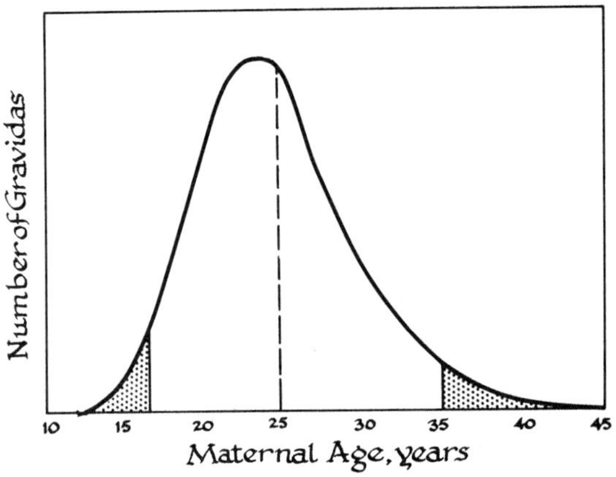


*Fig. 25.* Maternal age distribution in a large series of nulliparas, designating the mean age as 26 years, modal 24 years; 95 percent fall between 17 and 36 years.

(From Friedman EA, Sachtleben MR: Am J Obstet Gynecol 91:916, 1965a)

Our patients were, therefore, grouped into those younger than age 18, those between 18 and 35, and those older than 35 years. All patients were studied with reference to their course in labor, and the cervical dilatation–time and descent–time labor curves were constructed where possible. Of necessity some were deleted because insufficient numbers of determinations were available. This occurred either because labor had not been permitted (for example, elective cesarean section) or because the patient had arrived at the hospital too late in labor to permit reconstruction of the labor curves retrospectively.

### *Group Differences*

We wished to ascertain whether these groups were comparable in all factors other than maternal age. As indicated earlier, this was necessary so that subsequent analyses for the effect of age on the course of labor might be considered valid. To accomplish this, it was necessary to determine the composition of the subgroups in detail. The distributions of gestational age and infant birth weight were almost identical in all groups, between 83.8 and 85.0 percent of infants weighing between 2500 and 4000 g at birth. Similarly, the incidence of multiple birth was uniform. This was contrary to expectation in that increased twinning was expected with advancing maternal age.

There was an interesting and unexplained increase in the incidence of cephalopelvic disproportion with advancing age (2.0, 7.8, and 11.2 percent, respectively). This doubtfully implied a tendency for the pelvic configuration to change with time. It is not entirely impossible, of course, that this might occur, particularly with reference to osteoporotic changes. However, it seemed unlikely. It may suggest that our criteria for digital and radiographic evaluations change according to the patient's age. If this is true, serious biases are being introduced into our obstetric judgments, perhaps without our being completely aware of them.

With regard to fetal position in labor, the groups appeared comparable except for an increased incidence of breech presentation in the older group (8.3 percent as compared with 3.0 percent in the median group and 4.3 percent in the under-18 group). In addition, there was a slight increase in the number of occiput posterior positions in the elderly gravidas (28.1 percent versus 20.8 and 21.5 percent, respectively, in the median and younger groups). These differences were not statistically significant.

Factors known to influence the course of labor showed considerable differences in frequencies between the groups. Heavy sedation, for example, was given to 38.4 percent in the younger and 30.8 percent in the median age group. This contrasted sharply with 52.6 percent in the older age group. On the other hand, conduction anesthesia was administered to 31.2 percent of the younger, 17.4 percent of the median, and 24.7 percent of the older group. By further contrast, uterotonic stimulation was given to 34.0 percent of the adolescent subjects, as compared with 13.8 and 16.4 percent, respectively, in the other two groups. It was, therefore, determined that adjustments for these differences would have to be made part of any subsequent analysis in order for the results to be meaningful.

Breakdown by type of delivery demonstrated variations from 9.6 percent midforceps in the younger to 3.8 percent in the median, and a significant 18.7 percent in the older group. Strikingly, there were 20.6 percent cesarean sections among older patients as compared with 4.3 percent in the younger. When we reviewed the indications for the cesarean sections in the older category, we found about two-thirds in which the justifications were rather doubtful. It is likely that many would have delivered vaginally if they had been permitted to do so, reducing the cesarean section rate in these elderly gravidas to a reasonable figure of about 7 percent.

## *Labor Course*

Data derived from the graphic patterns of dilatation and descent (Table 16) showed that the course of labor in each of the three age groups was essentially identical, with the exception of the deceleration-phase and second-stage durations. Labor proceeded normally in general despite the deleterious factors that were found to be acting to bias the data against the older age group, including more heavy sedation and less uterotonic stimulation. However, we recognized that these uncorrected data need not necessarily have reflected the actual situation because we were not examining truly comparable groups. Each of them was heterogeneous in composition. Furthermore, it was possible that the limits we set were not sufficiently critical to point out significant deviations that might exist.

Because of the disparity among the groups under examination, we felt it essential to go further in order to verify or refute our observations. We idealized the data (see Chapter 7) by deleting all patients in whom complicating, hampering, or stimulating forces were at play. This excluded patients

*Table 16. LABOR DATA BY MATERNAL AGE*

| *Group* | *Latent Phase (hr)* | *Active Phase (hr)* | *Maximum Dilatation (cm/hr)* | *Deceleration Phase (hr)* | *Maximum Descent (cm/hr)* | *Second Stage (hr)* |
|---|---|---|---|---|---|---|
| Total series | | | | | | |
| Under 18 | 7.8±0.63 | 4.8±0.42 | 2.8±0.20 | 0.79±0.08 | 2.9±0.14 | 0.80±0.06* |
| Age 18–35 | 8.6±0.27 | 4.9±0.15 | 3.0±0.08 | 0.90±0.05 | 3.2±0.09 | 0.95±0.04 |
| Over 35 | 8.1±0.61 | 5.0±0.45 | 3.0±0.19 | 1.09±0.20 | 3.1±0.13 | 1.18±0.11* |
| Ideal labors | | | | | | |
| Under 18 | 5.1±0.56* | 3.4±0.23 | 3.4±0.33 | 0.52±0.05* | 3.6±0.30 | 0.72±0.07 |
| Age 18–35 | 7.1±0.28 | 3.4±0.11 | 3.5±0.13 | 0.70±0.05 | 3.6±0.16 | 0.76±0.04 |
| Over 35 | 5.4±0.69* | 2.8±0.23 | 4.2±0.45 | 0.42±0.04* | 3.8±0.32 | 0.83±0.14 |
| Matched pairs | | | | | | |
| Under 18 | 6.6±0.74 | 4.9±0.80 | 2.9±0.34 | 0.82±0.17 | 3.1±0.36 | 0.85±0.10 |
| Over 35 | 6.9±0.97 | 4.4±0.52 | 3.2±0.25 | 1.24±0.24 | 3.3±0.29 | 1.23±0.20 |

* Statistically significant, $p < 0.01$.

with factors such as large or premature babies, malpositions, malpresentations, disproportion, anesthesia in labor, excessive sedation, and uterotonic stimulation. It allowed us to derive somewhat more comparable groups for purposes of analysis. Data from ideal subseries within each of the maternal age groups showed that the latent and deceleration phases were foreshortened in both the younger and older gravidas, while the remaining phases and slopes were entirely within the normal range.

In our search for possible agents acting to produce these changes, we examined unstimulated and unsedated labors separately. We saw essentially complete resolution of the differences by this means, with the single exception of moderate prolongation of the second stage in the older age group. Comparison of groups stratified according to premature rupture of the membranes showed no difference except for similar trends in the deceleration phase and second stage. This was repeated again among patients who received conduction anesthesia.

From these data, we see that maternal age need not influence the course of labor deleteriously, except for some slight prolongation of the deceleration-phase and second-stage durations. When the material for the entire series was further stratified by maternal age on a biennial basis (Fig. 26), we verified that there were no hidden trends. The trend that was expected to occur in the deceleration-phase duration did not appear.

On the other hand, the second-stage tendency became more obvious (Fig. 27). This clear-cut prolongation of the second stage with progressing maternal age must not be magnified out of proportion, however. The entire range of variation is only about 45 minutes on the average. Therefore, this contributes very little to the total duration of labor. Except as far as it might contribute to the clinician's frustration in managing the second stage, this increment should not unduly lengthen labor.

As a last analytic process, we resorted to the statistical technique that involves matched pairs. This consists of matching gravidas according to all available information except the factor under surveillance, namely age. The data derived from these matched groups showed complete correspondence in the latent- and active-phase durations and the maximum slopes of dilatation and descent. At the same time, we again saw (Table 16) the expected increase in the deceleration-phase and second-stage durations among older gravidas.

Thus, we are unable to demonstrate any major alteration in the course of labor with advancing maternal age except for prolongation of the second stage. Nonetheless, the possibility still existed that abnormal labors may be occurring in unusual numbers. This phenomenon might be masked by dilution with otherwise normal cases. Similarly, we had eliminated some of the potentially abnormal cases by deleting those terminated by abdominal section prior to or early in labor.

Accordingly, we examined the case material to determine the presence of dysfunctional labor patterns as previously defined (see Chapter 8). Rather interesting data were obtained. The frequencies of abnormally prolonged

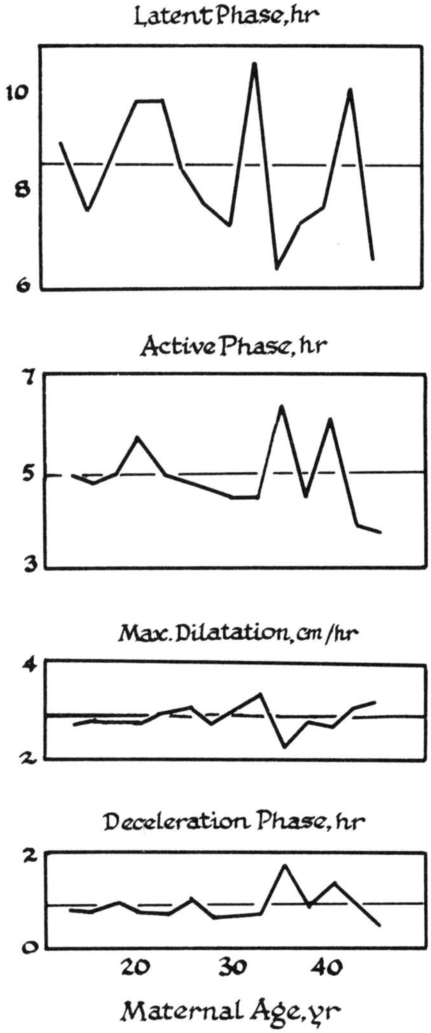


*Fig. 26.* Dilatation pattern data by maternal age for nulliparas grouped in 2-year age intervals, showing absence of any meaningful trends in any of these parameters with advancing age. The expected trend in the deceleration phase did not materialize.

latent phase, protracted active-phase dilatation, and protracted descent were comparable in all three groups. However, there was an impressive increase in the incidence of secondary arrest of dilatation, prolonged deceleration phase, and arrest of descent in the older-age category: the incidence of these three disorders totaled 11.4 percent, a difference statistically significant from the respective 4.9 and 5.2 percent incidence in the median- and younger-age gravidas. A similar finding has recently been reported from another source (Sokol et al, 1974a).

We had previously seen an unusually high frequency of use of heavy sedation in the older-age population. On this basis, we conjectured as to the possible relationship that this factor might have in yielding dysfunctional labor. It was of interest, therefore, to learn that in 89.2 percent of the older-

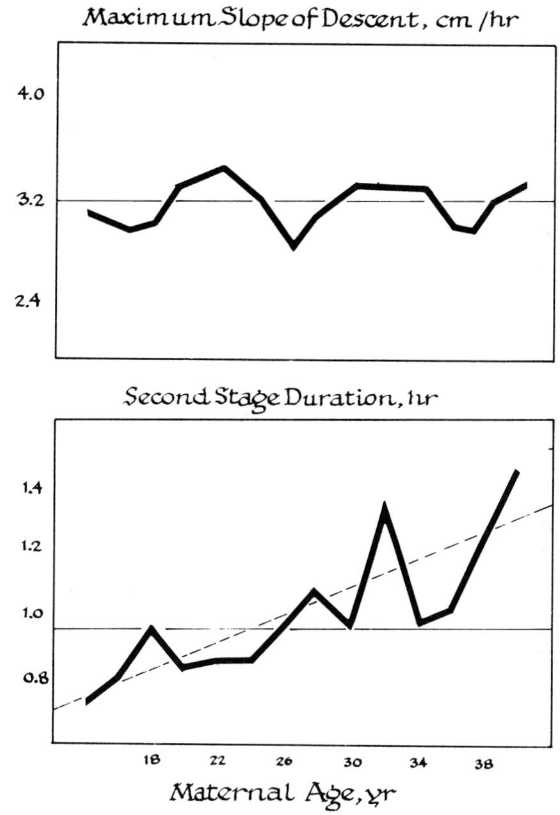


*Fig. 27.* Second-stage duration and maximum slope of descent in nulliparas as related to maternal age, grouped on an annual basis. There is a small but clear increase in second-stage length in older gravidas, totaling only 45 minutes in range.

age patients dysfunctional labor was associated with sedation in a post hoc relationship. The comparable incidence in the young group was 10.7 percent and in the median-age group, 10.3 percent. There was little doubt, therefore, that the increased numbers of dysfunctional labors in the older patients was somehow related to heavy sedation.

Additionally, the question of whether or not labors in older patients were more sensitive to sedation or conduction anesthesia was raised. It was determined that the frequency of dysfunctional labor patterns following these inhibitory factors was actually no higher than expected. It should be noted, however, that Sokol et al (1974a) found that dysfunctional patterns were more likely to occur in the older-age group after the administration of heavy sedation. They suggested, therefore, that labor progression in the elderly gravida is very sensitive to such agents.

The relationship between maternal age and labor has thus been examined in an objective manner using graphic techniques. No really important differences in the course of labor could be ascribed to advancing age, contrary to the widely held clinical impression that older patients have long labors. The single exception was a progressive increase in the second-stage duration.

However, this was a relatively small matter in the total picture of the course of labor.

## MATERNAL STATURE

The most extensive review of the relationship of maternal height and weight to various factors of pregnancy, labor, and delivery was that of Kaltreider (1963). This survey of nearly 19,000 patients yielded important and useful information. It showed, for example, that shorter patients had higher frequencies of preeclampsia, prematurity, perinatal loss, and cesarean section. Taller women were found to have larger babies. Heavier patients had more hypertension, diabetes, shoulder dystocia, and oversized babies. They also had the highest cesarean section rate. Lighter patients, on the other hand, had more anemia, premature babies, and cesarean sections. Overweight women—based on a normal range within one standard deviation of the mean weight according to height—were found to have more frequent hypertension, diabetes, shoulder dystocia, large babies, and cesarean sections. Underweight gravidas were more commonly anemic and had more premature infants and fewer large babies.

Labor was analyzed only from the point of view of two rather incompletely defined entities, namely, uterine inertia and labors lasting longer than 20 hours. Nevertheless, it was found that height did not affect the incidence of these disorders. Heavier patients, however, had had a greater incidence of uterine inertia, as did overweight women. With reference to prolonged labors, there seemed to be no correlation with either height or weight. The discrepancy between these two sets of findings was not readily explained.

It is clear that the question of the possible effect height and weight may have on the course of labor remains unanswered, although clarification is obviously necessary. Review of other reports in the obsteric literature reveals divided opinion, but the majority favor the concept that obesity is associated with uterine inertia.

### Group Limits

Utilizing our graphic approach, we tried to provide meaningful data on the relationship between maternal stature and the course of labor. Data were available on height, weight, cervical dilatation, and descent relationships in a large series of randomly selected nulliparas. The group was subdivided arbitrarily into thirds, according to the distribution of height: those shorter than 5 feet 2 inches tall, those between 5 feet 2 inches and just below 5 feet 4 inches, and those 5 feet 4 inches or taller.

Without specific regard for height correlation, the total group was independently and arbitrarily subdivided according to weight as well: those weighing less than 140 pounds, those between 140 and 159 pounds, and those weighing 160 pounds or more.

In addition, we considered the height–weight relationships, particularly for patients who were underweight or overweight. The distributions within the several height categories were examined and 95th-percentile ranges were determined on the basis of the distribution of two standard deviations from the mean. Thus for patients shorter than 5 feet 2 inches tall, those weighing less than 120 pounds at term were considered underweight while those weighing 155 pounds or more were designated overweight; the lower and upper limits in the median height group were 135 and 164 pounds, and in the tall group, 140 and 179 pounds, respectively.

## *Group Differences*

Specific trends for maternal age were detected among short patients. Among them, age and weight seemed to parallel each other. Lighter patients averaged 22.8 years of age; median, 25.0 years; heavy, 29.0 years. In more meaningful terms, underweight patients averaged 23.9 years of age, normal patients 24.6 years, and overweight patients 25.2 years.

It was of interest to note that prior obstetric experience varied among the groups. The incidence of prior abortion reflected the age trend we have just noted. Thinner patients had fewer prior abortions and heavier patients had many more (11.5 versus 33.3 percent). No similar trends were seen among average or tall patients. Relating height to ideal weight, we found 5.3 percent previous abortions in the underweight series and 16.7 percent in the overweight group.

Shorter patients demonstrated cephalopelvic disproportion in significantly greater numbers. There were 17.8 percent with disproportion among them, as contrasted with 9.4 percent for the nulliparous population at large. At the same time, there was a startling increase in the incidence of bony dystocia relative to weight within this group of short women. Among light patients, there was an incidence of 11.5 percent with disproportion; in the median weight group, 25.0 per cent; in the heavy group, 33.3 percent. In relative terms, underweight gravidas had 10.5 percent disproportion and overweight women, 22.2 percent.

This clear-cut trend for disproportion proved to be statistically quite significant. Similarly, the relative overall frequency of this condition in short patients was statistically validated. It was of further interest to note that within the median weight group, the trend was most pronounced. Disproportion was absent in tall patients but occurred in 10.0 percent of average-height patients and in 25.0 percent of short patients. These findings clearly verify Baird's contention that contracted pelves occur most commonly among short patients. There can be little question about this relationship.

Reports in the obstetric literature (Baird, 1953; Kasius et al, 1958) relate infant weight to maternal height. Taller mothers appeared to produce larger infants in general. A corollary is that the prematurity rate is lower among tall women. Our data also demonstrate that taller women have heavier babies overall. The average infant birth weight among short women was 3083 g; in the median height group, 3147 g; in the tall group, 3186 g.

In addition, there was a progressive increase in the incidence of large babies with advancing stature: 4.4 percent of infants born of the short-stature group weighed at least 4000 g, as compared with 8.7 percent born of tall women. No particular trend was noted with regard to the incidence of large babies in either the underweight or the overweight groups. This tended to nullify the significance of this relationship.

It is important to note, furthermore, that maternal weight acted as a much more significant factor in this regard. Our findings supported the general consensus that the smaller the mother, the greater the prematurity rate. This was seen especially in women of short stature. Among short, lightweight mothers, 7.7 percent delivered premature infants; none were delivered to short, overweight mothers. This relationship occurred to a lesser extent in average and tall patients. Underweight women bore 15.8 percent premature infants, overweight mothers 5.6 percent.

There can be little doubt that small mothers have biologically smaller infants. The average weight of infants born to lightweight mothers was 2913 g; to heavy mothers, 3170 g. Furthermore, the average weight of infants delivered to underweight mothers was 2945 g, as contrasted with an average weight of 3329 g for infants in the overweight series. Whether or not small infants born of small parents were premature from a functional point of view might be questioned, but our data cannot provide a definitive answer.

With regard to obstetric mechanisms, there seemed to be a consistent relationship between maternal weight and fetal position. The lighter the patient, the more likely for her infant to be in an occiput transverse (13.0 percent versus 7.9 percent for the heavier patients) or occiput posterior postion (23.9 percent contrasted with 13.2 percent). The incidence of malpositions or malpresentations did not seem to be affected by maternal stature in any way.

The phenomenon with reference to fetal position was totally unexplained. With this exception, the absence of correlation with abnormal presentations or positions confirms the previous findings by Kaltreider (1963). When examined with regard to relative height–weight relationships, the correlation referring to occiput transverse position disappeared. However, the relationship with occiput posterior positions was reconfirmed (21.1 percent in the underweight group, 16.7 percent in the overweight).

There seemed to be no meaningful trends with regard to sedation or the use of conduction anesthesia in labor in any of the height or weight subcategories. We inferred, therefore, that these factors were not acting to bring about any of the changes subsequently encountered in the labor data. Similarly, uterotonic agents were used in a rather uniform manner throughout. This coincidence made analysis of our data easier.

The time of membrane rupture was evenly distributed in the several subgroups. Initial cervical dilatation—a factor recognized to influence the duration of the latent phase (see Chapter 16)—was found to be further advanced in short, thin and tall, heavy gravidas. As to delivery outcome, the several modalities were normally dispersed. There were no unusual frequencies of labor complications other than the frequencies of labor dysfunction, which will be discussed further (see below).

### *Labor Course*

Based on analysis of the graphic patterns of labor, dilatation and descent data were evolved (Table 17). Trends were seen indicating more rapid active-phase dilatation and relatively shorter second stages with increasing maternal height. These were associated with progressively more rapid dilatation and descent slopes.

Trends with regard to increasing maternal weight, on the other hand, were not so clear-cut. There were tenuous tendencies toward increasing latent phase and shortening second stage with increasing maternal weight, but these were not as impressive as those seen with increasing height. It was apparent on more critical analysis that examining patients strictly according to absolute height or weight categories left much to be desired, because it was not possible in this way to define the relative influence of these two factors on labor.

By subgrouping patients into corresponding height–weight categories, unfortunately, we failed to shed much light on this complex problem. For example, it was found that among short patients, increasing weight resulted in decreasing latent and active phases as well as increasing maximum slopes of dilatation and descent. These trends were not duplicated among patients

*Table 17. LABOR DATA BY MATERNAL STATURE*

| Group | Latent Phase (hr) | Active Phase (hr) | Maximum Dilatation (cm/hr) | Deceleration Phase (hr) | Maximum Descent (cm/hr) | Second Stage (hr) |
|---|---|---|---|---|---|---|
| Height groups | | | | | | |
| Short | 9.0±1.12 | 5.0±0.46 | 2.7±0.22 | 0.74±0.08 | 2.9±0.26 | 1.04±0.13 |
| Medium | 8.1±0.84 | 4.4±0.43 | 3.0±0.20 | 0.76±0.08 | 3.0±0.20 | 0.87±0.09 |
| Tall | 9.2±1.14 | 3.8±0.77 | 3.4±0.38 | 0.75±0.10 | 3.2±0.30 | 0.84±0.11 |
| Weight groups | | | | | | |
| Light | 8.5±1.08 | 4.7±0.47 | 3.1±0.28 | 0.64±0.08 | 3.2±0.30 | 0.98±0.13 |
| Average | 8.3±0.74 | 5.7±0.69 | 2.5±0.18 | 0.87±0.09 | 2.8±0.22 | 0.90±0.09 |
| Heavy | 10.3±1.37 | 4.1±0.38 | 3.7±0.39* | 0.71±0.10 | 3.5±0.32 | 0.88±0.11 |
| Height–weight groups | | | | | | |
| Underweight | 5.5±0.78 | 3.3±0.37 | 3.6±0.50 | 0.49±0.07* | 3.8±0.48 | 0.94±0.15 |
| Normal | 8.8±0.67 | 5.3±0.42 | 2.8±0.31 | 0.82±0.06 | 3.0±0.33 | 0.94±0.08 |
| Overweight | 12.1±2.40 | 6.5±0.76 | 2.9±0.57 | 0.62±0.13 | 2.8±0.55 | 0.75±0.14 |

* Statistically significant, $p < 0.01$.

of average stature. Moreover, in tall patients, there was a clear-cut opposite trend in which the latent-phase and second-stage durations appeared to increase with maternal weight.

As to height variations, among lightweight patients, latent and active phases diminished, second stage decreased, and maximum slopes increased with advancing height. By contrast, among average-weight patients, the only significant trend observed was lengthening of the active phase with increasing height. In the heavy group, the latent phase appeared to be lengthened with increasing height. This combination of trends was most confusing and difficult to interpret.

Our observations can be summarized as follows: There is relative prolongation of the latent phase in both short, light patients and tall, heavy gravidas. Slightly built patients appear to have longer active phases. This is confirmed with reference to maximum slopes of dilatation and descent, because such light patients have the lowest mean slopes.

The labor course data for underweight and overweight patients were also examined (Table 17). We were able to demonstrate that obese patients have significantly longer latent and active phases overall. This was mirrored somewhat by an insignificant tendency toward slowing of the maximum slopes of dilatation and descent in these patients.

These relationships were also reflected in the high incidence of dysfunctional labor in both underweight and overweight gravidas (30.8 and 33.3 percent, respectively). Patterns of prolonged latent-phase and protraction disorders were most common, representing three quarters of all the aberrant labors encountered here. Thus, dysfunctional labor was surprisingly frequent at both ends of the spectrum of maternal stature. There were equivalent peak frequencies occurring in short, light women and in tall, heavy gravidas.

It was possible that other factors were acting to bring about these findings. For example, the initial cervical dilatation was not uniformly distributed. Relatively greater initial dilatation was seen in both the tall, light patients and in the short, heavy patients. This observation might have accounted in part for the latent-phase trends that were encountered, because there is a recognized correlation between latent-phase duration and initial cervical dilatation (see Chapter 16). Other less obvious factors might possibly account for the active-phase and maximum slope trends, but none was detected, except for somewhat more common use of excessive sedation during the active phase among short, light patients.

In abnormal height–weight categories, the incidence of dysfunctional labor took on an altogether different appearance. There were no aberrant labor patterns in the underweight patients; this contrasted sharply with 27.8 percent incidence in the overweight group. The correlation of labor dysfunction with obesity was statistically very significant. It confirmed Kaltreider's observations (1963).

We see, therefore, that weight affects labor in specific ways. This particularly applies to the ideal weight according to height. On average, overweight patients have significantly delayed progress in both the latent and active phases. Also, they have relatively higher frequencies of dysfunctional labors than underweight women or those of normal stature.

## *PARITY AND GRAVIDITY*

In several of our foregoing discussions on the various types of dysfunctional labor, it was suggested that prior obstetric experience might have been a determinant factor. We saw, for example, that more than the expected number of nulliparas with major labor aberrations had had prior abortions. There were simultaneous observations that many were older. It was reasonable to assume that the advanced age, particularly in women who developed arrest patterns, might account for the high rate of previous abortion, merely reflecting the greater opportunities for the older patient to conceive and to abort.

This might more reasonably explain the findings than the assumption that prior abortion somehow altered uterine physiology—or reflected an already altered physiologic mechanism—to produce or contribute to the production of dysfunctional labor in subsequent pregnancies. On the other hand, it could not be determined with any degree of certainty that this latter possibility did not exist. It became important, therefore, to determine whether or not gravidity actually influenced subsequent labor.

As to parity, we have already seen the great differences between the labors in nulliparas as compared with those in multiparas. Refinement of these data to indicate subtle changes with increasing parity was felt to be necessary.

In a large, randomly selected series of nulliparas (Friedman, 1955a), patients were examined according to whether or not they had had previous nonviable abortions. The labor courses were studied in detail. It was determined that the labor data for nulliparas who had had prior abortions were essentially identical with those of primigravid nulliparas (Table 18). Thus

*Table 18. LABOR DATA BY PARITY AND GRAVIDITY*

| *Group* | *Latent Phase (hr)* | *Active Phase (hr)* | *Maximum Dilatation (cm/hr)* | *Deceleration Phase (hr)* | *Maximum Descent (cm/hr)* | *Second Stage (hr)* |
|---|---|---|---|---|---|---|
| Gravidity | | | | | | |
| Primigravid nulliparas | 8.6±0.78 | 4.9±0.34 | 2.5±0.14 | 0.98±0.11 | 2.6±0.18 | 0.97±0.08 |
| Multigravid nulliparas | 8.4±0.95 | 4.8±0.60 | 2.6±0.30 | 0.95±0.20 | 2.7±0.26 | 0.94±0.19 |
| Parity | | | | | | |
| Para 0 | 8.6±0.27 | 4.9±0.15 | 3.0±0.08 | 0.90±0.05 | 3.2±0.10 | 0.95±0.04 |
| Para I | 5.4±0.27 | 2.2±0.11 | 5.4±0.22 | 0.23±0.03 | 5.7±0.26 | 0.27±0.02 |
| Para II | 5.4±0.38 | 2.2±0.14 | 5.9±0.31 | 0.22±0.03 | 5.9±0.30 | 0.20±0.02 |
| Para III | 5.0±0.39 | 2.0±0.15 | 6.7±0.54 | 0.16±0.02 | 6.5±0.44 | 0.20±0.02 |
| Para IV | 4.7±0.50 | 2.2±0.31 | 4.5±0.36 | 0.24±0.03 | 5.5±0.40 | 0.26±0.04 |
| Para V or more | 5.9±0.92 | 2.3±0.72 | 6.8±0.78 | 0.13±0.03 | 6.7±0.62 | 0.13±0.02 |

the tenuous clinical impression that rapid labors follow abortions could not be verified.

To ensure that the subgroups of nulliparas were comparable, we examined these cases more closely. It was clear that they were almost the same in terms of delivery distribution and the incidence of complicating features. A further subgroup, consisting of women who had had two or more prior abortions, was also examined in the same way. They, too, were found not to differ in any way from the mean nor from those who had had only one abortion or none at all.

The effect of parity was examined in another large series of multiparas (Friedman, 1956b) for comparison with nulliparas. Patients were grouped according to parity in order to evaluate the effect of increasing parity upon the course of labor. It has already been shown (Chapter 7) that the nulliparous labor curves differ considerably from the patterns in multiparas, the latter exhibiting shorter latent, active, and deceleration phases as well as shorter second stages and more steeply inclined slopes of dilatation and descent.

Breakdown of the labor data by parity is shown in Table 18. We recognized that the latent phase progressively shortens with succeeding pregnancies until the fourth, on average; then it elongates again. The changes in

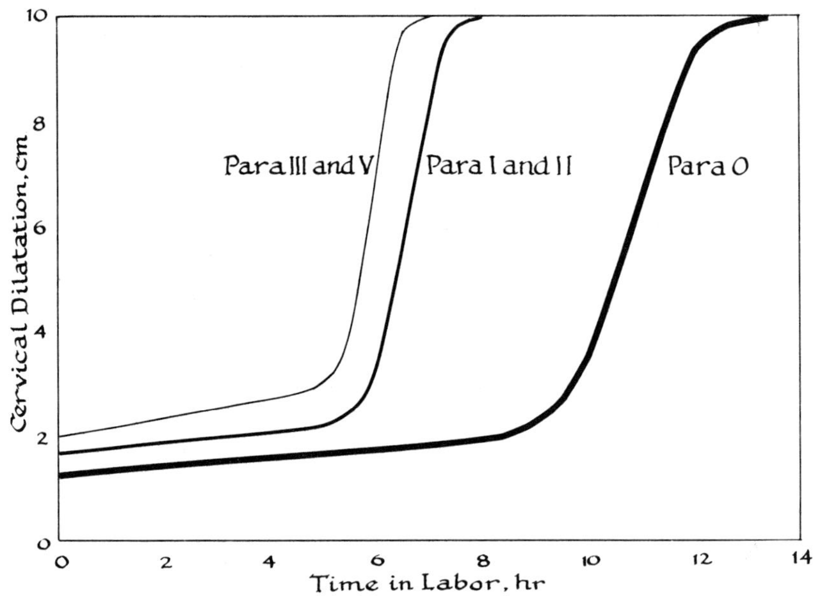


*Fig. 28.* Relation between parity and the pattern of cervical dilatation, showing marked shortening of latent-, active-, and deceleration-phase durations and concurrent increase of maximum slope with advancing parity. Data for Para IV patients, not illustrated, do not fall in line because they differ from other gravidas in factors that may alter the labor course. Descent trends are comparable.

latent phase, however, are not statistically significant. The duration of the active phase is remarkably stable with succeeding pregnancies after the first.

The mean maximum slopes of dilatation and descent increase steadily, and the deceleration-phase and second-stage durations decrease. The Para IV group presents an incongruous exception, perhaps explained by its special makeup (see below). The constancy of the active phase, in the face of a steepening maximum slope of dilatation and shortening deceleration phase, implies a probable lengthening of the evanescent acceleration phase with increasing parity.

The frequencies of complicating factors in these groups were entirely as expected, with the exception of the Para IV group. In this latter group were found abnormal numbers of occiput posterior positions (27 percent) and conduction anesthesias (17 percent). These may readily account for the discrepancies noted above in the progressive trends with advancing parity. Both malposition and conduction anesthesia are recognized to contribute toward flattening the maximum slopes and prolonging both the deceleration phase and second stage.

Correcting for discrepant inconsistencies between the groups, we succeeded in emphasizing and thereby corroborating the trends. Increasing parity thus produces shortening of the latent phase, deceleration phase, and second stage, together with steepening of the maximum slopes of dilatation and descent (Fig. 28). This is unassociated with any significant change in the duration of the active phase, suggesting prolongation of the acceleration phase.

A larger comparable study was undertaken to corroborate these findings (Friedman and Kroll, 1971b), utilizing a computer program to evaluate more than 10,000 gravidas. Computed and graphed data were found to be very similar with regard to distribution for all phases and slopes. In general, this intensive effort verified the findings described above.

# Fetal Factors

## CHAPTER 15

The smaller the fetus, the shorter the labor. This applies especially to the active phase and second stage and is reflected in progressively slower rates of dilatation and descent with increasing birth weights. With very small fetuses, however, two distinctive groups of labor patterns are discernible. These may represent gravidas whose labors began under quite different circumstances. Fetal position in vertex presentations does not seem to be a particularly important factor in affecting the course of labor, although occiput posterior and occiput transverse positions may be associated with some prolongation of the deceleration phase. Labor in breech presentations is about the same as in vertex presentations, with relatively minor differences perhaps accounted for on the basis of preselection of most potentially problematic cases for abdominal delivery. Face presentation, if unassociated with cephalopelvic disproportion, generally yields normal labor patterns. Brow presentation, on the other hand, usually results in prolongation of the deceleration phase and second stage. The descent process may be impeded; when this occurs, it suggests the likelihood that disproportion exists.

Our consideration of the factors that may affect the course of labor will continue here with discussions of the investigations relating to the possible effects of fetal factors. These include fetal size, position, and presentation. Other factors dealing with the fetus, such as its station and relationship to the pelvis, will be detailed in the section dealing with pelvic factors (Chapter 16); those relating to membrane status, multiple pregnancy, hydramnios, and placental site and weight will be reviewed under uterine factors (Chapter 17).

There is little doubt that the fetus does influence the course of labor, both directly and indirectly. It takes very little clinical experience to recognize the adverse effects of certain fetal malpositions and malpresentations. The matter of fetal size as it influences labor, however, is somewhat more subtle. The widely accepted clinical impression holds that large babies are associated with abnormal labors and small ones, with comparably more rapid labor.

Nevertheless, extremes of labor are seen in all infant weight categories. It is reasonable, therefore, to attempt to determine where the labor is consistently influenced by fetal size and, if it is, to determine its direction and magnitude. The same applies to issues relating to fetal position and presentation.

## *FETAL SIZE*

The relationship of fetal size to the course of labor has been studied extensively (Friedman and Sachtleben, 1969b). The course of labor was investigated by graphic techniques in large groups of term and premature labors. The groups were studied in depth in order to ensure that they were truly comparable with each other in factors other than infant weight.

### *Group Differences*

It was found that maternal age, for example, was essentially the same in the premature and term patients. Prior abortion, on the other hand, occurred in excessive numbers among patients who entered labor prematurely. The overall incidence of previous abortion among premature nulliparas was 20.2 percent (versus 12.4 percent among nulliparas being delivered at term) and in multiparas, 31.8 percent (25.4 percent at term).

Not unexpectedly, a diminished incidence of cephalopelvic disproportion was found in 0.6 percent of premature nulliparas, as compared with 7.8 percent at term (0.4 and 5.8 percent, respectively, in multiparas). Cases demonstrating disproportion were encountered exclusively in the largest weight premature category (and in the term group, of course).

Similarly, breech presentation occurred in high numbers among premature deliveries, as expected (7.8 percent in premature nulliparas and 14.7 percent in premature multiparas). There were more than twice the expected numbers of spontaneous rupture of the membranes prior to the onset of labor in the premature group (27.6 versus 11.8 percent in nulliparas and 32.6 versus 10.3 percent in multiparas).

The frequencies of uterotonic stimulation were essentially the same throughout. Sedation, however, was used much more sparingly in premature labors. This latter is consistent with the accepted practice based on risks attendant to premature infants from heavy sedation given to the mother.

## *Labor Course*

Labor data were derived from the premature and term groups; nulliparas and multiparas were considered separately (Table 19). In premature nulliparas, we encountered significant shortening of all phases of labor. The overall difference averaged 4.8 hours in total duration (the mean totals were 9.7 versus 14.5 hours). In addition to the shorter latent- and active-phase components of the first stage, maximum slopes of dilatation and descent were clearly increased and the second-stage duration diminished.

In multiparas, on the other hand, only active-phase duration and maximum slopes were affected. The total duration of premature labor in multiparas was only 0.6 hour shorter, on average, than comparable labors at term. Neither latent-phase nor second-stage duration was apparently influenced by prematurity in multiparas.

Among nulliparas whose labors were unaffected by enhancing or inhibiting factors—comprising an ideal labor group—essentially the same findings were duplicated. It was expected that limiting our observations to an ideal group of untampered labors would diminish or even eliminate any potential effect on labor of differences in patient makeup.

Specifically, we were concerned that such extraneous differences as diminished sedation and less disproportion in the prematures might serve to distort the data. Both these factors have previously been shown to affect the course of labor significantly (see Chapters 16 and 19). Since the relationships persisted, we felt it necessary to stratify the data to correct for these effects. When this was done, however, the differences persisted, although they were somewhat diminished quantitatively.

Dilatation and descent patterns were examined according to infant weight groupings in 500-g increments (Table 20). Clear-cut trends were encountered. We found, for example, that there were statistically significant progressive prolongations in the active-phase, deceleration-phase, and second-stage durations with increasing birth weight in nulliparas. Simultaneously,

*Table 19.* *LABOR DATA BY FETAL MATURITY*

| *Group* | *Latent Phase (hr)* | *Active Phase (hr)* | *Maximum Dilatation (cm/hr)* | *Deceleration Phase (hr)* | *Maximum Descent (cm/hr)* | *Second Stage (hr)* |
|---|---|---|---|---|---|---|
| Nulliparas | | | | | | |
| Term | 8.6±0.27 | 4.9±0.15 | 3.0±0.08 | 0.90±0.05 | 3.2±0.10 | 0.95±0.04 |
| Premature | 6.8±0.32* | 3.0±0.12* | 4.6±0.16* | 0.52±0.03* | 4.8±0.18* | 0.56±0.02 |
| Ideal Nulliparas | | | | | | |
| Term | 7.1±0.28 | 3.4±0.11 | 3.5±0.13 | 0.70±0.05 | 3.6±0.15 | 0.76±0.04 |
| Premature | 5.8±0.46* | 2.6±0.10* | 4.9±0.24* | 0.34±0.03* | 4.7±0.28* | 0.51±0.03* |
| Multiparas | | | | | | |
| Term | 5.3±0.19 | 2.2±0.07 | 5.7±0.16 | 0.23±0.01 | 6.0±0.20 | 0.24±0.01 |
| Premature | 4.9±0.21 | 1.8±0.04* | 6.8±0.20* | 0.22±0.01 | 6.8±0.24* | 0.23±0.01 |

* Statistically significant, $p < 0.01$.

*Table 20. LABOR DATA BY BIRTH WEIGHT (grams)*

| Group | Latent Phase (hr) | Active Phase* (hr) | Maximum Dilatation* (cm/hr) | Deceleration Phase† (hr) | Maximum Descent* (cm/hr) | Second Stage† (hr) |
|---|---|---|---|---|---|---|
| Nulliparas | | | | | | |
| 1000–1499 | 7.2±0.79 | 2.5±0.12 | 5.2±0.42 | 0.29±0.03 | 5.4±0.48 | 0.50±0.09 |
| 1500–1999 | 6.7±0.68 | 3.1±0.40 | 4.8±0.44 | 0.41±0.04 | 5.0±0.46 | 0.57±0.05 |
| 2000–2499 | 6.9±0.50 | 3.7±0.20 | 3.8±0.26 | 0.62±0.05 | 4.0±0.30 | 0.70±0.04 |
| 2500–2999 | 9.5±1.08 | 4.6±0.46 | 3.4±0.35 | 0.70±0.04 | 3.8±0.32 | 0.96±0.15 |
| 3000–3499 | 7.9±0.59 | 4.2±0.30 | 3.0±0.18 | 0.72±0.02 | 3.4±0.22 | 0.94±0.08 |
| 3500–3999 | 8.5±0.99 | 5.0±0.51 | 2.9±0.28 | 0.90±0.11 | 3.0±0.30 | 1.08±0.14 |
| 4000+ | 6.9±0.97 | 6.0±0.86 | 2.3±0.22 | 0.94±0.10 | 2.8±0.28 | 1.02±0.12 |
| Multiparas | | | | | | |
| 1000–1499 | 5.0±0.48 | 1.9±0.14 | 7.3±0.55 | 0.20±0.03 | 6.8±0.52 | 0.24±0.03 |
| 1500–1999 | 4.8±0.40 | 1.8±0.12 | 7.0±0.46 | 0.22±0.02 | 6.6±0.50 | 0.28±0.06 |
| 2000–2499 | 4.7±0.33 | 1.8±0.08 | 6.6±0.39 | 0.22±0.02 | 6.6±0.46 | 0.20±0.03 |
| 2500–2999 | 5.5±0.49 | 2.1±0.13 | 5.9±0.39 | 0.17±0.04 | 6.2±0.40 | 0.12±0.02 |
| 3000–3499 | 5.5±0.27 | 2.0±0.10 | 6.2±0.26 | 0.20±0.02 | 5.8±0.32 | 0.24±0.02 |
| 3500–3999 | 4.7±0.29 | 2.2±0.14 | 5.6±0.36 | 0.26±0.03 | 5.5±0.33 | 0.23±0.02 |
| 4000+ | 5.5±0.98 | 2.5±0.22 | 4.9±0.74 | 0.23±0.04 | 5.0±0.60 | 0.33±0.10 |

* Statistically significant trends, $p < 0.01$, for both nulliparas and multiparas.
† Statistically significant trend, $p < 0.01$, for nulliparas only.

the maximum slopes of dilatation and descent progressively diminished among these nulliparas.

In multiparas, only the active phase showed this tendency to prolong with increasing fetal size, together with progressively slowing maximum slopes of dilatation and descent. In both nulliparas and multiparas, the latent-phase correlations could not be verified. The relationship between fetal weight and the active-phase duration and maximum slopes of dilatation and descent, however, was very evident (Fig. 29).

Major aberrant dysfunctional labor patterns occurred rather commonly. There were 11.2 percent abnormal labors in premature nulliparas and 9.6 percent in premature multiparas. In the nulliparous series, only protracted active-phase dilatation was encountered in excessive numbers (7.6 versus 3.6 percent expected). This contrasted with the normal relative frequency of other forms of dysfunctional labor in this group.

In multiparas, on the other hand, the incidence of dysfunctional labor patterns was nearly 12 times the expected frequencies at term. These multiparas included large numbers of patients with prolonged latent-phase, protraction, and arrest disorders. These findings clearly indicate that aberrant labor patterns can and do occur in premature labors. Moreover, aberrant patterns are found in especially large numbers in multiparas.

The finding that dysfunctional labors occurred so frequently among premature births, particularly in multiparas, appeared to contradict the data purporting that the course of labor in this group was significantly more rapid, particularly in the active phase. This suggested the possibility that we were dealing with a heterogeneous group of labors, some of which were

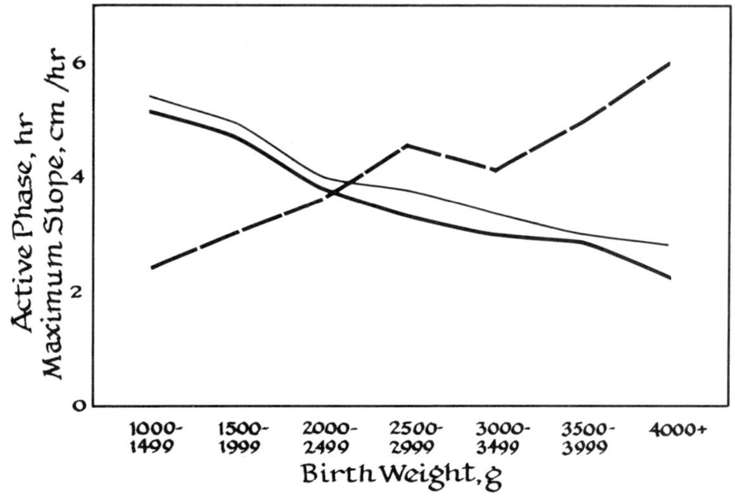


*Fig. 29.* Birth weight of infants delivered of nulliparas as related to duration of active phase (*broken line*) and maximum slopes of dilatation (*heavy line*) and descent (*light line*), illustrating clear trends toward longer, slower active phase and descent progression with larger babies. The same trends exist in multiparas. No latent-phase relationship is demonstrable.

dysfunctional and therefore abnormally slow, while others were contrastingly rather rapid.

Closer examination of our data for active-phase durations according to birth weight in 500-g increment groups yielded material of considerable interest (Fig. 30). The distribution of active-phase durations among term multiparas presented a single modal peak at 1.5 hours. This is identical with material previously demonstrated in unselected multiparas (Friedman, 1956b). When we examined the distribution curves for smaller birthweight groups, significant differences began to appear.

In the largest premature group (2000 to 2499 g), for example, we found the beginning of a distortion in the distribution pattern, suggesting a deviation from normal distribution. Progressing into the 1500 to 1999-g subseries, we saw a distinct secondary peak appearing at about 2.5 hours. This new peak became dominant in the 1000 to 1499-g group.

This indicated rather clearly that there were two distinctly characteristic varieties of labors. The two separate hypothetical populations are defined by the superimposed distribution curves shown in Figure 30 for the 1000 to 1499-g group. Similar observations were seen among nulliparas, but the relationships were less clear-cut.

It appears likely, therefore, that two dissimilar forms of labor are associated with infants of small size. We could distinguish no differences in pre-

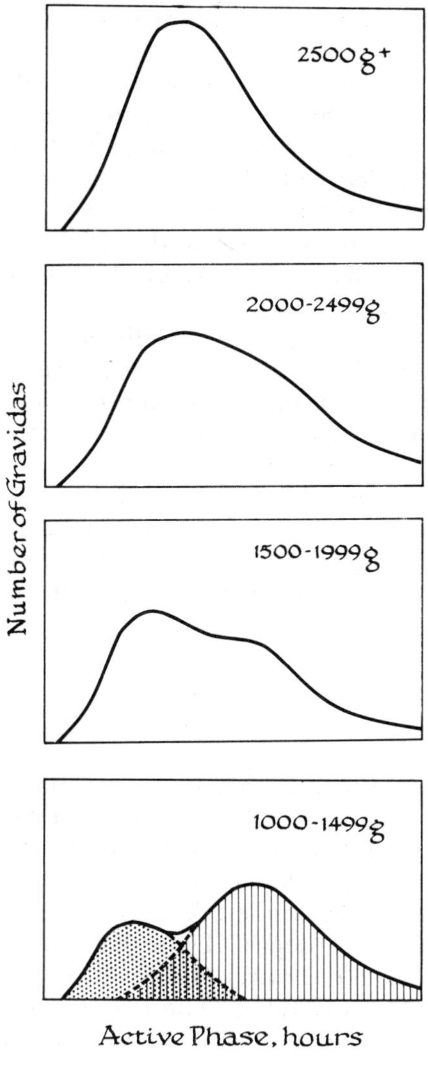


*Fig. 30.* Distribution of data on active-phase duration among multiparas grouped by infant birth weight in 500-g increments. Somewhat skewed, but essentially normal (Gaussian) unimodal distribution is seen in term infants weighing 2500 g or more. Distortion from normality increases progressively with diminishing birth weight until it is clear that there is a bimodal distribution among labors associated with infants weighing less than 1500 g. This suggests two distinctive populations of gravidas (see text).

labor maternal soft-tissue preparation between these groups. There were no differences in initial cervical dilatation, effacement, or fetal station at the onset of labor. Therefore, they were indistinguishable prospectively.

However, the two varieties became disparate as the active phase evolved. The more normal group, characterized by more rapid evolution of the active phase, could readily be distinguished from the less normal or dysfunctional variety. The incidence of the dysfunctional labor patterns appeared to be inversely related to the infant weight. Fewest dysfunctional patterns occurred in term infants and most occurred in labors that resulted in infants weighing less than 1500 g.

It is likely that these two distinctive labor groups represent separate populations of patients who are undergoing labor under different conditions. The characteristics of these conditions are probably unique for the premature labor pattern. The more rapid variety, for example, is likely to be associated with conditions that make rapid progress feasible. These include minimal resistance by maternal soft parts coupled with efficient, strong myometrial contractions. Dysfunctional patterns, on the other hand, seem to reflect less favorable conditions, such as resistant, inelastic, and unyielding cervical and vaginal tissues together with inefficient, weak, or dyskinetic uterine contractions.

The more normal labors might be considered to have been influenced to begin by an intrinsic and optimal mechanism. Here, all factors in the myometrium and soft tissues are in readiness for the process. The more abnormal variety is perhaps triggered into action by extrinsic factors in the presence of unsuitable uterine and soft-tissue prelabor preparation.

We do not know what factor or constellation of factors causes labor to begin. Nonetheless, we seem to be confronted here with labors that begin with factors either ideally suited for progression of normal active-phase labor patterns, on the one hand, or quite unfavorable and therefore producing relatively more abnormal patterns, on the other.

## *FETAL POSITION*

Among patients with dysfunctional labor patterns, we have seen an increased incidence of minor malposition (see Chapters 10–12). These especially include occiput posterior and occiput transverse mechanisms. It was important, therefore, to try to define the potential influence of fetal position on the course of labor. Detailed investigations were undertaken (Friedman, 1955a; Friedman, 1956b) to analyze material in depth. These have been supplemented (Friedman and Kroll, 1972) by a computer assessment of the labors in a series of patients exceeding 10,000 in number. The material derived in this manner was largely corroborative of the results of the earlier studies.

Previous studies on labor patterns associated with several fetal positions in vertex presentations were not able to document any specific gross effects or correlations between the occurrence of these minor malpositions and abnormal labor. We saw slight prolongations of the deceleration phase of the first stage; these proved to be statistically significant only in multiparas. The increased frequency of dystocic factors occurring in conjunction with occiput posterior positions has, of course, been verified (Anderson, 1965; King, 1957; Sokol et al, 1975). However, one may conjecture that such dystocias may originate in the abnormality of the pelvis in which they occur. The implication of this concept is that minor malpositions may actually be the result of the labor abnormalities or of underlying factors producing the dystocic pattern, rather than their cause.

## *Group Differences*

Before we could accept the trends in labor data as meaningful, it was imperative we ascertained that the several subgroups were indeed comparable in other respects. When we examined the patients with occiput posterior positions, for example, it was determined that conduction anesthesia had been administered in 23 percent, an unusually high frequency. Moreover, cephalopelvic disproportion coexisted in 12 percent, also a high frequency. Dysfunctional labor patterns were determined to be present in 17 percent. These are all statistically significant differences from those expected in the normal nulliparous population.

Patients with persistent occiput transverse positions differed from normal nulliparas in the same way. Excessive numbers were found to have been given conduction anesthesia (27 percent) or to have had associated bony dystocia (15 percent). Analogously, 24 percent exhibited disordered labors.

## *Labor Course*

These differences notwithstanding, the labor data derived from nulliparas (Table 21) showed only moderately prolonged durations of active and deceleration phases and second stage in association with both occiput posterior and occiput transverse positions. Neither the latent phase nor the slopes of dilatation or descent were affected.

When we stratified the groups so as to examine only those ideal labors untampered by exogenous influences, we derived data suggesting that these minor malpositions do not influence the course of labor directly. Labor in association with occiput posterior and occiput transverse positions was not significantly different in any measurable way from labor in comparable ideal nulliparas.

Therefore, although these malpositions may be associated with cephalopelvic disproportion and other inhibitory influences, they themselves cannot be implicated as etiologic or contributory factors in the development of ab-

*Table 21. LABOR DATA BY FETAL POSITION IN VERTEX PRESENTATION*

| *Group* | *Latent Phase (hr)* | *Active Phase (hr)* | *Maximum Dilatation (cm/hr)* | *Deceleration Phase (hr)* | *Maximum Descent (cm/hr)* | *Second Stage (hr)* |
|---|---|---|---|---|---|---|
| Nulliparas | | | | | | |
| Occiput anterior | 6.3±0.27 | 4.6±0.15 | 3.0±0.09 | 0.78±0.05 | 3.3±0.09 | 1.08±0.06 |
| Occiput posterior | 6.5±0.48 | 6.3±0.46* | 2.8±0.20 | 1.30±0.21* | 3.0±0.22 | 1.35±0.10* |
| Occiput transverse | 6.6±0.52 | 6.0±0.48* | 2.6±0.22 | 1.35±0.23* | 2.8±0.25 | 1.36±0.12* |
| Multiparas | | | | | | |
| Occiput anterior | 4.6±0.20 | 2.3±0.08 | 5.7±0.18 | 0.32±0.05 | 6.3±0.19 | 0.34±0.05 |
| Occiput posterior | 5.0±0.49 | 2.5±0.22 | 5.4±0.38 | 0.48±0.06* | 5.9±0.32 | 0.39±0.08 |
| Occiput transverse | 5.2±0.50 | 2.7±0.25 | 5.4±0.40 | 0.52±0.06* | 5.6±0.34 | 0.40±0.09 |

* Statistically significant, $p < 0.01$.

normal labor patterns. Except for the slight residual prolongation of the deceleration phase (which was not statistically significant), the composite labor curves for these patients were determined to be normal in all respects.

Comparable findings (Table 21) were seen in multiparas. The course of labor was determined to be entirely normal, with the exception of prolongation of the deceleration phase on average. This latter finding proved to be statistically significant. As with the nulliparas, however, it was clear that the subgroup compositions were not comparable.

Multiparas with occiput posterior positions, for example, had been heavily sedated in 24.0 percent and those with occiput transverse, in 22.4 percent —both significantly increased frequencies, as compared with the occiput anterior group. Contrary to the findings in nulliparas, there was no increase in frequency of conduction anesthesia in multiparas. Other factors were also comparable.

Correcting for the differences in the distribution of sedation did not erase the significant prolongation of the deceleration phase. Therefore, occiput posterior and occiput transverse positions in multiparas were not implicated as causative in abnormal labors and, except for the prolongation in the deceleration phase, they were associated with a normal labor pattern.

## *BREECH PRESENTATION*

There has been a growing apprehension among obstetricians regarding vaginal delivery of fetuses presenting by the breech. Concerns are justifiably based on the demonstrated risks (Abroms et al, 1973; Alexopoulos, 1973; Rovinsky et al, 1973). These concerns have been expressed in a clear-cut trend toward cesarean section. Indeed, in some areas abdominal delivery is now being done electively for breech delivery at or near term without even awaiting the onset of labor. This practice may not be defensible, particularly in view of the fact that spontaneous conversions to vertex presentation do occur (Scheer and Nubar, 1976) as term approaches.

Nonetheless, as the indications for cesarean section for breech presentation become more and more liberalized, experience with and observations of labor in such cases diminish. It is of even greater importance, therefore, that we understand the course of labor in these patients. Heretofore, obstetric reports dealing with breech presentation were largely preoccupied with management of the delivery. Labor factors have rarely been dealt with in such evaluations. Results of superficial analyses dealing with total duration of labor or duration of the first stage have failed to reveal consistent differences between labors with breech presentation and those with vertex presentation (Calkins, 1955b; Dunn et al, 1965; Hall et al, 1965). Ill-defined statements inferring good prognosis from normal progress (usually not otherwise clarified) appear throughout the obstetric literature (Brenner et al, 1974).

Recognizing the basic difficulty in assessing fetopelvic relationships in the breech presentation and accepting the fact that criteria based on trial labors are essentially nonexistent, we have taken advantage of the availability of techniques for assessing labor progress under these circumstances. This matter becomes rather academic if pelvic inadequacy is obvious, but it may provide valuable information when clinical and radiographic pelvimetry do not offer definitive answers.

It has been stated that the trial of labor in the breech presentation is a trial of the type of labor (Vartan, 1959). If this premise is acceptable, it becomes imperative to find a means for quantitative assessment and characterization of the labor in these cases. Recognizing the need for critical determination of progress, we undertook to explore the graphic analytic techniques we have described earlier (see Chapter 7) as applied to patients with breech presentation.

A large group of relevant nulliparas and multiparas who were allowed to labor at term was studied extensively. Those with insufficient information to allow adequate graphing of the dilatation and descent curves were omitted, including patients who were subjected to cesarean section early in their course. Our material showed a preponderance of nulliparas, who comprised 45.3 percent; this contrasted with the 30 percent incidence of nulliparity in our gravid population. Other investigators have reported similar findings, indicating that breech presentation occurs more frequently among nulliparas.

### *Group Differences*

Maternal age and prior obstetric experience, however, were normally distributed. Gestational age and infant weight data were somewhat different from normal in that we had selected this series by limiting our observations to term births.

Some degree of fetopelvic disproportion was encountered in 15.4 percent of nulliparas and 1.8 percent of multiparas; the corresponding rates for vertex presentation were 7.8 and 5.8 percent, respectively. That disproportion occurred in twice the usual frequency in nulliparas may or may not reflect clinical hyperacuity in regard to evaluation of the fetopelvic relationships when the breech presents. Thus, even minimal discrepancies would tend to be classified as disproportionate. Indeed, the incidence of disproportion among nulliparas might have been increased even more had the patients subjected to elective cesarean section been retained for purposes of calculation. In multiparas, on the other hand, there appears to have been less concern in this regard, the incidence of disproportion being much lower than anticipated.

With regard to fetal position, about one-half presented in the sacrum transverse position (52 percent in nulliparas and 48 percent in multiparas). Most of the remaining were in the sacrum anterior position (33 and 42 percent, respectively). As to infant weight, the tendency for multiparas to have larger babies was not unexpected. There were 10.9 percent of infants delivered of multiparas, which infants weighed 4000 g or more, as contrasted with a general average of 5.8 percent in multiparas with vertex presentation. This undoubtedly also reflected selection methods. Nearly two-thirds presented as frank breech (66 percent nulliparas and 62 percent multiparas).

The distribution of rupture of the membranes was interesting in that almost twice the expected incidence of premature or early rupture occurred. In more than one-third of cases, the membranes had ruptured at or before the onset of labor (37.6 percent in both nulliparas and multiparas, as contrasted with 21.3 and 19.5 percent expected). This fact should be kept in mind for future reference so that its potential influence on the course of labor may be considered.

Along the same lines, use of uterotonic stimulation and heavy sedation were both encountered in greater frequencies than ordinarily seen with vertex presentation. For example, oxytocin was administered to 23 percent of nulliparas and 16 percent of multiparas (versus 14 and 11 percent expected). Excessive sedation was noted in 41 percent of nulliparas and 26 percent of multiparas (31 and 14 percent normally). Unsedated patients, on the other hand, were encountered in average numbers in nulliparas (3.3 versus 3.8 percent expected), but occurred in nearly four times the expected incidence in multiparas. The frequency of unsedated multiparas was 15.4 percent, as contrasted with 4.2 percent in the multipara with vertex presentation.

## *Labor Course*

Separate graphic analyses were carried out on nulliparas and multiparas with breech presentation (Table 22). We found that the nulliparous breech labor is quite comparable to its vertex counterpart, with the exception of significant foreshortening of the latent phase. In multiparas, on the other hand, the latent phases are comparable, but there appears to be uniform

*Table 22.* *LABOR DATA IN BREECH PRESENTATION*

| *Group* | *Latent Phase (hr)* | *Active Phase (hr)* | *Maximum Dilatation (cm/hr)* | *Deceleration Phase (hr)* | *Maximum Descent (cm/hr)* | *Second Stage (hr)* |
|---|---|---|---|---|---|---|
| Nulliparas | | | | | | |
| Vertex | 8.6±0.27 | 4.9±0.15 | 3.0±0.08 | 0.90±0.05 | 3.2±0.09 | 0.95±0.04 |
| Breech | 6.8±0.54* | 5.3±0.47 | 2.9±0.24 | 0.98±0.11 | 3.1±0.20 | 0.96±0.08 |
| Ideal Nulliparas | | | | | | |
| Vertex | 7.1±0.28 | 3.4±0.11 | 3.5±0.13 | 0.70±0.05 | 3.6±0.16 | 0.76±0.04 |
| Breech | 6.4±0.66 | 3.7±0.32 | 3.7±0.42 | 0.77±0.17 | 3.6±0.33 | 0.80±0.11 |
| Multiparas | | | | | | |
| Vertex | 5.3±0.19 | 2.2±0.07 | 5.7±0.16 | 0.23±0.01 | 6.0±0.20 | 0.24±0.01 |
| Breech | 5.0±0.43 | 2.6±0.17† | 5.0±0.30† | 0.43±0.04* | 5.2±0.32† | 0.36±0.04* |

* Statistically significant, $p < 0.01$.
† Borderline significance, $0.01 < p < 0.05$.

lengthening of all other portions of labor with concomitant decreases in the maximum slopes of dilatation and descent.

In order for us to determine if the differences encountered are inherent in the breech presentation or might instead reflect factors other than presentation, it was necessary to stratify these data into relevant subgroups. Variations with advancing parity, for example, emphasize the persistent relative deceleration-phase prolongation.

As to the labor patterns associated with the several types of breech presentation, the course of labor in each was nearly identical. The single exception appears among nulliparous footling breeches. Here we see foreshortening of the deceleration phase and second stage, but this is only of borderline significance. The same tendency is encountered among multiparas, but the differences are not statistically significant. Additionally, we find some lengthening of deceleration phase and second stage in conjunction with frank breech presentations in multiparas.

It is possible that the data referring to incomplete breeches may merely reflect the greater preponderance of active intervention in cases where the fetal extremities are presenting outside the introitus. Under these circumstances, the temptation to effect timely delivery might play a role in dictating management. In frank breech presentations, inhibitory factors may be at play. The position of the breech, however, appears to have no demonstrably consistent differential effect on the course of labor.

We undertook to search for factors that might influence labor progress in the breech. This was felt to be especially relevant because this series was composed entirely of term births. Accordingly, we examined subgroups by increments of infant weight. Significant trends were uncovered in this way.

With increasing fetal weight, there is lengthening of the active and deceleration phases as well as of the second-stage duration in nulliparas. Simultaneously, there is progressive diminution in the maximum slopes of dilatation and descent.

These trends are similar to those seen earlier in vertex presentations with increasing fetal weight (see above). While the tendencies appear to occur in the same direction, their magnitude is somewhat less in breech presentations, however. Among multiparas, comparable analyses did not uncover like trends.

Initial cervical dilatation as a determinant factor (see Chapter 16) was also considered important for analytic purposes. This factor has been used as an ingredient in the scoring system that was devised to help prognosticate the outcome for breech deliveries (Zatuchni and Andros, 1965). Among labors with vertex presentation, clear-cut foreshortening of the duration of labor has been described as an accompaniment of increasing prelabor cervical dilatation. The same is seen in breech presentations. In addition to the especially apparent effect in latent-phase durations, the active phase is similarly affected, but to a lesser extent. This probably reflects only acceleration-phase foreshortening, because the maximum slope of dilatation remains essentially constant.

Among multiparas, correlation with prelabor cervical dilation is somewhat different. Of course, there is the expected progressive shortening of the latent phase with advancing initial dilatation. However, there is a counterbalancing and significant lengthening of the active and deceleration phases as well as the second-stage duration, together with flattening of the maximum slopes of dilatation and descent.

Because these findings were unexpected, it became important to determine whether factors other than the status of the cervix at the onset of labor played a role in producing them. Closer scrutiny of the subgroups by initial dilatation did not provide any explanation in the form of increased frequencies of deleterious factors or agents. Only the factor of the breech presentation itself remained to explain the observed changes in the active phase and second stage.

As mentioned earlier, it was necessary to introduce correction techniques to account for the numbers of breech labors with early rupture of the membranes. This was done because it has previously been shown that the latent phase is shorter in patients whose membranes rupture spontaneously before or at the onset of labor (see Chapter 17). It was found that patients whose membranes had ruptured after the onset of labor had an average latent phase that was nearly identical with the latent-phase duration in the comparable gravid population with vertex presentation. Thus, simple correction alone completely erases the significant foreshortening of the latent phase encountered among nulliparous breech labors.

Similarly, we had noted earlier that uterotonic stimulation and excessive sedation were used significantly more often with breech presentation than with vertex presentation. Accordingly, corrections had to be made for these factors as well because of the known effect they have on the course of labor. The simplest and most effective technique for providing such correction was that of idealization (see Chapter 7).

Idealization was accomplished merely by omitting those cases presenting with significant abnormalities (such as cephalopelvic disproportion) and by omitting the patients whose labors had been inhibited or stimulated (by heavy sedation, oxytocin stimulation, and conduction anesthesia). Those ideal labors remaining among nulliparas with breech presentation were then available for direct comparison to like patients with vertex presentation. The labor courses for both groups of patients (Table 22) were essentially identical. Although the latent phase proved to be still somewhat shorter among those with breech labors, the difference was no longer significant.

Fetal station at the onset of labor was also examined because of the recognized effect that prelabor engagement appeared to have on the course of labor (see Chapter 16). Analysis of breech labors grouped according to this factor showed the existence of trends identical with those seen in vertex presentation. There was foreshortening of all phases of labor with descending station.

This observation should be stressed in passing. It is generally agreed that estimations of fetal station in breech presentation are more difficult to make

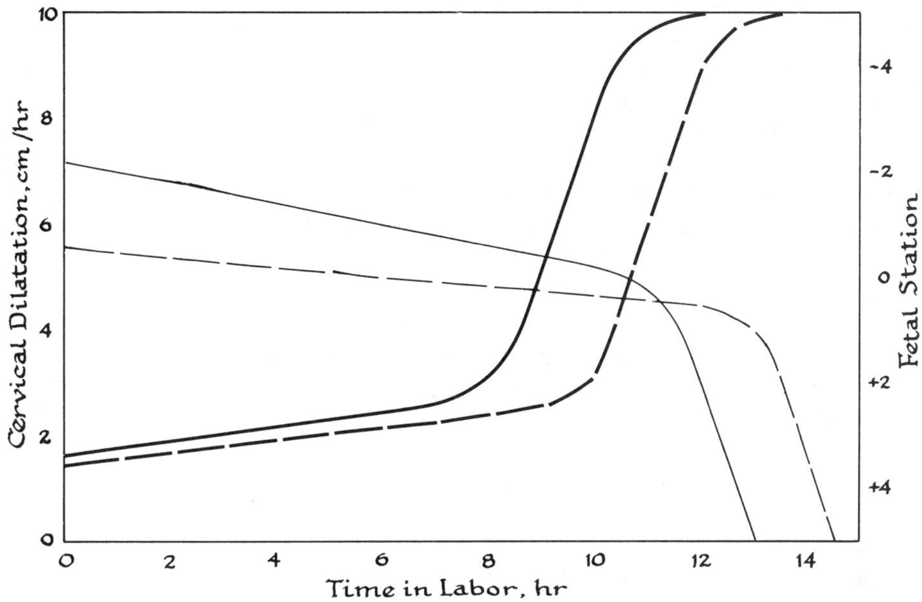


*Fig. 31.* Comparison of labor course in nulliparas with breech presentation (*solid lines*) with that in comparable vertex presentation (*broken lines*), showing their relatively higher station at the onset of labor and subsequent earlier progress in terminating the latent phase and in effecting descent. The same trends are seen in multiparas and may be explained on the basis of preselection of cases with guarded fetopelvic relationships for abdominal delivery.

than in vertex presentation and likely to be less accurate. While this is undoubtedly true to some extent, determination of station in breech presentation is still obviously very important for its usefulness in helping the clinician evaluate and predict the course of labor in these patients.

Progression of fetal descent in breech labors is different from that in vertex labors in several important ways (Fig. 31). Most obvious is the difference in initial station. Breech labors tend to begin with much higher levels of station at their onset. It is generally alleged that the high fetal presenting part in breech labor is a serious problem. It is said to represent a condition in which the prognosis for vaginal delivery is guarded.

Our observations here suggest that this contention is not necessarily correct. Despite the high station commonly seen, there is rapid acceleration of descent, starting with the onset of the active phase in most instances. This correlation of descent with dilatation parallels the findings in vertex labors.

In nulliparas, the average station at the onset of labor is —2.1; comparable vertex labors in nulliparas begin at station —0.5, on the average. In multiparas, the average initial station in breech labor is —2.7; in vertex, —1.3. Similarly, at the onset of the active phase, nulliparous breech labors average —0.7 station (vertex +0.4) and multiparous labors, —1.6 (vertex —0.3).

Still more importantly, at the onset of the second stage, breech labors in nulliparas average +2.8 (comparable vertex +3.5) and in multiparas, +3.7 (vertex +3.4). The differences in station seen early in labor no longer appear to apply by the time the second stage is entered.

Dysfunctional labor patterns as defined by aberrations of the dilatation and descent curves were frequent in breech labors. This was rather unexpected, in view of the essential normality of the mean graphic labor data. Abnormal labors were encountered in significantly excessive numbers in both nulliparas and multiparas with breech presentation. This verified data reported by others (Todd and Steer, 1963). The incidence of labor disorders was 29.7 percent overall; this was significantly greater than the 17.2 percent expected in comparably constituted vertex labors. The most commonly encountered dysfunctions were protraction disorders.

We examined these patients still more critically and contrasted them with their vertex counterparts in order to try to uncover factors that give rise to these disorders. We found that there were excessive numbers of large babies delivered of mothers who developed dysfunctional labors with breech presentation. In all, there were 11.1 percent of infants who weighed more than 4000 g in this group, as contrasted with 3.3 percent in nulliparous breech labors in general. In addition, two-thirds of these gravidas had been excessively sedated in the latent or early active phase. Other factors, including maternal age, fetopelvic disproportion, breech position, or type of presentation, were not unusually distributed here.

However, it is most important to point out that most of the nulliparous breech labors associated with fetopelvic disproportion did develop a major labor aberration. Similarly, all infants weighing 4000 g or more were delivered following a dysfunctional labor. In actuality, no normal nulliparous breech labor produced an infant of this size. Moreover, among labors with infants weighing 3500 g or greater, more than three-quarters of the patients developed labor dysfunction. This correlation, therefore, appears to be undeniable.

Further evidence of the ominous nature of dysfunctional patterns appearing in the presence of breech presentation was available in the delivery results. A total of 41 percent of such patients were delivered by cesarean section. Among normal breech labor, by contrast, the total cesarean section rate was 8.9 percent. This form of trial labor appears to be reasonable and conservative. Support for this contention exists in the absence of perinatal loss among such patients. These data become all the more meaningful when one considers that patients with documented fetopelvic disproportion of even relatively minor degree were not considered here because they were delivered by cesarean section before or soon after the onset of labor.

A more recent and much more extensive analysis of breech labors (Friedman and Kroll, 1972) has verified these findings. By means of a computer program, analysis was carried out in depth, and breech presentations were found to be associated with essentially normal labor progression overall. The only significant deviations from labors in comparable vertex presentations were diminished maximum slopes of dilatation and descent. In addition, there were slight prolongations of the active and deceleration phases, but these were only of borderline statistical significance.

The breech labor data were somewhat paradoxical in that the low maximum slope of dilatation was found to be associated with an essentially normal active-phase duration. This implied that the unmeasured portion of the active phase, namely the acceleration phase, was compensatorily foreshortened. Since the acceleration-phase duration generally reflects latent-phase progression, the relatively short latent-phase durations seen among patients with breech presentation should be expected to be followed by similarly diminished acceleration phases.

The overall effect of these trends is a labor characterized by normal latent phase, short acceleration phase, slowed maximum slopes of dilatation and descent, and minimally prolonged deceleration phase. These add together to produce a first stage of normal duration. When coupled with an average second stage, these events result in a total labor of normal length among gravidas with breech presentation.

Labor in the breech presentation appears to reflect the efficiency of the mechanism just as it does in the vertex presentation. If the fetus is large and the pelvis relatively small, dysfunctional patterns can be expected to develop. Whenever a major labor aberration appears under these circumstances, it should serve to alert the obstetric attendant to the potentially serious nature of the situation. If suitable evaluation is undertaken, previously unrecognized fetopelvic disproportion may be uncovered. The real value of the dilatation and descent patterns in this regard is obvious.

## *FACE PRESENTATION*

Continuing our interest in determining the effects of fetal factors on the course of labor, we next address ourselves to labors associated with face presentation. It is recognized that the widest engaging diameter in face presentation is the trachelobregmatic diameter. When the forward leading edge of the presenting face is at the level of the ischial spines, this diameter is still usually well above the inlet. The face generally engages in the transverse position and then undergoes internal rotation similar to that of the vertex presentation.

There is general agreement that a persistent mentum posterior presentation is best resolved by cesarean section, especially if it occurs in association with cephalopelvic disproportion. Rates of spontaneous deliveries with face presentation have been reported as high as 90 percent. The associated perinatal mortality, however, is about twice that of the vertex presentation, even discounting the influence of prematurity and fetal abnormality.

It becomes imperative, therefore, that we study the course of labor in association with face presentation so as to characterize the type of labor associated with this complication and to recognize problems as they arise. In this way, we may be able to improve the results among those patients who are allowed to experience labor under these circumstances.

A study has been carried out (Dede and Friedman, 1963a) for this purpose. A series of cases was investigated retrospectively in order to evaluate the labor progression. Data on the labor course were determined by means of graphic analytic methods (see Chapter 7). The data obtained in this manner were available for comparison with corresponding data from gravidas with vertex presentation.

## *Group Differences*

Examination of the study population showed an interesting preponderance of older gravidas. It was noteworthy that 8.0 percent were more than 40 years of age. This was more than twice the expected incidence of 3.4 percent. Although this distribution represented an apparent weighting toward the older-age category, statistical significance could not be elicited because of the relatively small numbers of patients involved.

Similarly, there were no real differences between these cases and the general population with vertex presentations as to parity, despite a suggestion of an increased number of multiparas. There were 72.7 percent multiparas among patients with face presentation and 61.0 percent with vertex presentation. On the other hand, the number of grand multiparas with parity of five or more was about the same as expected (4.5 versus 3.0 percent). These findings tended to confirm the contention that maternal age and parity had some relationship to the development of the face presentation.

The distribution of pelvic types showed nearly three times the expected incidence of platypelloid pelves (5.7 versus 2.0 percent). Moreover, significant differences existed with regard to the incidence of relative cephalopelvic disproportion. There were 14.8 percent of gravidas with bony dystocia, as contrasted with an expected incidence of 7.8 percent in nulliparas and 2.7 percent in the overall gravid population. The correlation of face presentation with disproportion has been well documented (Chen and Wei, 1960).

Important disturbances of the normal pelvic anatomy were found in 9.1 percent. These may have predisposed the fetus to malpresentation. They included leiomyomata uteri, bicornuate uterus, oblique axis of the uterus, ovarian mass, precedent uterine suspension, markedly relaxed pelvic supports, and endometriosis. One can only conjecture as to the mechanism by which such anatomic distortions might bring about the face presentation.

There were a considerable number of premature infants. Fully 25.0 percent of neonates weighed less than 2500 g. The expected incidence in comparable vertex presentations was 9.8 percent for the study. The clear-cut relationship between face presentation and prematurity is firmly established.

At the same time, large fetal size was considered to be an etiologic factor in 11.4 percent because the infant weighed more than 4000 g at birth. Fetal anomalies included anencephaly, short umbilical cord, and cervical extensor hypertonus.

*Labor Course*

The labor patterns were studied in those patients with face presentation who were permitted to labor. Needless to say, many had been subjected to cesarean section; these were generally indicated by the face presentation itself —especially if found in the mentum posterior position—or by the associated fetopelvic disproportion. Among those remaining, progressive cervical dilatation and fetal descent in labor provided useful information to characterize the course of labor to be expected here (Table 23).

Face presentation did not appear to affect the course of labor to any significant degree in either nulliparas or multiparas. The findings were essentially the same as those of comparable vertex presentations.

These observations were contrary to the generally held clinical impression, exemplified by the frequent statements in the literature, that face presentations are associated with prolonged labors. Because of this apparent discrepancy, we sought to subject the data to further stratification in order to determine whether or not some concealed factors might be acting to correct or compensate for any inhibitory effects on these labors from the face presentation.

A tangential inquiry was undertaken to determine if inclusion of very small babies in this series might have counteracted the effects of large infants presenting by the face. Accordingly, all infants weighing less than 2500 g were studied separately from those weighing 2500 g or more. The data derived in this way indicated a statistically insignificant, but nonetheless definite, trend toward longer durations of latent, active, and deceleration phases and second-stage durations in both nulliparas and multiparas with larger babies. Indeed, the results were quite similar to those seen with large babies delivered in vertex presentation (see above). The trends were of the same magnitude and in the same direction.

In a similar way, we attempted to demonstrate the suggested influence of cephalopelvic disproportion in this group. Those with disproportion were omitted, and the remaining labors were found to resemble those with vertex presentation much more closely. This reconfirmed the close association between bony dystocia and abnormal labor courses (see Chapter 16).

*Table 23. LABOR DATA IN FACE PRESENTATION*

| *Group* | *Latent Phase (hr)* | *Active Phase (hr)* | *Maximum Dilatation (cm/hr)* | *Deceleration Phase (hr)* | *Maximum Descent (cm/hr)* | *Second Stage (hr)* |
|---|---|---|---|---|---|---|
| Nulliparas | | | | | | |
| Vertex | 8.6±0.27 | 4.9±0.15 | 3.0±0.08 | 0.90±0.05 | 3.2±0.09 | 0.95±0.04 |
| Face | 10.9±2.63 | 4.9±0.89 | 2.6±0.41 | 1.26±0.69 | 3.0±0.38 | 1.30±0.43 |
| Multiparas | | | | | | |
| Vertex | 5.3±0.19 | 2.2±0.07 | 5.7±0.16 | 0.23±0.01 | 6.0±0.20 | 0.29±0.01 |
| Face | 5.4±0.64 | 3.1±0.55 | 4.6±0.51 | 0.33±0.07 | 5.3±0.54 | 0.19±0.03* |

* Statistically significant, $p < 0.01$.

Factors known to affect the course of labor in vertex presentation were found to act in like manner here. Protraction of the course of both the latent and active phases occurred in association with excessive sedation, for example. Stimulation of labor with oxytocin augmented labor, especially in the active phase, and speeded the maximum slopes of dilatation and descent. The frequencies of these factors among labors complicated by face presentation was essentially the same as in vertex presentation. When suitable statistical corrections were made for these factors, the data were not altered to any extent.

Other factors known to influence the course of labor, such as inadequate prelabor cervical preparation or conduction anesthesia, occurred in negligible numbers. The time the membranes were ruptured was also distributed normally. Thus, it would appear that the labor data must be accepted as demonstrating that face presentation per se does not adversely affect labor progression. Nonetheless, factors known to affect the course of labor in vertex presentation will act in essentially the same way in association with face presentation.

It is suggested that progress in labor is not influenced by the face presentation but rather by the clinical milieu in which it occurs. This applies particularly to the fetopelvic relationships. Bony disproportion, as demonstrated objectively by pelvimetric studies and inferentially by the delivery of large infants and the need for operative intervention to effect delivery, seems to be the prime offending factor. Correcting the labor data for associated disproportion permits one to interpret the findings to indicate that face presentation does not contribute to the production of abnormal patterns of labor progress as defined by the course of cervical dilatation and fetal descent.

## *BROW PRESENTATION*

Brow presentation usually occurs as a transitional form that undergoes spontaneous conversion to face or vertex presentation. Only occasionally does it persist as a brow presentation throughout labor. Its impact on labor has not clearly been characterized, but it is generally considered to yield a prolonged, complicated, or abnormal labor progression. Notwithstanding, spontaneous vaginal delivery has been observed as often as 74 percent (Posner et al, 1957). As a consequence, it is generally accepted that the gravida with brow presentation should be permitted a trial of labor (Jacobson and Johnson, 1962). This practice stresses the need for clearer understanding of the labor course to be expected under these conditions.

Therefore, a study was undertaken (Meltzer et al, 1968) for purposes of ascertaining dilatation and descent progression in labors complicated by brow presentation. In addition to our attempts to evaluate each case retrospectively in order to discover any factors that might be etiologic in the development of the brow presentation, we evolved graphic labor data by the methods described earlier (see Chapter 7) for comparison with similar gravid women with vertex presentation.

## *Group Differences*

Maternal age distribution was about as expected, but there was a slight increase in the frequency of nulliparas (41.0 versus 35.0 percent). Although not statistically significant, the increased numbers of nulliparas lend tenuous support to the relationship that has been suggested to exist between brow presentation and parity. Indeed, there were 7.1 percent grand multiparas as compared with 3.0 percent expected in women with vertex presentations.

Cephalopelvic disproportion was detected by clinical and radiographic evaluation in 10.9 percent; this contrasted with 2.7 percent in comparable gravidas with vertex presentation. Among nulliparas, the incidence of disproportion was 20.3 percent, whereas only 7.8 percent was expected. On this basis, there can be little doubt of an association between cephalopelvic disproportion and brow presentation.

The incidence of small infants was unexpectedly high. In all, 14.2 percent of neonates weighed less than 2500 g; the expected incidence was 9.5 percent. Furthermore, among nulliparas, 20.4 percent of infants were premature at birth. At the other extreme, there was no increase in the frequency of infants weighing more than 4000 g. The 3.7 percent incidence was the same as in the vertex population.

## *Labor Course*

The labor patterns of patients delivering with persistent brow presentation (Table 24) differed somewhat from those of gravidas with vertex presentation. Specifically, progression in the pelvic division (see Chapter 7) was adversely affected. There was some negligible slowing of the rate of dilatation in the active phase in nulliparas, but this proved to be not statistically significant. There was significant lengthening of the second-stage duration in both nulliparas and multiparas. In multiparas, the deceleration-phase duration was clearly lengthened as well. The average maximum rate of descent was slowed in association with brow presentation.

These findings are in general agreement with the widely held clinical impressions that labor in association with brow presentation tends to be somewhat slowed, especially in its pelvic division from the beginning of the deceleration phase onward. The findings verify that the generally larger presenting diameters in brow presentation, although not necessarily interfering with the dilatation function, may deleteriously affect descent and second-stage progress.

Because fetal size and disproportion were not homogeneously distributed between the brow and vertex groups, these populations of patients were not truly comparable. The data derived from them, therefore, could not be relied

*Table 24.* *LABOR DATA IN BROW PRESENTATION*

| Group | Latent Phase (hr) | Active Phase (hr) | Maximum Dilatation (cm/hr) | Deceleration Phase (hr) | Maximum Descent (cm/hr) | Second Stage (hr) |
|---|---|---|---|---|---|---|
| Nulliparas | | | | | | |
| Vertex | 8.6±0.27 | 4.9±0.15 | 3.0±0.08 | 0.90±0.05 | 3.2±0.09 | 0.95±0.04 |
| Brow | 7.5±0.74 | 4.8±0.50 | 2.6±0.19 | 0.73±0.11 | 2.5±0.22* | 1.35±0.17† |
| Multiparas | | | | | | |
| Vertex | 5.3±0.19 | 2.2±0.07 | 5.7±0.16 | 0.23±0.01 | 6.0±0.20 | 0.24±0.01 |
| Brow | 5.4±0.46 | 2.6±0.28 | 5.6±0.44 | 0.36±0.04* | 5.1±0.36† | 0.43±0.06* |
| Matched Nulliparas | | | | | | |
| Vertex | 7.9±0.79 | 4.5±0.56 | 2.9±0.36 | 0.62±0.12 | 3.0±0.32 | 0.64±0.10 |
| Brow | 8.1±1.13 | 4.7±0.76 | 2.8±0.26 | 0.76±0.18 | 2.1±0.30† | 1.46±0.25* |
| Matched Multiparas | | | | | | |
| Vertex | 5.3±0.60 | 2.4±0.31 | 5.4±0.45 | 0.25±0.06 | 5.8±0.40 | 0.22±0.03 |
| Brow | 5.0±0.51 | 3.0±0.47 | 5.4±0.66 | 0.42±0.08 | 4.6±0.48† | 0.49±0.07* |

* Statistically significant, $p < 0.01$.
† Borderline significance, $0.01 < p < 0.05$.

upon for purposes of statistical comparison. When we omitted those infants weighing less than 2500 g we felt we had for examination a more realistic series of labors with brow presentation. By so doing, we obtained a series of labors characterized by greater flattening of the maximum slopes of both dilatation and descent.

Moreover, patients with documented cephalopelvic disproportion showed these changes to an even greater extent. The findings expected to occur in association with excessive sedation, namely, still slower dilatation and descent as well as further prolongation of the second stage, were encountered. Conduction anesthesia, when administered, was associated with persistent slowing in active-phase dilatation and further retarded descent.

These data, therefore, confirm that factors known to affect the course of labor in vertex presentation will behave in much the same manner with brow presentation, but perhaps exert their influence to a greater degree. We might infer on this basis that the course of labor has been influenced not so much by the brow presentation itself, but more likely, by related conditions giving rise to relative fetopelvic disproportion. These in turn yield the brow presentation. In addition to obvious factors of intrinsically constricted pelvic diameters and enlarged fetal diameters, we may cite combinations of positional variations (such as deflexion), inherently poor uterine powers (dysfunctional labor), and exogenously depressed motive forces (excessive sedation and conduction anesthesia).

Unlike the face presentation data, however, corrections for associated disproportion and other inhibitory factors do not provide the entire answer in that there remains a residual change in dilatation and descent data. This is seen (Table 24) when pairs of cases are matched and studied for labor progression. Matching is accomplished by ensuring comparability of maternal and gestational age, gravidity, parity, fetal weight, analgesia, anesthesia, uterotonic stimulation, prelabor cervical dilatation and fetal station, status of the membranes, and cephalopelvic relationships. These matched cases showed significant prolongation of the second stage as well as moderate delays in deceleration-phase duration in both nulliparas and multiparas with brow presentation. The diminution in maximum slope of descent was impressive in these labors.

Dysfunctional labor patterns as previously defined (see Chapter 8) were encountered in 30.5 percent of gravidas with brow presentation. This is an excessively high frequency. Among nulliparas, the incidence was 42.0 percent and in multiparas, 22.1 percent.

The most common aberrations encountered were the arrest disorders. They occurred in decreasing frequency in the following order: most often, arrest of descent, then secondary arrest of dilatation, and least frequently, prolonged deceleration phase. They accounted for more than three-quarters of the dysfunctional labor patterns among these patients.

These patterns are recognized to occur in association with cephalopelvic disproportion. The high incidence of disproportionate cases with brow presentation clearly accounts for the common occurrence of arrest patterns in these labors.

Brow presentation thus appears to prolong the deceleration phase and second-stage progression somewhat. The effects of other labor-inhibiting factors appear to be exaggerated in the presence of brow presentation. Cephalopelvic disproportion is commonly associated with brow presentation and will frequently result in a dysfunctional labor pattern, particularly one of the arrest disorders.

It is important to reemphasize that arrest in the active phase or in the second stage connotes disproportion. Whenever these patterns are encountered in association with brow presentation (exactly analogous to vertex presentation), disproportion must be suspected to exist and should be documented or ruled out by objective means. Further trial of labor under these circumstances should not be permitted to occur unless one is reasonably certain that disproportion is not present to impede further progress.

# Pelvic Factors

## CHAPTER 16

The degree of soft-tissue preparation achieved prior to the onset of labor significantly alters the course of labor. The greater the prelabor cervical dilatation, for example, the shorter the latent and acceleration phases. Fetal station at the onset of labor is likewise related to the subsequent course of labor. Lower stations are generally associated with shorter latent and acceleration phases. Station achieved by the beginning of the active phase influences the rest of the labor course. Fetal station may be a useful indicator of disproportion or disordered labor patterns; the higher the station, the greater the probability of these problems. Prelabor cervical dilatation is correlated with prelabor fetal station, but their effects on labor are both independent and augmentative (or compensatory). The labor course also reflects the present or absence of cephalopelvic disproportion; extrapolation of the expected graphic course in the active phase can be used for purposes of defining a trial of labor under these circumstances. The course of labor serves as a valuable prognostic index.

Conditions prevailing in the pelvis before labor begins play a large role in the labor that follows. There is little doubt that the greater the degree of prelabor soft-tissue preparation, for example, the more expeditiously will the labor evolve. We have already seen (Chapter 9) how clearly the latent-phase duration reflects this principle. In this chapter, we will try to quantitate the effect on labor of prelabor status as related to the cervical dilatation and the fetal station that have been achieved up to the onset of labor. We will also examine the influence exerted on the course of labor by the fetopelvic relationship.

## *PRELABOR CERVICAL DILATATION*

Prelabor preparation of the cervix by softening, effacement, and dilatation is recognized to be a pertinent factor influencing the course of labor. Calkins (1934, 1941, 1944, 1955a) used clinical evaluations of the cervical consistency, effacement, and dilatation at the beginning of labor to predict the duration of labor. By allowing additional time in labor according to the existence of unfavorable characteristics, he derived a rough index (see Chapter 2) for use as a guide in detecting and assessing labors of unusual total length. However, his approach was unable to characterize the specific effects on the progress in labor brought about by the condition of the cervix.

In Chapter 9, we alluded to the apparent cause–effect relationship found to exist between the unripe cervix—characterized by excessive firmness and lack of effacement and dilatation—and prolongation of the predilatational latent phase of the first stage of labor. We were able to implicate the unprepared cervix as a potential etiologic factor in the development of abnormal prolongation of the latent phase in about 7 percent of the gravid population. In a more extensive series of nulliparas who developed pathologic prolongation of the latent phase (Friedman and Sachtleben, 1961a), poor prelabor cervical preparation was found to exist in 18 percent overall.

Qualitative correlations of the association between prolonged latent-phase disorders and an unfavorable state of cervical preparedness were well documented. They clearly verified the earlier findings of Calkins. Nonetheless, this issue deserved clarification, particularly with regard to the degree of quantitative variation that could be anticipated with progressively greater prelabor preparation.

In order to achieve this objective, a prospective study was carried out on two simultaneously consecutive series of nulliparas and multiparas at term (Friedman and Sachtleben, 1962b). Each patient was followed in labor with frequent, careful evaluations of cervical dilatation and fetal station, as previously detailed (see Chapter 7). Data collections were continued until adequate dilatation and descent curves were obtained in 500 nulliparas and 500 multiparas. Curves were considered to be adequate if evaluations of dilatation and descent were available from the beginning of labor and were done in sufficient numbers to permit us to trace both dilatation and descent adequately.

Cases were stratified according to initial cervical dilatation into those with prelabor dilatation of less than 1 cm and with features suggesting unpreparedness, those with dilatation of more than 1 cm but less than 2 cm, and those with 2 cm of cervical dilatation or greater. A majority of both series (62.0 percent nulliparas and 59.4 percent multiparas) fell into the middle group, with dilatation between 1 and 2 cm at the onset of labor.

## *Group Differences*

The several subgroups were reasonably comparable with reference to age, gravidity, parity, fetal position, and infant weight. Delivery frequencies were normally distributed, with the possible exceptions of excessive numbers of cesarean sections in nulliparas who began labor with unripe cervix (5.0 percent versus 1.3 percent in the average prelabor dilatation group) and of midforceps procedures in the corresponding multiparas (5.4 versus 1.8 percent). The unusual frequency of abdominal deliveries in those nulliparas with negligible prelabor cervical preparation was statistically significant. The excess of multiparous midforceps operations, on the other hand, could not be verified statistically.

Factors known to influence the course of labor were also investigated. Fetopelvic disproportion, for example, was encountered in 8.0 percent of nulliparas with unripe cervix and in 9.7 percent of those with dilatation between 1 and 2 cm, but in only 1.1 percent of the remaining nulliparas. Comparable findings were not encountered in the multiparas. Early excessive sedative-analgesic medication was encountered in larger numbers than expected among nulliparas with unripe cervix (18.0 percent versus 8.0 percent in the median dilatation group); the same trend, but to a lesser extent, was seen in multiparas.

Oxytocin infusions were administered in about equal numbers in essentially all groups, with only one exception. This exception appeared in multiparas beginning labor with 2 cm of dilatation or greater; among them, 18.7 percent had been stimulated with uterotonic agents. This large number reflected the elective inductions that were done in multiparas with particularly favorable cervix. Conduction peridural anesthesias were distributed in equivalent numbers throughout.

## *Labor Course*

Labor data were derived by analysis of the component phases of the dilatation and descent curves obtained in these several groups of patients (Table 25). The degree of initial dilatation of the cervix was significantly associated with latent-phase duration. This was not unexpected in view of the previously cited evidence (see Chapter 9). A possible influence of the cervix on the duration of the active phase was also encountered in both nulliparas and multiparas (statistically significant in the former only). This effect persisted into the deceleration phase as well, but could not be verified statistically. It was also reflected in the maximum slope of dilatation, but not in the slope of descent.

A more extensive stratification of the data (Table 26) according to finer subdivisions of initial cervical dilatation was accomplished. The data derived from this operation illustrated these relationships even more cogently. Clear-cut progressive diminution in the durations of latent and active phases was seen with increasing prelabor dilatation. Neither the maximum slopes

*Table 25.* LABOR DATA BY PRELABOR CERVICAL DILATATION

| Group | Latent Phase (hr) | Active Phase (hr) | Maximum Dilatation (cm/hr) | Deceleration Phase (hr) | Maximum Descent (cm/hr) | Second Stage (hr) |
|---|---|---|---|---|---|---|
| Nulliparas | | | | | | |
| 0.0–0.9 | 11.1±0.65* | 6.2±0.43* | 2.6±0.16 | 1.16±0.19 | 3.0±0.14 | 0.91±0.07 |
| 1.0–1.9 | 8.6±0.29* | 4.9±0.18* | 3.0±0.10 | 0.90±0.06 | 3.2±0.11 | 0.95±0.05 |
| 2.0 or greater | 5.9±0.44* | 3.8±0.19* | 3.2±0.20 | 0.75±0.07 | 3.1±0.16 | 1.07±0.10 |
| Multiparas | | | | | | |
| 0.0–0.9 | 7.7±0.94* | 2.3±0.30 | 6.7±0.73 | 0.18±0.03 | 5.8±0.34 | 0.21±0.02 |
| 1.0–1.9 | 5.3±0.20* | 2.2±0.07 | 5.7±0.17 | 0.23±0.01 | 6.0±0.22 | 0.29±0.01 |
| 2.0 or greater | 4.0±0.21* | 1.9±0.08 | 5.8±0.27 | 0.21±0.02 | 6.0±0.40 | 0.22±0.01 |

* Statistically significant trend, $p < 0.01$.

*Table 26.* LATENT AND ACTIVE PHASE TRENDS BY DILATATION AT ONSET OF LABOR*

| Prelabor Cervical Dilatation (cm) | Nulliparas | | Multiparas | |
|---|---|---|---|---|
| | LATENT PHASE (HR) | ACTIVE PHASE (HR) | LATENT PHASE (HR) | ACTIVE PHASE (HR) |
| 0.0–0.5 | 11.6±0.83 | 6.4±0.52 | 8.7±1.30 | 2.4±0.43 |
| 0.6–0.9 | 9.9±0.91 | 6.0±0.77 | 5.5±0.90 | 2.3±0.30 |
| 1.0–1.9 | 8.6±0.29 | 4.9±0.18 | 5.3±0.20 | 2.2±0.07 |
| 2.0–2.9 | 6.6±0.64 | 4.1±0.27 | 4.0±0.42 | 1.9±0.20 |
| 3.0–3.9 | 4.9±0.60 | 3.6±0.33 | 4.2±0.28 | 1.9±0.11 |
| 4.0 or greater | 4.5±0.91 | 3.1±0.37 | 3.4±0.39 | 1.5±0.14 |

* All trends statistically significant, $p < 0.01$.

of dilatation and descent nor the durations of deceleration phase and second stage varied with the status of the cervix at the beginning of labor.

It was reasonable to assume, therefore, that the acceleration portion of the active phase was primarily involved here. This assumption is based on the apparently paradoxical fact that the active-phase duration is related to cervical preparedness, but the maximum slope of dilatation and duration of deceleration phase do not change with increasing prelabor cervical dilatation. Thus, the acceleration phase is functionally related to the latent phase as far as its response to the influence of prelabor preparation is concerned.

These data are shown graphically in Figure 32. Several composite cervical dilatation patterns are shown, representing the average of homogeneous groups of nulliparous labors according to the degree of cervical dilatation achieved before labor began. We see the obvious correlations of the latent- and active-phase durations with the status of the cervix. In addition, we can recognize the progressive foreshortening of the acceleration phase with increasing initial cervical dilatation.

We have clearly demonstrated that the duration of the latent phase is

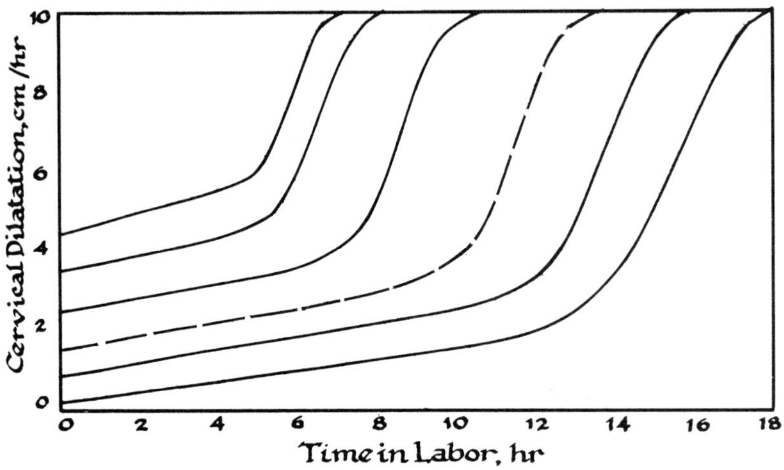


*Fig. 32.* Effect of prelabor preparation of the cervix in nulliparas on the subsequent course of dilatation in labor, showing the composite dilatation patterns according to the degree of initial cervical dilatation. Patients with the most frequently occurring condition (beginning labor with 1 to 2 cm of dilatation) followed the curve previously shown for nulliparas in general (*broken line*). The more favorable the cervix at the onset of labor, the shorter the latent and acceleration phases. The unprepared cervix yields prolonged latent and acceleration phases. The descent curve and the remainder of the dilatation pattern reflects no comparable effect.
(From Friedman EA, Sachtleben MR: Am J Obstet Gynecol 84:933, 1962)

inversely related to the dilatation of the cervix at the onset of labor. This relationship in nulliparas can be quantified by the parabolic expression*

$$y = 11.7 - 2.79x + 0.23x^2$$

in which $x$ represents initial dilatation in centimeters and $y$, the duration of the latent phase in hours. This relationship is expressed graphically in Figure 33. The regression curve for active-phase duration as related to prelabor cervical preparation is essentially linear and can be expressed by the equation

$$y = 6.5 - 0.81x$$

* Parabolic regression curves were derived by the method of least squares, in which the constants of the curve

$$y = a + bx + cx^2$$

are defined by solution of the simultaneous equations

$$\Sigma y = na + b\Sigma x + c\Sigma x^2$$
$$\Sigma xy = a\Sigma x + b\Sigma x^2 + c\Sigma x^3$$
$$\Sigma x^2 y = a\Sigma x^2 + b\Sigma x^3 + c\Sigma x^4$$

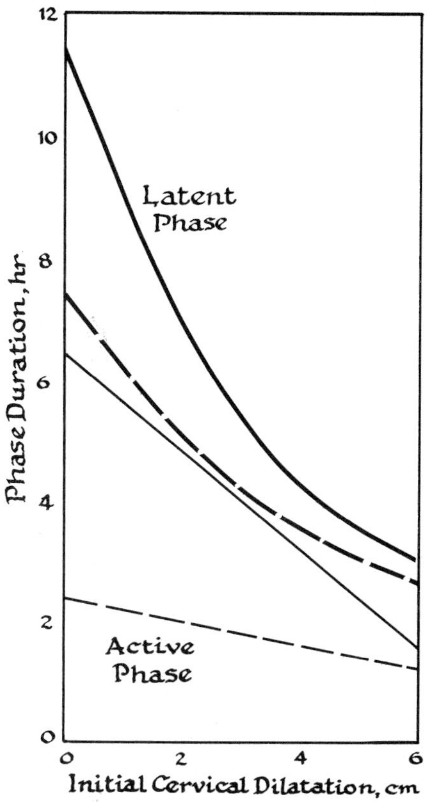


*Fig. 33.* Effect of initial cervical dilatation on duration of latent and active phases in nulliparas (*solid lines*) and multiparas (*broken lines*). There are very clear trends, expressed by regression equations in the text, for these measurable intervals to be shorter in association with greater prelabor dilatation. The relationships do not hold for the later phases of the dilatation curve or for descent.

Corresponding curvilinear equations for multiparous data giving latent- and active-phase variations, respectively, according to initial dilatation are

$$y = 7.5 - 1.39x + 0.10x^2$$
$$y = 2.5 - 0.23x$$

These expressions may be combined to given an accurate representation of the expected total duration of the first stage of labor by summating latent-phase and active-phase equivalents, as follows:

$$\text{For nulliparas, } y = 18.2 - 3.60x + 0.23x^2$$
$$\text{For multiparas, } y = 10.0 - 1.62x + 0.10x^2$$

For an estimate of the anticipated total duration of the entire labor as it refers back to initial dilatation, one need merely add to the derived solution a quantity equivalent to the average length of the second stage.

When using these equations, one should keep in mind that they are based on the best mathematical mean of the data and therefore represent only

*Table 27. LIMITS OF NORMAL BY PRELABOR DILATATION**

| *Prelabor Cervical Dilatation (cm)* | *Nulliparas* | | *Multiparas* | |
|---|---|---|---|---|
| | LATENT PHASE (HR) | ACTIVE PHASE (HR) | LATENT PHASE (HR) | ACTIVE PHASE (HR) |
| 0.0–0.5 | 19.2 | 11.4 | 16.1 | 5.0 |
| 0.6–0.9 | 14.8 | 10.7 | 10.1 | 3.9 |
| 1.0–1.9 | 15.4 | 8.8 | 8.8 | 3.3 |
| 2.0–2.9 | 12.0 | 6.0 | 7.6 | 3.5 |
| 3.0–3.9 | 8.2 | 5.2 | 7.1 | 2.9 |
| 4.0 or greater | 7.9 | 4.1 | 5.7 | 2.3 |

* Based on 95th percentile values of distribution curve.

coarse averages. The solution of any particular point on the curve gives a value for rough comparison only and should not be interpreted as a fixed requirement. By calculating the relative error* of each subgroup, it has been determined that any single observation may be incorrect by an average factor of as much as 34 percent in either direction.

These data have additional usefulness in permitting us to derive statistical maxima for the latent- and active-phase durations (as well as total first-stage duration) based on the 95th percentile distribution. This is analogous to the method used for deriving statistical maxima for the several components of the dilatation and descent curves for use in defining abnormal labor (see Chapter 8). Here we can focus our attention more critically on expected phase durations according to the factor of prelabor dilatation of the cervix.

The data derived for this purpose are shown in Table 27. They may prove useful in assessing abnormal states in a manner that is more sophisticated than the simplistic approach detailed in Chapter 8. We can recognize, for example, that the range of normality for first-stage duration in nulliparas extends from 30 hours in conjunction with an unprepared cervix (less than 0.6 cm of dilatation at the onset of labor) to 12 hours with initial dilatation of 4 cm or greater. The comparable range in multiparas is from 21 to 8 hours.

We have thus derived definitive quantitations of the influence of initial cervical dilatation on the course of labor. This material is based on the assumption that the several subgroups are comparable in all respects except, of course, the initial dilatation of the cervix. The inference is that no other pertinent factor is playing a role in producing the effects that are encountered. Earlier, we saw that the groups were not entirely homogeneous in composition, however. Nulliparas with more favorable cervix had relatively

* The mean square error is the error whose square is the mean of the squares of all the errors:

$$m = \pm\sqrt{\frac{\Sigma d^2}{n-1}}$$

The relative error is this mean error divided by the mean.

fewer problem pelves. Those with unprepared cervix tended to be more heavily sedated. Multiparas with advanced cervical dilatation at onset of labor were more often stimulated with oxytocin infusion than those in corresponding subgroups with less initial cervical dilatation.

In order to verify or refute those relationships we had previously uncovered, therefore, it was necessary to make suitable corrections. This was done by means of stratifications of the subpopulations. No noteworthy changes occurred as a consequence of such statistical manipulations. For example, only a negligible foreshortening of latent- and active-phase durations was brought about by entirely omitting patients with bony dystocia and those who were heavily sedated from the group of nulliparas with favorable cervix. Similar deletions in other corresponding groups of nulliparas produced changes of almost the same magnitude and in the same direction.

Corrections for the excessive numbers of oxytocin administrations in multiparas with favorable prelabor cervix lengthened the latent-phase duration and decreased the maximum slope of dilatation, but again these changes were insignificant. The active-phase duration did not change at all. Equivalent variations occurred when the other multiparous groups were subjected to the same procedure.

These data are presented to quantitate the influence of cervical dilatation at the onset of labor on the subsequent course of labor. They serve to provide a measure of the effect of the state of prelabor preparedness of the cervix. We have clearly demonstrated that shorter labors result in those gravidas who begin labor with more favorable cervical dilatation. The specific effect appears to be in the foreshortening of the latent and the acceleration phases of the first stage of labor. Mathematical expressions are set forth along with statistical maxima to aid in the application of these data to both the management of the individual parturient and the investigation of other factors that may potentially affect the labor process.

## *FETAL STATION*

Continuing our efforts to determine how labor is affected by prelabor soft-tissue preparation, we endeavored to determine the influence of fetal station (Friedman and Sachtleben, 1965d) . The apparent relationship between cervical dilatation and station has previously been discussed (Chapters 6 and 7) , together with a general description of the expected pattern of descent in normal labor. Our prime interest here was to ascertain whether the course of labor was somehow influenced by the degree of engagement that the fetus had reached by the time labor began.

The importance of this pursuit lies in the acknowledged likelihood that the unengaged fetal head at the onset of labor, especially in the nullipara, is commonly associated with cephalopelvic disproportion (Auer and Simmons, 1949; Burke et al, 1958; Friedman and Sachtleben, 1965d) . Contrary opinions (Stipp, 1969; Weekes and Flynn, 1975) have stirred a controversy worthy of resolution. Indeed, Weekes and Flynn even assert that the fetal head in most nulliparas may not engage between 36 and 38 weeks of gestation, contrary to common belief.

Our extensive analysis of station data tends to confirm that engagement is not a universal phenomenon in nulliparas (Table 28). On the average, the fetal head in nulliparas has descended to 0.5 cm cephalad to the plane of the ischial spines (station −0.5). Whereas the modal (most frequently occurring or peak value of the distribution curve) is zero station, the majority of nulliparas begin labor with stations above zero, although relatively few are actually out of the pelvis. The cephalad limit is −2.8, based on the 95th percentile of the distribution curve of station values. This signifies that it is exceedingly unusual for the nullipara to begin labor with a fetal station higher than −3, but deep engagement is the exception, not the rule.

*Table 28. PROGRESSION OF FETAL STATION IN LABOR*

| | *Mean* | $SE_m$* | *Limit*† |
|---|---|---|---|
| Nulliparas | | | |
| Onset of latent phase | −0.5 | 0.06 | −2.8 |
| Onset of active phase | +0.4 | 0.06 | −1.7 |
| Midmaximum slope | +1.1 | 0.07 | −1.0 |
| Onset of deceleration phase | +2.0 | 0.09 | −0.1 |
| Onset of second stage | +3.4 | 0.10 | +0.8 |
| Multiparas | | | |
| Onset of latent phase | −1.3 | 0.11 | −4.0 |
| Onset of active phase | −0.3 | 0.09 | −3.1 |
| Midmaximum slope | +0.6 | 0.10 | −2.1 |
| Onset of deceleration phase | +1.8 | 0.14 | −0.6 |
| Onset of second stage | +3.4 | 0.16 | +0.3 |

* Standard error of mean.
† Cephalad value equal to twice the standard deviation greater than the mean, $p = 0.05$.

By contrast, the majority of nulliparas have a well-engaged fetal presenting part by the time the active phase of labor has begun. The mean station at the onset of the acceleration phase is +0.4 and the 95th percentile cephalad limit is −1.7. By the time the deceleration phase of dilatation has been reached, essentially all normal nulliparas have deeply engaged fetuses: mean station +2.0, cephalad limit, station zero. These data are accentuated when second stage begins: mean station +3.4, limit +0.8.

It is generally accepted that multiparas rarely present with an engaged fetal presenting part at the onset of labor. This is clearly verified in our series (Table 28). Again, however, most have engaged by the beginning of the active phase and very few remain unengaged when the deceleration phase starts. We have already seen that the failure of descent to begin and continue uninterruptedly from the beginning of the deceleration phase onward is a serious abnormality of labor progression (Chapter 11). At the same time, we recognize now that, contrary to accepted obstetric concepts, the lack of engagement in nulliparas until well into the active phase of dilatation is not as unusual as might be expected. It is, therefore, not necessarily the ominous sign we once thought it was. Nevertheless, it is still worthy of our critical attention.

## *Index of Disproportion*

Just as the cervical dilatation at the onset of labor is reflected in the course of the labor that follows (see above), the prelabor station also appears to influence subsequent labor events. We examined a large group of gravidas who presented with sufficient data on both station and cervical dilatation from the onset of labor, for purposes of critical analysis (Friedman and Sachtleben, 1965d). Patients were grouped according to the station of the presenting part at the onset of labor, at the onset of the active phase (the beginning of the acceleration phase), and at the onset of the deceleration phase. Composite data on cervical dilatation patterns were collected from these subgroups to yield information on the course of labor as it relates to fetal station.

Examining the several subgroups for make-up, we verified their relative uniformity with regard to such factors as maternal age, previous obstetric experience, gestational duration, fetal size, presentation, and position. The incidence of fetopelvic disproportion in nulliparas, however, was unevenly distributed. Whereas the overall incidence was 7.5 percent, lack of engagement at the onset of labor was associated with disproportion in 10.7 percent; this contrasted with an incidence of 4.4 percent when the fetal presenting part was engaged.

The clear-cut correlation between cephalopelvic disproportion and high

*Table 29. FETOPELVIC DISPROPORTION AS RELATED TO FETAL STATION*

| | *Frequency of Disproportion (%)* | | |
|---|---|---|---|
| *Fetal Station* | At Onset of Labor | At Onset of Active Phase | At Onset of Deceleration Phase |
| −3 | 38.5 | * | * |
| −2 | 12.5 | 28.9 | * |
| −1 | 6.1 | 10.0 | * |
| 0 | 6.4 | 10.8 | 18.2 |
| +1 | 0.0 | 2.5 | 9.1 |
| +2 | 0.0 | 0.0 | 5.9 |
| +3 | * | * | 4.8 |
| All unengaged | 10.7 | 12.8 | 15.4 |
| All engaged | 4.4 | 6.2 | 6.0 |
| All +1 or lower | 0.0 | 1.8 | 5.4 |

* Numbers insufficient for frequencies to be meaningful.

station was corroborated (Table 29). Verification was encountered even though many gravidas with high degrees of disproportion were undoubtedly eliminated from consideration because they had been delivered by cesarean section at or before the onset of labor (that is, they were not considered for evaluation because their dilatation and descent curves never evolved fully). The frequency of disproportion falls rapidly with descending initial fetal station. The lower the station at the onset of labor, the less likely will be the need for cesarean section.

Essentially the same relationship was found for fetal station at the onset of the active phase. Here disproportion occurred at a rate of 11.8 percent for cases with initial stations of zero and above, as contrasted with 1.8 percent for those below this level. At the onset of the deceleration phase, the distribution of disproportion was also similar.

It is of interest to note that there were documented instances of significant disproportion in which the forward leading edge of the presenting part had progressed to very low levels in the pelvis. In general, these fell into the category of protracted descent (Chapter 10) or arrest of descent (Chapter 11). In some of these, the descent may have been more apparent than real, consisting of progressive molding and impacting of the fetal head deeper and deeper into the pelvis. The obvious relevance of this phenomenon to clinical practice will be discussed further in Chapter 21. A similar association of cephalopelvic disproportion with very high initial stations (—2 or above) was encountered among multiparas, although the numbers of such cases were small. Whereas the overall incidence of disproportion among multiparas was 1.2 percent, it occurred in 3.5 percent of those presenting with high stations at the onset of labor. High fetal station at the onset of the active phase was even more critical, but disproportion occurred only in those patients with fetal presenting parts at station —3 or higher.

The relationship of prelabor fetal station to cervical dilatation was also of special interest. We found that patients who begin labor with fetal heads at high station generally have lesser degrees of initial cervical dilatation as well. This was particularly marked in multiparas. Thus, it is possible that the trends we saw in the labor course with advancing station (see below) may be referable in part at least to the condition of the cervix in these cases. By the same token, the delivery outcome that is clearly affected by the course of labor—as described by the dilatation pattern—may also be influenced to a significant degree by the descent pattern. This has been cogently illustrated in our discussions dealing with abnormal descent patterns (see Chapters 10 and 11).

### *Labor Course*

The influence of the initial fetal station on the course of labor has been studied in depth (Table 30). Rather interesting trends were demonstrated. The latent-phase duration is clearly shorter in both nulliparas and multiparas if labor begins with low-level fetal stations. When statistical corrections are

*Table 30. LABOR DATA BY STATION AT ONSET OF LABOR*

| *Station* | *Latent Phase* (hr)* | *Active Phase* (hr)* | *Maximum Dilatation (cm/hr)* | *Deceleration Phase (hr)* | *Maximum Descent (cm/hr)* | *Second Stage (hr)* |
|---|---|---|---|---|---|---|
| Nulliparas | | | | | | |
| −3 | 14.0±2.43 | 5.7±1.34 | 2.9±0.45 | 0.68±0.17 | 3.1±0.50 | 0.71±0.11 |
| −2 | 11.6±1.04 | 6.0±0.60 | 2.6±0.27 | 0.79±0.08 | 2.8±0.32 | 0.98±0.13 |
| −1 | 9.7±0.66 | 4.8±0.27 | 2.7±0.19 | 0.83±0.08 | 2.8±0.28 | 0.92±0.08 |
| 0 | 8.4±0.61 | 4.5±0.39 | 3.1±0.20 | 0.71±0.06 | 3.0±0.24 | 0.96±0.08 |
| +1 | 8.4±0.87 | 4.2±0.50 | 3.0±0.27 | 0.89±0.16 | 3.2±0.30 | 0.96±0.14 |
| +2 and +3 | 7.8±1.74 | 4.8±1.14 | 2.9±0.40 | 0.87±0.14 | 3.0±0.44 | 0.94±0.20 |
| Multiparas | | | | | | |
| −4 and −5 | 10.0±3.76 | 2.9±0.59 | 5.2±0.93 | 0.33±0.11 | 5.0±0.84 | 0.29±0.07 |
| −3 | 5.7±0.78 | 3.4±0.84 | 5.9±1.07 | 0.19±0.04 | 5.6±0.92 | 0.22±0.05 |
| −2 | 5.4±0.59 | 2.7±0.32 | 5.1±0.81 | 0.32±0.12 | 5.4±0.90 | 0.19±0.02 |
| −1 | 5.8±0.75 | 1.8±0.13 | 6.2±0.41 | 0.13±0.02 | 5.8±0.52 | 0.19±0.02 |
| 0 | 4.6±0.56 | 1.7±0.12 | 6.1±0.50 | 0.17±0.02 | 6.0±0.55 | 0.21±0.02 |
| +1 and +2 | 2.9±0.46 | 1.6±0.31 | 6.7±1.89 | 0.15±0.04 | 6.2±0.99 | 0.16±0.05 |

* Statistically significant data by analysis of trends, $p < 0.01$.

made for the aforementioned differences in initial cervical dilatation among these groups, the trends are not altered to any significant degree. Thus, we cannot explain these findings away on the basis of differences in prelabor cervical dilatation. These clear-cut trends between initial fetal station and subsequent latent-phase duration are illustrated graphically in Figure 34.

A similar trend holds for the duration of the active phase as it relates to station at the onset of labor, although the relationship is not nearly so strong as with latent-phase durations. The active phase diminishes in length as station progresses caudally with a fair degree of consistency. The inconsistencies at both extremes (that is, at high and at low stations) seem to be due to the instability brought about by the relatively small numbers of cases involved. The maximum slopes of dilatation and descent as well as the durations of the deceleration phase and second stage all remain essentially constant regardless of the preceding fetal station at labor onset. In view of these latter findings, one may plausibly conclude that the active-phase trend reflects changes in the acceleration phase duration only. We have previously seen that the latent and acceleration phases respond to various influences in much the same way (Friedman and Sachtleben, 1962b); this is verified here once again.

Since advancing station at the onset of labor does not seem to affect any of the later parts of labor (after the latent and acceleration phases), we may assume that its effect on the course of labor is transitory at best. Approaching this concept from a dynamic point of view, we must take into account that station is not static during the course of labor. Indeed, progressive change must necessarily occur as labor advances (see above and Chapter 6). Theoretically, the expected changes in station may themselves affect subsequent labor patterns. If high station, for example, results in slow labor, correcting

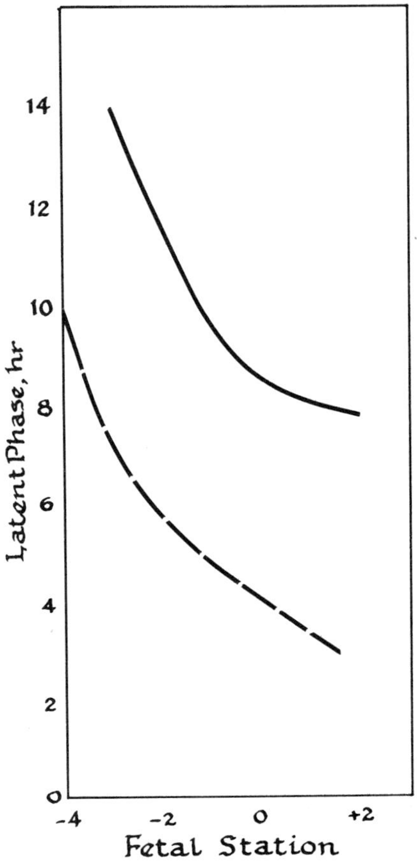


*Fig. 34.* Effect of fetal station at the onset of labor on latent-phase duration in nulliparas (*solid line*) and multiparas (*broken line*), showing obvious trends toward progressive lengthening at higher initial stations.

(From Friedman EA, Sachtleben MR: Am J Obstet Gynecol 93:532, 1965)

the station should be expected to enhance progress. Therefore, it becomes important to study the course of labor as it bears on the fetal station at various specified intervals after the onset of labor. One such given point is that which marks the end of the latent phase and the beginning of the active phase of cervical dilatation. Data are available on fetal station observations to help us determine whether or not labor reflects this factor (Table 31).

Fetal station in the active phase fails to show any specific tendency to influence latent-phase durations. This probably reflects the dynamic phenomenon to which we have just alluded. Patients grouped by fetal station at the onset of the active phase are likely to be heterogeneous in regard to foregoing fetal station at the onset of labor. On the other hand, their homogeneity is demonstrated by the rather clear-cut trend for the active-phase duration to diminish progressively with lower stations. This is shown by the regression curves in Figure 35. At the same time, the maximum slope of dilatation increases progressively, although this trend is inconsistent in multiparas. Similarly, the deceleration phase and second stage shorten. These

*Table 31. LABOR DATA BY STATION AT ONSET OF ACTIVE PHASE*

| *Station* | *Latent Phase (hr)* | *Active Phase* (hr)* | *Maximum Dilatation* (cm/hr)* | *Deceleration Phase* (hr)* | *Maximum Descent* (cm/hr)* | *Second Stage (hr)* |
|---|---|---|---|---|---|---|
| Nulliparas | | | | | | |
| −2 and −3 | 8.4±1.02 | 7.7±0.62 | 1.8±0.40 | 1.30±0.26 | 2.1±0.44 | 2.00±0.22 |
| −1 | 8.5±0.82 | 5.1±0.47 | 2.7±0.22 | 0.96±0.19 | 2.5±0.36 | 0.95±0.13 |
| 0 | 9.2±0.69 | 5.0±0.34 | 2.9±0.17 | 0.77±0.06 | 2.9±0.22 | 1.03±0.09 |
| +1 | 8.9±0.73 | 3.7±0.27 | 3.4±0.26 | 0.66±0.07 | 3.3±0.30 | 0.86±0.07 |
| +2 | 7.8±0.99 | 3.6±0.33 | 3.4±0.36 | 0.63±0.07 | 3.6±0.40 | 0.72±0.10 |
| +3 | 6.2±1.10 | 3.8±0.55 | 3.6±0.43 | 0.57±0.18 | 3.8±0.44 | 0.67±0.16 |
| Multiparas | | | | | | |
| −3 and −4 | 6.4±0.82 | 3.5±1.19 | 4.0±0.52 | 0.29±0.07 | 4.5±0.60 | 0.34±0.15 |
| −2 | 3.3±0.40 | 2.5±0.38 | 5.0±0.65 | 0.34±0.12 | 5.2±0.62 | 0.32±0.05 |
| −1 | 4.9±0.42 | 2.0±0.16 | 6.4±0.59 | 0.23±0.03 | 6.0±0.60 | 0.25±0.04 |
| 0 | 6.1±0.66 | 2.4±0.19 | 6.0±0.34 | 0.23±0.03 | 6.0±0.44 | 0.25±0.03 |
| +1 | 6.0±0.80 | 1.9±0.20 | 6.7±0.64 | 0.18±0.04 | 6.6±0.64 | 0.18±0.02 |
| +2 and +3 | 5.1±1.04 | 1.8±0.25 | 6.2±0.79 | 0.17±0.02 | 6.8±0.80 | 0.20±0.03 |

* Statistically significant trends, $p < 0.01$.

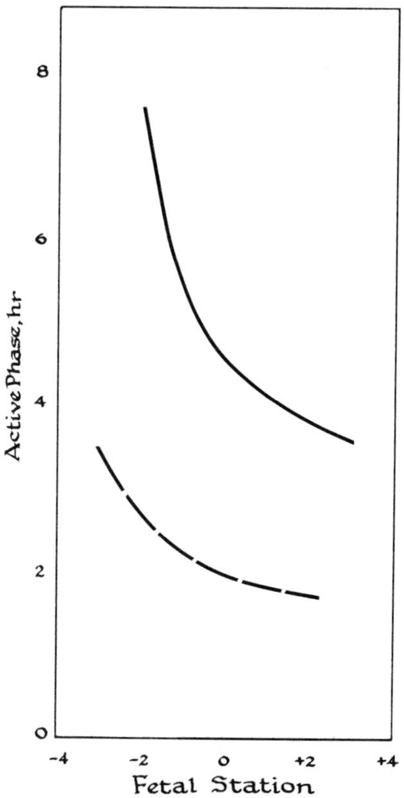


*Fig. 35.* Relationship between the fetal station that has been attained by the time labor reaches the beginning of the active phase and the subsequent duration of that active phase in nulliparas (*solid line*) and multiparas (*broken line*), clearly showing the trend for the active phase to be longer in duration in conjunction with higher stations.

*Table 32.* LABOR DATA BY STATION AT ONSET OF DECELERATION PHASE

| Station | Latent Phase (hr) | Active Phase (hr) | Maximum Dilatation (cm/hr) | Deceleration Phase* (hr) | Maximum Descent* (cm/hr) | Second Stage* (hr) |
|---|---|---|---|---|---|---|
| Nulliparas | | | | | | |
| 0 and −1 | 7.0±1.16 | 5.4±0.40 | 2.7±0.38 | 1.50±0.10 | 2.4±0.40 | 1.37±0.09 |
| +1 | 8.5±0.90 | 5.1±0.56 | 2.6±0.50 | 1.44±0.12 | 2.9±0.46 | 1.12±0.06 |
| +2 | 8.0±0.62 | 6.3±0.26 | 2.6±0.32 | 1.40±0.07 | 3.4±0.38 | 1.16±0.05 |
| +3 and +4 | 8.9±0.58 | 5.3±0.40 | 2.7±0.28 | 1.07±0.07 | 3.8±0.32 | 1.07±0.05 |
| Multiparas | | | | | | |
| 0 and −1 | 5.0±1.13 | 3.1±0.37 | 3.0±0.40 | 0.46±0.09 | 4.4±0.48 | 0.35±0.09 |
| +1 | 5.5±0.81 | 3.3±0.85 | 4.8±0.78 | 0.34±0.17 | 5.8±0.80 | 0.25±0.04 |
| +2 | 5.4±0.76 | 2.4±0.22 | 4.4±0.37 | 0.29+0.05 | 6.2±0.40 | 0.26±0.04 |
| +3 | 5.7±0.66 | 3.0±0.44 | 4.1±0.52 | 0.29±0.07 | 6.6±0.54 | 0.18±0.03 |

* Statistically significant trends, $p < 0.01$.

trends are all statistically verifiable. Therefore, while station at the onset of labor affects only the latent and acceleration phases, fetal station at the onset of the active phase clearly influences the rest of labor.

Grouping patients according to the station at the onset of the deceleration phase (Table 32) provides the expected effect on the duration of the deceleration phase and the second stage. Of special interest is the progressive shift in the slope of descent. As before, it is not surprising that neither the latent phase nor that part of the active phase preceding deceleration is affected. The dynamic principle just expressed appears to apply here as well.

*Table 33.* DYSFUNCTIONAL LABOR BY STATION IN NULLIPARAS

| Station | All Dysfunctional Labors* (%) | Prolonged Latent Phase (%) | Protraction Disorders† (%) | Arrest Disorders† (%) |
|---|---|---|---|---|
| At onset of labor | | | | |
| −2 and −3 | 29.8 | 16.4 | 14.7 | 11.4 |
| −1 | 20.4 | 6.1 | 12.2 | 5.1 |
| 0 | 14.5 | 2.7 | 9.1 | 6.3 |
| +1 | 11.4 | 5.7 | 8.6 | 2.9 |
| +2 and +3 | 14.3 | 7.1 | 7.1 | 0.0 |
| At onset of active phase | | | | |
| −1 to −3 | 23.4 | 4.3 | 14.9 | 10.6 |
| 0 | 19.8 | 5.4 | 10.8 | 8.2 |
| +1 | 11.3 | 6.3 | 6.3 | 1.3 |
| +2 and +3 | 11.8 | 5.9 | 5.9 | 0.0 |
| Total incidence | 18.9 | 6.1 | 10.9 | 7.1 |

* Discrepancies in total percentages occur because more than one labor aberration may occur in individual labors.
† Statistically significant trends, $p < 0.01$.

### *Index of Dysfunctional Labor*

Because the fetal station appeared to be related in some way to the course of subsequent labor, it was conjectured that it might also serve as an index of disordered labor. Breakdown of relevant case material by fetal station at the onset of labor (Table 33) did show an association among nulliparas. There were significantly more dysfunctional patterns in association with high station. The incidence decreased progressively with lower fetal stations. Clear-cut trends were seen for both protraction and arrest patterns. Similar trends, although not statistically significant, occurred with regard to the incidence of prolonged latent-phase abnormalities. These findings were not duplicated in multiparas.

Examination of these data by station at the onset of the active phase in nulliparas (Table 33) yields the same trends with reference to the incidence of protraction and arrest patterns. However, the frequencies of prolonged latent phase are clearly unaffected. Here again, we see the effect that might be expected on the basis of dynamic change in fetal station. Thus, with the exception of latent-phase abnormalities, the differences in outlook among nulliparas predicated on station at the onset of the active phase are impressive. The prognostic value of station as it applies to subsequent disordered labor, however, does not hold for multiparas (if unengaged, 7.8 percent developed dysfunctional patterns and if engaged, 10.1 percent).

Station of the fetal presenting part influences the progression of labor. This effect is transitory, varying with changes in the station itself. Speculation on and fuller discussion of the factors that bring about these changes are beyond our scope. It is unclear, of course, whether the relationship we see is one of cause and effect, either directly or remotely. We need not enter on a series of polemics on theoretical mechanistic considerations dealing with engagement and descent and how these might influence labor. What is important is that the relationship exists and may be useful and practical for ongoing evaluations of the patient in labor. Knowledge of this relationship may serve as an additional and potentially valuable tool for clinical study.

When the fetal head remains high in the pelvis at the beginning of labor, the labor that follows is generally but not invariably associated with a long latent phase. If this condition persists into the active phase, the active phase will often be prolonged also. Similarly, if still present in the deceleration phase, the last part of the first stage as well as the second stage will likewise tend to be prolonged. On the other hand, high fetal heads that descend rapidly into the pelvis need not necessarily be associated with abnormal labor progress. This is confirmed by the relatively good dilatation patterns encountered with low stations in the active phase. These occur without regard for the foregoing descent pattern. Thus, any deleterious effect that high fetal station may have on labor appears to be remediable. The adverse effect is reversed if the station is correctable sometime during the course of the labor.

### *Interrelationship with Cervical Dilatation*

Fetal station at the onset of labor has been shown to correlate well with the duration of the latent phase (see above). A similar relationship exists with reference to the degree of cervical dilatation at the onset of labor. Moreover, fetal station and cervical dilatation are not independent variables (Friedman and Sachtleben, 1965d). Therefore, it becomes necessary to clarify the relative effects that these two factors, station and dilatation, have on each other and on labor.

Data were compiled for analysis by detailing the progressive changes of station and cervical dilatation with elapsed time in labor. Patients were grouped according to initial fetal station and cervical dilatation simultaneously so as to allow intensive study of the effects of these factors upon the course and outcome of labor. We directed our attention to elucidating the relationship between cervical dilatation and station, first at the onset of labor and then at the onset of the active phase of dilatation. We have just shown that the fetal station at these two points in labor bears directly upon the course of the ensuing portion of labor. As a natural extension of these studies, information on the relationship between dilatation and station and their relative influences on the course of labor were forthcoming.

On average, initial cervical dilatation in nulliparas was found to be 1.5 cm; the average initial station, —0.5. In multiparas, initial dilatation averaged 1.9 cm and initial station, —1.3. When the data for average cervical dilatation at the onset of labor is compiled according to subgroupings by initial fetal station (Table 34), a clear relationship is demonstrated. Greater initial dilatation appears to be the rule with more deeply engaged presenting parts at the onset of labor; the corollary is also true—that there is less dilatation at higher stations. This is somewhat less obvious in nulliparas than in multiparas (the trend is statistically significant in multiparas but not in nulliparas).

There is nearly a linear change in mean dilatation with advancing station in multiparas (Fig. 36), paralleled to a degree in nulliparas. The same

*Table 34. RELATION BETWEEN DILATATION AND STATION*

| *Fetal Station* | *Cervical Dilatation (cm) at Onset of Labor* | | *Cervical Dilatation (cm) at Onset of Active Phase* | |
|---|---|---|---|---|
| | NULLIPARAS | MULTIPARAS* | NULLIPARAS | MULTIPARAS |
| —3 and above | 1.3 | 1.7 | — | 2.5 |
| —2 | 1.6 | 1.9 | 1.9 | 2.5 |
| —1 | 1.8 | 2.1 | 2.3 | 2.5 |
| 0 | 1.8 | 2.3 | 2.5 | 2.8 |
| +1 | 1.8 | 2.7 | 2.9 | 3.1 |
| +2 and below | — | — | 2.7 | 3.1 |
| Total | 1.5 | 1.9 | 2.6 | 2.8 |

* Statistically significant trend, $p < 0.01$.

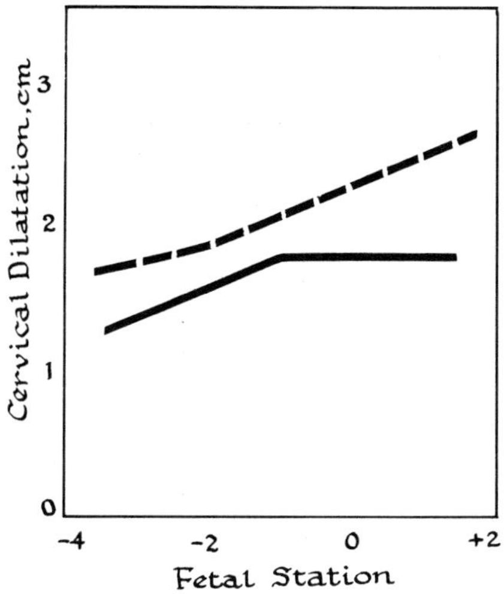


*Fig. 36.* Correlation between cervical dilatation and fetal station at the onset of labor in nulliparas (*solid line*) and multiparas (*broken line*). The demonstration of an almost linear relationship among multiparas implies that dilatation and station may be mutually interdependent among them; interdependence may also exist in nulliparas, but not for those beginning labor with dilatation greater than 1.5 cm or station −1 or lower.
(From Friedman EA, Sachtleben MR: Am J Obstet Gynecol 93:539, 1965)

general tendencies occur at the onset of the active phase: greater degrees of cervical dilatation exist in conjunction with lower fetal stations.

We see now that station and dilatation are interrelated. Both must be taken into account simultaneously in studying their relative effects on labor. A matrix can be created by stratifying case material by both station and dilatation to determine the latent-phase duration of the population within each cell. When this is done, we find interesting and characteristic trends (Table 35). The bidimensionality of these trends is important to recognize. The latent phase is clearly longer at high stations and with small degrees of cervical dilatation. It is successively shorter with lower stations and greater dilatation.

These data are best examined by keeping one of the variables constant.

*Table 35. LATENT-PHASE DURATION BY STATION AND DILATATION AT ONSET OF LABOR**

| *Cervical Dilatation (cm)* | *Fetal Station* | | | | | | |
|---|---|---|---|---|---|---|---|
| | −3 | −2 | −1 | 0 | +1 | +2 | +3 |
| 0.0–0.4 | | (16.3) | (17.3) | 10.8 | 9.3 | (8.0) | |
| 0.5–0.9 | (20.8) | 12.6 | 11.9 | 10.0 | 8.2 | (10.2) | |
| 1.0–1.4 | (18.6) | (14.3) | 10.2 | 8.7 | 7.6 | (10.0) | (2.0) |
| 1.5–1.9 | (15.6) | 12.0 | 8.8 | 8.2 | 8.2 | 6.5 | (4.5) |
| 2.0–2.9 | (11.5) | (10.9) | 8.3 | 8.0 | (8.3) | (3.5) | |
| 3.0–3.9 | | (5.8) | (6.9) | 5.8 | (5.5) | | |
| 4.0–4.9 | | (6.0) | | (3.3) | (4.0) | | |
| 5.0+ | | | (4.8) | | | | |

* Data are expressed in hours and apply to nulliparas only; parentheses indicate subgroups of insignificant size.

For example, we may peruse the latent phase data for the tier of information dealing with advancing fetal station (from −3 to +3) associated with fixed initial cervical dilatation of, say, 1.5 to 1.9 cm. As we read across this row of figures, it is immediately transparent that there is progressive diminution in the latent-phase duration. Each row of figures diminishes progressively with advancing station. By the same token, the vertical axis indicates similar comparable trends with advancing cervical dilatation when the station is maintained constant. These data imply a degree of independence with regard to the influence of both fetal station and cervical dilatation on the duration of the latent phase. The trends are definitive and statistically significant.

Data for active-phase duration are strikingly similar as they relate to the effect of station and dilatation at the onset of the active phase (Table 36). Not unexpectedly, we see more rapid progress with lower station, greater dilatation, or both. Once again, we can verify that the effects of station and dilatation are independent of each other.

*Table 36. ACTIVE-PHASE DURATION BY STATION AND DILATATION AT ONSET OF ACTIVE PHASE**

| *Cervical Dilatation (cm)* | *Fetal Station* | | | | | |
|---|---|---|---|---|---|---|
| | −2 | −1 | 0 | +1 | +2 | +3 |
| <2.0 | (15.4) | (7.3) | 6.8 | 5.6 | (4.9) | (4.7) |
| 2.0–2.9 | (9.8) | 5.6 | 5.2 | 4.8 | 4.2 | (4.3) |
| 3.0–3.9 | (8.0) | 4.5 | 4.9 | 3.4 | (2.7) | (3.4) |
| 4.0+ | | (4.5) | 3.2 | 3.2 | (2.0) | (1.9) |

* Data for nulliparas expressed in hours; parentheses indicate subgroups of insignificant size.

In addition to the above, fetal station at the onset of the active phase also appears to influence the maximum slopes of dilatation and of descent, but these are not statistically significant trends. Neither the deceleration-phase duration nor the length of the second stage seems to be comparably affected in any consistent way.

It is of particular interest here that relationships exist between (1) initial cervical dilatation and initial fetal station, (2) cervical dilatation and the course of labor, and (3) fetal station and the labor course. These three relationships can be demonstrated graphically in a three-dimensional perspective presentation (Fig. 37). This presentation shows the prolongation of the latent phase in association with higher stations of the fetal presenting part and with smaller degrees of cervical dilatation at the onset of labor. With lower station, larger initial dilatation, or both, the latent phase is relatively foreshortened.

Examining Figure 37, we can intuitively visualize the material falling into three major groups. There is an optimal group with average latent-phase

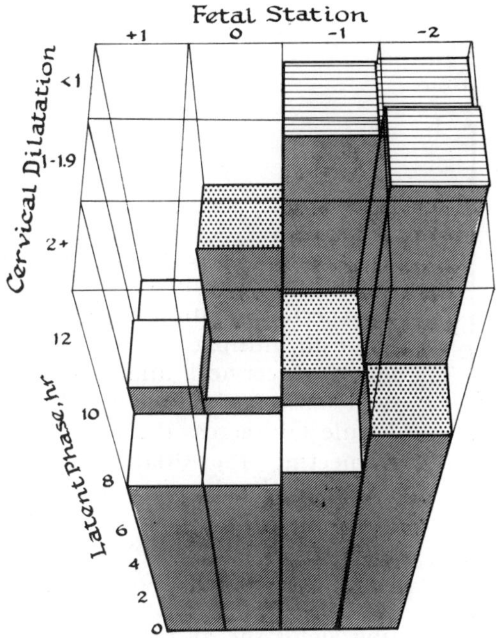


*Fig. 37.* Three-dimensional perspective to demonstrate how initial fetal station (*horizontal axis*) and cervical dilatation (*deep axis*) act alone and in concert to affect the duration of the latent phase (*vertical axis*) in nulliparas. Three roughly homogeneous levels of response are seen: relatively prolonged latent phases in association with high station, little dilatation, or both (*cross-hatched bars*); median-range lengths with lower stations, more dilatation, or both (*stippled bars*); foreshortened latent phases with low station, much dilatation, or both at the onset of labor (*white bars*).
(From Friedman, EA, Sachtleben MR: Am J Obstet Gynecol 93:541, 1965)

duration of about 8 hours; a middle group at 10 hours; and a potentially abnormal group at about 13 hours in length. This last is associated with high station and small initial dilatation; by contrast, the group characterized by relatively short latent phases is associated with low station and ample dilatation. Adequate dilatation may thus compensate for high station. Similarly, low station may compensate for small dilatation. Once again, we can recognize that the effects of these factors are independent.

This material can also be represented by a nomographic device (Fig. 38). This is useful for determining what the approximate duration of the latent phase ought to be, on the basis of cervical dilatation and fetal station at the onset of labor. With the aid of a ruler, a nomogram enables one to read the value of a dependent variable when the values of two or more independent variables are given. Knowing the dilatation and station, one readily obtains the expected latent-phase duration. As a prognostic device, this gives one a reasonable idea of what may be expected of a given labor.

Partial dependency has been shown to exist between cervical dilatation and fetal station. Tendencies are found for lower presenting stations to be associated with larger cervical dilatation at both the onset of labor and the onset of the active phase. These relationships are especially noteworthy in multiparas and to a lesser extent, in nulliparas. The course of labor is affected in well-defined directions by either factor acting in an apparently independent manner with regard to the other. In fact, dilatation and station appear to be mutually compensatory (when one is salutary and the other

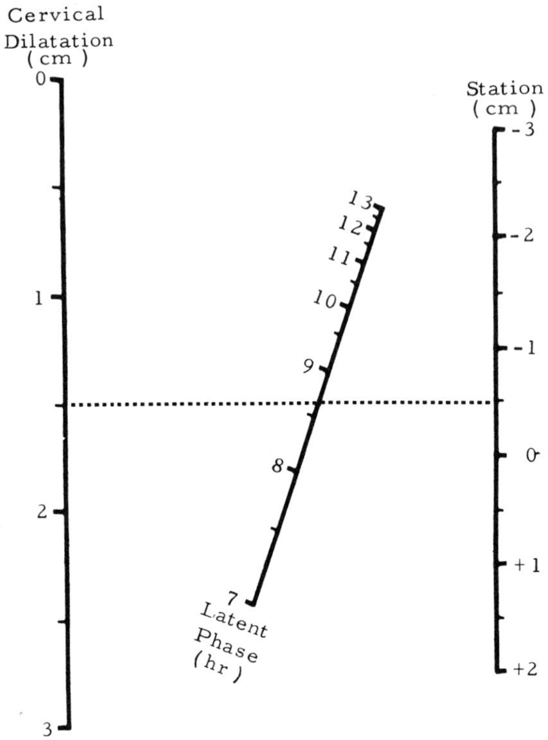


*Fig. 38.* Nomographic aid for obtaining approximate projection of expected duration of the latent phase in nulliparas based on estimates of cervical dilatation and fetal station at the onset of labor. A rule laid across the nomogram connecting the dilatation (*left scale*) with the station (*right scale*) will intersect the center scale to give the information on latent-phase duration that is sought. The broken horizontal line yields the average values for all three parameters.

(From Friedman EA, Sachtleben MR: Am J Obstet Gynecol 93:541, 1965)

unfavorable) or augmentative (when both are choice or both are disadvantageous) with regard to their influence on labor progression.

## *FETOPELVIC RELATIONSHIP*

Disproportion between the bony pelvis and the fetus is often associated with abnormal labor (Friedman, 1957a). Indeed, the appearance of a disordered labor can serve as a prognostic index. This has been dealt with at length in Chapter 12. When an arrest pattern develops, for example, its appearance should encourage the clinician to evaluate the fetopelvic relationship.

Because of the apparent close association between bony dystocia and labor progression, we conjectured that the labor pattern could be utilized to help define a suitable clinical trial of labor. Normal labors follow well-defined patterns of dilatation and of descent (Chapter 7). Therefore, in cases where the lower limb of these curves is established and active dilatation or descent is occurring, subsequent events should be predictable. The curves may be projected forward in time because the maximum slopes of dilatation and descent are essentially linear. For a particular labor that has entered the active phase of dilatation, for example, one may anticipate full dilatation after a specific number of hours. When this will occur is dependent on the previously established rate of cervical dilatation. This general principle was applied for purposes of establishing a meaningful tool for assessing expected labor progression.

## *Formulating a Trial of Labor*

We began with the hypothesis that normal labors describe characteristic dilatation and descent curves. From these, we formulated expressions for the extrapolation of the curve of an incompletely dilated cervix or an incompletely descended fetal presenting part. The material that follows will address itself to the dilatation phenomenon, but the same basic concept applies for descent as well.

For a labor that has entered the active phase under observation and in which the maximum slope is definable (that is, two or more observations within the phase of maximum slope have been obtained), the active-phase slope may be projected on the time abscissa as a straight-line extension to a point representing anticipated full dilatation (Fig. 39). If we add to this a factor representing the deceleration-phase duration, we obtain the time when the second stage should normally begin. Adding another suitable interval for the duration of the second stage, we derive that time when delivery should take place. Either of these projections may be used to define normal progress and to delimit the proper duration of an adequate trial of labor, but the former is more practical.

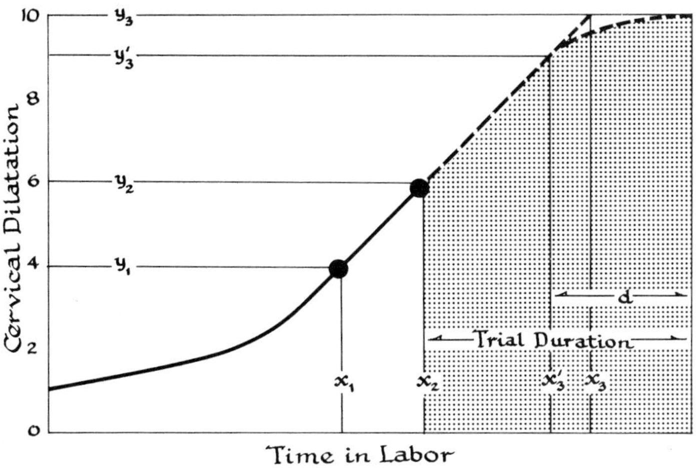


*Fig. 39.* Defining a clinical trial of labor based on the foregoing course of cervical dilatation in the active phase of a given patient. Projecting the linear maximum slope line upward on the time scale gives the clinician an objective measurement of the kind of progress the gravida should be expected to experience. The text provides means for calculating the theoretical limits for such a trial, but it is generally very easily solvable by graphic means.

(From Friedman EA: Obstet Gynecol 10:2, 1957)

The trial of labor formulated in this way may be expressed simply in mathematical terms, using the principle of geometric linear extrapolation. Referring to Figure 39, we find at time $x_2$ (the point of reference) that the cervical dilatation curve has entered the phase of maximum slope. The slope is defined by two points, $x_1y_1$ and $x_2y_2$, respectively. The slope may be expressed in centimeters per hour as

$$m = \frac{y_2 - y_1}{x_2 - x_1}$$

This is also the slope of the theoretical linear progression of the curve. If it continued to full dilatation, the curve would arrive at time $x_3$. Thus, the slope of the projected line can be expressed as

$$m = \frac{y_3 - y_2}{x_3 - x_2}$$

Equating these and solving for the unknown $x_3$, we derive

$$x_3 = \frac{x_2\,(y_3 - y_1) \;-\; x_1\,(y_3 - y_2)}{y_2 - y_1}$$

At time $x_3$, therefore, full dilatation is expected. The duration of a trial of labor starting at time $x_2$ might be the interval $x_3 - x_2$. This, of course, assumes linear projection up to full cervical dilatation. The normally occurring deceleration phase, however, must be taken into account. This modifies the duration of a trial of labor to

$$x_3 - x_2 + d$$

The quantity $d$ is variable, but for practical purposes in a labor trial, it may be taken as the upper limit of the normal deceleration phase. For nulliparas, this is 3.3 hours and for multiparas, 0.9 hour.

These time factors cannot be added directly to that of projected full dilatation because the duration of the deceleration phase is timed from its onset —usually at 8.5 to 9.0 cm of dilatation—to the beginning of the second stage. It is reasonable, therefore, to project the active-phase dilatation curve to only 9 cm for the purpose of determining the proper duration of a trial of labor. If $y_3 = 9.0$ cm, then

$$x'_3 = \frac{x_2\,(9.0 - y_1) \;-\; x_1\,(9.0 - y_2)}{y_2 - y_1}$$

This proves to be a rather useful formula for these objectives. We may utilize it to determine the interval required to attain 9 cm of dilatation

$(x'_3 - x_2)$, and add the deceleration factor $d$ to derive a theoretically accurate working value for the maximum length of time needed in a normally progressing labor to achieve full cervical dilatation. This, then, is the duration of a trial of labor in the first stage. It is noteworthy that the computed trial duration varies inversely with the slope; that is, the slower the rate of dilatation, the longer the trial required.

An example may clarify the practical usefulness of this formulation. A nullipara in labor, having begun labor at 12 o'clock midnight, is examined at intervals after admission (Fig. 39). At 5 A.M. the cervix is 1 cm dilated; at 9 A.M., 2 cm; at 11 A.M., 4 cm; at 1 P.M., 6 cm. It is apparent by 1 P.M. (and in retrospect even at 11 A.M.) that the active phase of dilatation has been entered. Progress should be expected to continue in a straight line. The points of importance are $x_1y_1$ (11.0 hours, 4.0 cm) and $x_2y_2$ (13.0 hours, 6.0 cm). Substituting these into the formula gives the following:

$$x'_3 = \frac{13.0\ (9.0 - 4.0)\ - 11.0\ (9.0 - 6.0)}{6.0 - 4.0} = 16.0 \text{ hours}$$

This corresponds to 4 P.M. The duration of the trial of labor then is $x'_3$ (16.0 hours) minus $x_2$ (13.0 hours) plus factor $d$ (3.3 hours), to give a total of 6.3 hours. During this interval, full cervical dilatation should normally be reached. Since our point of reference is time $x_2$ or 1 P.M., the trial will not be concluded until 7:20 P.M. It is, parenthetically, of some importance to keep units comparable in these calculations. For example, time should be in integer hours and decimal fractions (not minutes), and cervical dilatation should be in centimeters.

It is clearly a superfluous refinement to solve this formula as shown for every given case. Merely projecting the maximum slope curve forward in the manner described will provide the same information by graphic means. We formulated the mathematical definition, however, so that we might assess its applicability to clinical problems. What we desired was specific clinical criteria for defining the adequacy of a trial of labor in association with cephalopelvic disproportion. Of course, the problem of bony disproportion is only one of several that may be studied by means of a delimited test of labor.

## *Labor Course*

Extensive investigations have been carried out (Ince and Young, 1940; Jacobs, 1942; Pettit et al, 1936; Thomas, 1935; Thomas et al, 1939) to determine the course of labor among patients with cephalopelvic disproportion who were allowed to labor. In general it was agreed that disordered and prolonged labors were common. To explore this matter in somewhat more depth, we undertook to study a large series of nulliparas at term with objective documentation of disproportion (Friedman, 1957a; Sogolow and Friedman, 1967). Documentation took the form of digital and radiographic cephalopelvimetry, primarily following the tenets of Caldwell and Moloy (1933; Caldwell et al, 1939; Moloy and Steer, 1950) and the techniques of Ball (1936a, b, 1950; Ball and Marchbanks, 1935; Friedman and Taylor, 1969; Klapholz, 1975; Friedman, 1976b).

Utilizing the formulation for trial of labor as defined above, we were able to assess expected progression and to detect and categorize any deviations that were found. Three major classes of progression in labor were encountered:

1. Those that followed the expected projection of the labor curve (designated group A),
2. Those who developed protraction disorders subsequently (group B), and and
3. Those with later arrest of dilatation or arrest of descent (group C).

Group A cases were normal in all respects in that the labor pattern followed the expected course as defined by the formula. Ensuing observations fell either on the projected curve or to its left. It was of interest that normal labor frequently did evolve in association with clearly documented bony disproportion. Moreover, normal progression served as a very good prognostic sign under these circumstances. Labors falling into group B were clearly abnormal due to the occurrence of significant distortions in progression, characterized specifically by protraction disorders. In addition, major prolongations of the deceleration phase occurred rather commonly in this group. Group C was composed of cases with overtly documented arrest patterns in which subsequent observations fell far to the right of the extrapolated curve. This proved to be a uniformly ominous sign. The relative incidence of these labor patterns among our series of patients with cephalopelvic disproportion was: group A, 24.3 percent; group B, 40.6 percent; group C, 35.2 percent.

Notwithstanding the shortcomings of radiographic pelvimetry, the groups were analyzed to determine the incidence of numerically absolute disproportion among them. It was found that group A possessed relatively few cases, whereas groups B and (especially) C contained significantly more. In passing from the normal to the abnormal labor groups, therefore, one finds a trend toward higher degrees of disproportion. Moreover, although no real distinction could be detected among the groups with regard to location of pelvic contracture, whether inlet or midpelvic, there was a slight tendency for midpelvic problems to concentrate in group B and inlet problems, in Group C. These observations lent support to the contention that a disordered labor pattern may reflect the presence of bony dystocia and that disproportion may be expected to give rise to an abnormal dilatation or descent curve.

Graphic analysis of the labor patterns described by nulliparas with disproportion shows striking differences from comparable nulliparas with adequate pelves (Table 37). Whereas the average latent phase is almost the

*Table 37. LABOR DATA WITH CEPHALOPELVIC DISPROPORTION*

| *Group* | *Latent Phase (hr)* | *Active Phase (hr)* | *Maximum Dilatation (cm/hr)* | *Deceleration Phase (hr)* | *Maximum Descent (cm/hr)* | *Second Stage (hr)* |
|---|---|---|---|---|---|---|
| A: Normal labor projection | 9.5±0.94 | 5.9±0.49 | 2.3 ±0.19 | 0.82±0.17 | 2.6 ±0.22 | 1.0±0.20 |
| B: Protraction disorder | 7.7±0.52 | 10.6±0.38 | 1.8 ±0.12 | 5.2 ±0.37 | 1.6 ±0.19 | 3.1±0.32 |
| C: Arrest disorder | 10.3±0.78 | 13.4±0.67 | 0.72±0.07 | 9.6 ±0.52 | 0.70±0.08 | 4.4±0.48 |
| Nulliparas with disproportion | 9.1±0.39 | 10.0±0.36 | 1.5 ±0.08 | 6.0 ±0.31 | 1.4 ±0.08 | 2.9±0.30 |
| Nulliparas without disproportion | 8.6±0.27 | 4.9±0.15 | 3.0 ±0.08 | 0.90±0.05 | 3.2 ±0.10 | 1.0±0.04 |

same as expected, all the rest of labor is not. Significant prolongations of active- and deceleration-phase durations are obvious, together with diminution of the maximum slopes of dilatation and descent. These deviations from normal become still more apparent in those labors characterized by protraction or arrest disorders (groups B and C), as shown in Table 37. Except for the latent-phase duration, all are statistically significant differences from data in patients with adequate cephalopelvic relationships. Most impressively, the deceleration phase and second stage are uniformly and markedly prolonged. Much of this prolongation is undoubtedly attributable to the long intervals of arrested progress in many of these labors, averaging 6.1 hours overall. There can be little doubt from these data that labor is adversely affected by cephalopelvic disproportion.

## *Delivery Results*

Other important findings in our studies concerned the ultimate outcome of the labor. There were remarkable differences between the delivery frequencies in the several groups (Table 38). Patients whose labor patterns fell into group A because they progressed along the extrapolated dilatation and descent curves were delivered by cesarean section in only 5.2 percent. This is especially impressive because all of the patients in this group had clearly documented cephalopelvic disproportion. Group B labors with protraction disorders were concluded by cesarean section in 36.4 percent and by mid-

*Table 38. DELIVERY AFTER LABOR WITH DISPROPORTION*

| *Group* | *Cesarean Section (%)* | *Midforceps (%)* | *Low Forceps and Spontaneous (%)* |
|---|---|---|---|
| A: Normal projection | 5.2 | 15.8 | 79.0 |
| B: Protraction disorder | 36.4 | 39.6 | 24.0 |
| C: Arrest disorder | 98.8 | 1.2 | 0.0 |

forceps in 39.6 percent. In sharp contrast, labors in group C with arrest disorders were terminated by cesarean section in 98.8 percent and by midforceps in 1.2 percent. Indeed, no patient with a demonstrated arrest pattern was able to deliver normally, regardless of the measures utilized trying to effect further dilatation or descent. These data are statistically very significant.

It is clear from these observations that arrest patterns occurring in conjunction with cephalopelvic disproportion demand cesarean section. The probability of atraumatic vaginal delivery under these circumstances is so small as not to warrant the attempt. Moreover, the adverse effects on the fetus of such attempts (see below and Chapter 23) strongly interdicts them. One word of caution is essential here. The prognostic value of arrest patterns in association with disproportion should not be misconstrued to imply that all arrested labors occur with bony dystocia. There are many remediable conditions that produce these same abnormal patterns (see Chapter 11). In the absence of disproportion, the prognosis is much more optimistic.

### *Fetal Outcome*

With regard to perinatal mortality, there was a concentration of fetal deaths in patients in group B with protraction disorders. Most of these were associated with potentially traumatic operative vaginal delivery. Recent evidence has accumulated (Chapter 23) to show that adverse effects on the fetus as well as the surviving infant result from both the abnormal labor patterns and the trauma of delivery, especially when they occur in combination.

Among the deleterious effects encountered were increased mortality and neonatal depression (Friedman et al, 1969b; Friedman and Sachtleben, 1971; Friedman, 1973c), as well as neurologic and developmental disorders (Friedman et al, 1969c, 1977). The overriding importance of such observations cannot be too strongly stressed, therefore.

We have seen how the use of a device for determining the expected course of dilatation and descent on the basis of what has transpired up to any given point permits us to classify the ensuing portion of labor according to how closely the anticipated curve is followed. By mathematical or graphic means, we determine when the second stage ought to occur. This practical tool establishes the approximate required duration for a trial of labor and simultaneously assesses the progression to indicate whether or not it is acceptably normal.

Labors with normal patterns do rather well, 95 percent delivering vaginally despite the documented disproportion. At the other extreme, labors developing an arrest pattern are almost uniformly terminated by cesarean section. It is clear that the labor pattern can be utilized as a prognostic index. There is a very close correlation between high degrees of disproportion and arrested progress. Arrest patterns are not only a frequent finding in association with bony disproportion, but they are expected. We may further infer that when arrest disorders occur, the disproportion will probably be such a significant obstructive factor that operative delivery by cesarean section will be required. On the other hand, labors exhibiting normal progression as defined here should be expected to delivery uneventfully (with few exceptions).

# Uterine Factors

## CHAPTER 17

Amniotomy cannot be objectively shown to speed the course of labor, clinical impressions notwithstanding. Labor associated with multiple pregnancy is usually of normal average length as a result of the combination of foreshortened latent phase (probably due to advanced prelabor cervical dilatation) and lengthened active phase (the rate of dilatation and descent perhaps slowed by uterine overdistention). Hydramnios, in contrast, affects labor negligibly, if at all. Similarly, neither placental site and weight nor leiomyomata uteri have any demonstrable influence on the course of labor.

Our interest in factors that may affect the course of labor will turn here to variables dealing with intrinsic uterine conditions in pregnancy. These include the status of the chorioamniotic membranes, uterine overdistention as manifested by multiple pregnancy and hydramnios, the site and weight of the placenta, and leiomyomata uteri. While the subject matter of this chapter is varied, it deals with items of some relevance nevertheless. Information on the labor patterns that can be expected to occur under these circumstances is important to the clinician who is faced with practical problems of evaluation and management. To this end, it is necessary to review the available data.

### *STATUS OF THE MEMBRANES*

There is a generally accepted clinical impression that amniotomy stimulates labor in progress. The experimental evidence to support this contention just does not exist. Nevertheless, the conviction with which it is held is almost unshakable. It appears to derive from our collective inability to divorce the recognized effect of amniotomy in initiating labor under appropriate circumstances from its poorly defined effect in augmenting labors that are already in progress. There can be little question that amniotomy in selected cases is effective for inducing labor. However, its stimulatory effects after labor has begun are undocumented.

Contributing to our misapprehension in this regard, amniotomy done routinely after labor is established—that is, late in latent phase of the first stage—will almost invariably be followed by more rapid progress, as evidenced by the ensuing cervical dilatation. Active dilatation must necessarily take place eventually in all normal labors (see Chapter 7). It must occur in the course of the natural evolution of labor from the latent to the active phase. Recognizing this, we might question whether or not such acceleration would have occurred if the membranes had been left intact.

There is, of course, a documented and predictable upswing in the rate of dilatation at the beginning of the active phase. Moreover, the basic criteria widely used for proceeding with elective rupture of the membranes in labor are the very same features that characterize the beginning of the active phase. Such features include increasing amplitude, frequency and regularization of uterine contractions, and softening, effacement, and beginning dilatation of the cervix. When such conditions exist, active dilatation should be expected to occur very soon.

Needless to say, the ensuing progress can mistakenly be ascribed to anything done to or for the patient at that time (provided it is not inhibitory, of course). Since it is common practice to rupture the membranes at about this time for purposes of stimulating the labor and thereby effecting some progress (recall that the patient in the latent phase has not yet made any significant progress in dilatation to this point), the ensuing rapid progression repeatedly reinforces our erroneous impression of its effectiveness.

Practical and theoretical considerations of this question have been weighed in the past. In 1940, King reviewed reports dealing with almost 15,000 patients with early rupture of the membranes. Although he did not differentiate between spontaneous rupture and surgical amniotomy, he could not show any differences in total duration of labor as a consequence of this event. In a somewhat more controlled study, Keetel et al (1940) also showed no significant differences in labor progression according to membrane status. Several studies did show that labor following premature spontaneous rupture of the membranes tended to be more rapid than expected.

Of special interest was the report by Calkins (1958) verifying that premature spontaneous rupture of the membranes is often followed by markedly shorter labors; at the same time, rupture after labor is already established generally failed to show any effect. As to its use in the treatment of arrested labor progress, Calkins went on to admonish that amniotomy does not yield consistent results. We have already seen the ineffectiveness of this ostensibly stimulatory device as a treatment for disordered labors (Chapters 10 and 11).

Pioneer tocodynamometric studies (Murphy, 1947; Reynolds et al, 1954) showed that early spontaneous rupture of the membranes had no significant immediate effect on uterine tonus or labor progression. This was countered, however, by other reports (Caldeyro-Barcia and Heller, 1961) claiming that the uterine work required to effect cervical dilatation in oxytocin-induced labors was less if the membranes were ruptured than if intact (in 6 and 10 cases, respectively). Although this observation was open to question because it involved small numbers of unmatched cases, it is still widely cited as evidence to support the value of amniotomy for augmenting spontaneous uterine activity (even though the observations were based on oxytocin-induced labors). Actually, more recent objective investigations on uterine contractions in spontaneous labors, originating from the same clinical laboratory (Krapohl et al, 1970), found no differences before or after membrane rupture.

In order to try to resolve the controversy, objective studies of labor progression were undertaken (Friedman and Sachtleben, 1963c). The results of these investigations form the basis for asserting that amniotomy actually has no consistent effect on labor in progress. Widely held clinical impressions notwithstanding, amniotomy appears to be highly overrated as a means for augmenting labor.

### *Labor Course*

Experimental design for determining the influence of the membranes on labor progress presented a problem. Random selection of successive gravidas for assignment to groups in which the membranes were either to be ruptured or left intact is clearly impractical. For example, it would be limited by patients admitted with membranes already ruptured (in excess of 20 percent), by those in doubtful or false labor because of the recognized hazards of prolonged rupture of membranes (another 10 percent or more), by patients admitted for elective cesarean section, by those with obstetric conditions militating against amniotomy such as floating presenting part, breech presentation, prematurity, and possible placenta previa, and by those with conditions requiring amniotomy, including abruptio placentae, fetal distress, and hydramnios (at least 10 percent). Those gravidas arriving for obstetric care near the end of the first stage or later in labor would also not be suitable candidates for study. Of those remaining, some assigned to the intact membrane group might rupture the membranes spontaneously and hopelessly confound the experimental design.

It was necessary, therefore, to approach the problem from a different point of view. A time interval was designated during which obstetricians were encouraged to rupture the membranes at the earliest convenience after the patient was admitted to the hospital, except in those cases in which the membranes had already ruptured spontaneously or in which amniotomy was specifically contraindicated. A subsequent interval was designated during which a restrictive policy prevailed prohibiting the performance of amniotomy as completely as possible. This was intended to supply data on the effect of leaving membranes intact. A third permissive interval followed for purposes of verifying the information obtained from the first period. The results of these consecutive studies provided useful information on the course of labor as it relates to the status of the membranes during the several phases of labor.

The groups were essentially identical with regard to parity, age, infant weight, fetal presentation and position, types of delivery, and perinatal results. There were recognizable management differences that undoubtedly reflected the attitude of the physicians during the restrictive period: uterotonic stimulation was given relatively more often, while heavy sedation occurred less often. Whereas these differences were not statistically significant, it was felt that they had to be taken into account because they may have weighted the corresponding labor courses somewhat.

The labor data derived from representative subgroups according to membrane status (Table 39) showed no real differences, even to suggest that leaving membranes intact might be inhibitory. Interestingly, the maximum slopes of dilatation and descent in multiparas were actually significantly greater in association with intact membranes. Based on such preliminary data, the status of the membranes did not seem to influence the course of labor. Any alleged deleterious effect of unruptured membranes could not be confirmed.

*Table 39.* *LABOR DATA BY MEMBRANE STATUS*

| *Group* | *Latent Phase (hr)* | *Active Phase (hr)* | *Maximum Dilatation (cm/hr)* | *Deceleration Phase (hr)* | *Maximum Descent (cm/hr)* | *Second Stage (hr)* |
|---|---|---|---|---|---|---|
| Nulliparas | | | | | | |
| Early rupture | 8.9±0.35 | 5.0±0.19 | 3.1±0.10 | 0.95±0.07 | 3.2±0.12 | 1.02±0.04 |
| Late rupture | 8.6±0.60 | 4.8±0.32 | 3.1±0.22 | 0.96±0.08 | 3.3±0.18 | 0.93±0.07 |
| Ideal Nulliparas | | | | | | |
| Early rupture | 7.2±0.38 | 3.4±0.14 | 3.8±0.17 | 0.72±0.06 | 3.8±0.20 | 0.78±0.06 |
| Late rupture | 6.6±0.88 | 3.3±0.23 | 3.8±0.32 | 0.68±0.07 | 3.9±0.28 | 0.74±0.08 |
| Multiparas | | | | | | |
| Early rupture | 5.6±0.23 | 2.3±0.08 | 5.4±0.18 | 0.25±0.02 | 5.8±0.22 | 0.25±0.01 |
| Late rupture | 6.1±0.36 | 2.1±0.16 | 7.3±0.44* | 0.25±0.05 | 7.7±0.39* | 0.21±0.02 |

* Statistically significant, $p < 0.01$.

We recognized earlier that there might have been some underlying bias inherent in the intact membrane group because uterotonic stimulation had been used more often and heavy sedation less. Accordingly, it was felt necessary to provide statistical corrections to adjust for these possible influences. The parallel series were made more comparable by "idealizing" them (see Chapter 7). This entailed deleting those cases associated with use of oxytocin and heavy sedation as well as those with disproportion, malposition, malpresentation, multiple pregnancy, and conduction anesthesia. These unhampered and unstimulated gravidas represented essentially normal parturition. The course of their labors (Table 39) were on average identical throughout. This clearly demonstrated that the factors of stimulation and relatively less heavy sedation did not falsely correct for a possible detrimental effect from intact membranes.

To focus still more closely upon the problem, we grouped the material according to the precise phase in which the membranes ruptured (Fig. 40). In nulliparas, it was found that latent-phase durations were essentially normal when the membranes ruptured at or before the onset of labor. There was an obvious trend toward significant lengthening of the latent phase

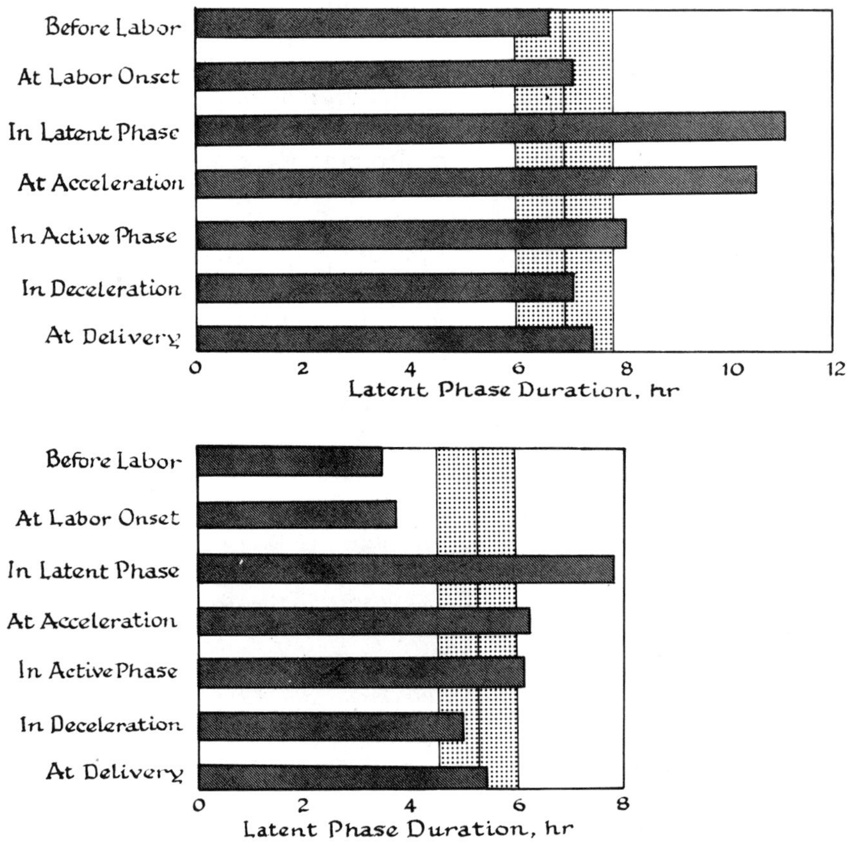


*Fig. 40.* Association between the time in labor when rupture of the membranes occurs and the duration of the latent phase in nulliparas (*upper frame*) and multiparas (*lower frame*). Means and 95th percentiles are shown (*stippled*) to emphasize significant deviations from expected. Prolongation of the latent phase is seen in nulliparas whose membranes rupture during the latent or acceleration phase; at no other time is there any apparent effect in lengthening or shortening the latent phase, except in those multiparas whose membranes rupture at or before the onset of labor. Preselection accounts for these differences (see text).

when the membranes ruptured during the latent phase or at its termination in the acceleration phase. The latent phase returned to normal on the average, with membranes ruptured subsequently. Similar trends were seen with multiparas, although rupture of the membranes at or before the onset of labor was also associated with significant foreshortening of the latent phase in general.

It is of special interest that no obvious trends were encountered in the durations of the active and deceleration phases and second stage or in the maximum slopes of dilatation and descent. These data remained almost constant in all subgroups. The only exception was in the second-stage duration among nulliparas. Foreshortening of small but significant magnitude occurred if the membranes ruptured during the deceleration phase. The magnitude of this effect was so small, however, as not to influence the overall duration of labor meaningfully. These observations show that there is essentially no correlative relationship between rupture of the membranes and the course of active-phase or second-stage progression.

Amniotomy in the latent phase is seemingly detrimental to the course of labor, since it is associated with significant prolongations of the latent phase. More rationally, we might conjecture that the membranes were often ruptured during the latent phase for the specific purpose of stimulating an already prolonged latent phase. Indeed, this proves to be the case. In most instances the latent phase was already prolonged at the time the amniotomy was undertaken. This contention is supported by our finding that the latent phase is also prolonged in association with rupture during the acceleration phase. It is inconceivable that the duration of the latent phase could have been affected retroactively. Furthermore, when the data were examined by spontaneous versus artificial rupture of the membranes in the latent phase, the average duration was reduced to normal (8.8 hours) among those with spontaneous rupture; average duration increased still further (to 13.5 hours) among gravidas subjected to amniotomy during the latent phase.

As a further refinement, two series of patients were matched according to many relevant characteristics, including parity, gravidity, gestational age, fetal weight and position, pelvis, type and depth of analgesia, anesthesia, and oxytocic stimulation. One of each pair had the membranes ruptured at or before the onset of labor, and the other, in the deceleration phase or second stage. The labor data of these pairs were identical in all respects, except for latent-phase duration. While the differences were not statistically significant, the latent phase was somewhat shorter among gravidas with membranes ruptured before labor developed actively. When corrections were applied for the differential distribution of prelabor changes in the cervix, this difference was reduced considerably.

Aside from latent phase effects, there was no demonstrably consistent adverse effect on the course of the rest of labor from rupturing the membranes or leaving them intact. With the advent of universal application of internal fetal monitoring, this issue will undoubtedly become moot, since current procedures require that the membranes be ruptured for purposes of applying the electrode to the fetal scalp. However, as technology advances and more sophisticated noninvasive external monitoring facilities are developed, the issue may well be raised again.

Moreover, the results of these studies also show that amniotomy is ineffectual as a therapeutic procedure in consistently abbreviating any of the phases of labor. The foreshortening of the latent phase seen in association with rupture of the membranes at the onset of labor appears to be based on natural selection of cases. This is exemplified by the large number of patients in this group who begin labor with advanced cervical dilatation. It is possible that the intrinsic forces of intrauterine pressure may be directed against the unsupported and unprotected membrane overlying the partially dilated cervix at the onset of labor. This would tend to cause the membranes to rupture selectively in these cases. If this were true, the foreshortening of the latent phase should not be ascribed to the status of the membranes, but rather to the prior preparation of the cervix. The influence of prelabor cervical dilatation on the duration of the latent phase has been well documented (see Chapter 16).

Regardless of the underlying basis for the shortening of the latent phase in association with spontaneous membrane rupture at or before labor, there can be no rational justification for assuming that artificial rupture of the membranes at this time will do likewise. In actuality, our studies have shown that the labors that follow inductions by amniotomy are identical in all details to comparable labors that begin spontaneously without amniotomy (when matched case-for-case according to prelabor status of the cervix).

## *MULTIPLE PREGNANCY*

There is a diversity of opinion concerning the course of labor with multiple pregnancy. Eastman (1961) postulated that because initial cervical dilatation is often considerable in these cases, the ensuing labor should be expected to be short. Since labors in twin gestations tend on average to be normal in duration, it logically follows that progression must be relatively slowed. Objective data in support of this hypothesis are now available (Friedman and Sachtleben, 1964a). The graphic method for studying the labor phenomenon has made it possible to elucidate subtle variations in the clinical pattern as applied to patients whose labor is complicated by uterine overdistention due to plural pregnancy. The same technique has been used in parallel studies of uterine overdistention resulting from hydramnios (see below).

### *Labor Course*

A large population of patients with twin and triplet gestations was studied (Friedman and Sachtleben, 1964a). The make-up of this group differed somewhat from the average gravid population. The mean age in this group was about as expected, but there was an increase in higher parities among the multiparas. The incidence of low birth weights was considerably increased, corresponding to previously reported data (Little and Friedman, 1958a) documenting the correlation of high prematurity rate with plural pregnancy. Similarly, breech presentations were common, reflecting the high prematurity rate.

As to factors known to influence the course of labor, cephalopelvic disproportion was rare. However, heavy sedation had been administered in somewhat increased numbers; the potential effect of this factor on the course of labor, therefore, had to be taken into account. Uterotonic stimulation had been used sparingly. Although the incidence of uterotonic augmentation was not excessive for our gravid population, it was felt that this factor might have corrected any deleterious effect that uterine overdistention exerted on the course of labor. Thus, this factor had to be accounted for as well.

Critical analysis of the labor data (Fig. 41, Table 40) revealed important differences between singleton and multiple pregnancies. In both nulliparas and multiparas, there were significant foreshortenings of the latent phase. In the active phase, the maximum slopes of dilatation were essentially identical. This was offset, however, by slight and statistically insignificant prolongation of the active-phase duration. The deceleration phase was similarly prolonged, especially in multiparas in whom it reached statistical significance. The absolute magnitude of the deceleration phase prolongation did not completely account for the overall prolongation of the active phase. This

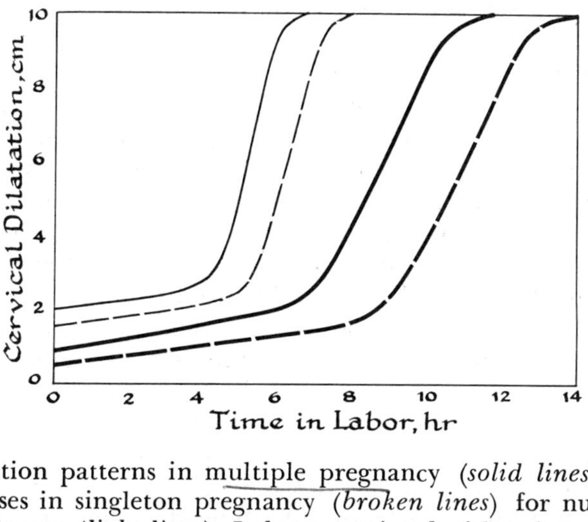


*Fig. 41.* Dilatation patterns in multiple pregnancy (*solid lines*), as compared with labor courses in singleton pregnancy (*broken lines*) for nulliparas (*heavy lines*) and multiparas (*light lines*). Labors associated with twins are characterized by longer latent phase and a slightly lengthened active phase based on longer acceleration and deceleration components (but essentially unaltered phase of maximum slope). Not illustrated are the somewhat longer second stage and diminished maximum slope of descent.

*Table 40. LABOR DATA IN MULTIPLE PREGNANCY*

| *Pregnancy Groups* | *Latent Phase (hr)* | *Active Phase (hr)* | *Maximum Dilatation (cm/hr)* | *Deceleration Phase (hr)* | *Maximum Descent (cm/hr)* | *Second Stage (hr)* |
|---|---|---|---|---|---|---|
| Nulliparas | | | | | | |
| Singleton | 8.6±0.27 | 4.9±0.15 | 3.0±0.08 | 0.90±0.05 | 3.2±0.10 | 0.95±0.04 |
| Multiple | 6.2±0.82* | 5.4±0.51 | 3.0±0.40 | 1.26±0.26 | 2.7±0.42 | 1.05±0.16 |
| Multiparas | | | | | | |
| Singleton | 5.3±0.19 | 2.2±0.07 | 5.7±0.16 | 0.23±0.01 | 6.0±0.20 | 0.24±0.01 |
| Multiple | 4.0±0.39* | 2.6±0.27 | 5.5±0.36 | 0.42±0.05* | 4.7±0.40* | 0.39±0.04* |

* Statistically significant, $p < 0.01$.

implied that the acceleration phase of the active phase was also prolonged. These alterations were carried into the second stage and were reflected in the maximum slope of descent as well.

These paradoxical data indicated that labor in multiple pregnancy was associated with both shortened latent phase and lengthened active phase and second stage. Furthermore, the total duration of labor overall tended to be shorter with twin pregnancies than with singleton pregnancies. The larger magnitude of the foreshortening in the latent phase overshadowed the relatively smaller prolongation of the active phase and second stage. The total length of the average nulliparous labor with twins was 12.7 hours and with singleton pregnancies, 14.5 hours; multiparas with twins averaged 7.0 hours in labor and those with singleton pregnancies, 7.8 hours. Although these differences were not statistically significant, they showed that previous studies based solely on total duration of the first stage were perhaps misleading and lent themselves to misinterpretation.

Additionally, it was felt necessary to verify that the changes seen in the labor patterns were specifically related to degrees of uterine overdistention. In order to determine the relative effect of gradations in overdistention, we classified patients according to total infant weight. It was assumed this might provide a rough measure of the amount of uterine stretching that had been attained. This was especially relevant in view of the large numbers of premature infants in this series. It was conjectured that the mere presence of a multiple pregnancy did not necessarily mean that there was physiologic overdistention present. It was, unfortunately, impossible to take into account the total volume of the uterus by including the amount of amniotic fluid present. Subjective estimates of volume are acknowledged to be grossly inaccurate.

Data were grouped (Table 41) according to combined fetal weight in 1000-g increments. Composite labor data showed no specific changes in durations of latent phase with increasing uterine distention. However, there were definite trends in active-phase progression. With increasing birth weight, there was prolongation of the active and deceleration phases, together with

*Table 41. LABOR DATA BY INCREASING COMBINED TWIN INFANT WEIGHT*

| *Infant Weight (g)* | *Latent Phase (hr)* | *Active Phase* (hr)* | *Maximum Dilatation* (cm/hr)* | *Deceleration Phase* (hr)* | *Maximum Descent* (cm/hr)* | *Second Stage (hr)* |
|---|---|---|---|---|---|---|
| Nulliparas | | | | | | |
| <4000 | 7.1±1.82 | 4.1±0.56 | 3.4±0.62 | 0.54±0.09 | 3.7±0.58 | 0.49±0.08 |
| 4000–4999 | 4.5±0.69 | 5.0±0.91 | 3.3±0.85 | 1.71±0.60 | 3.4±0.68 | 1.26±0.34 |
| 5000+ | 7.8±1.77 | 6.7±0.89 | 2.5±0.43 | 1.28±0.26 | 2.8±0.50 | 1.14±0.19 |
| Multiparas | | | | | | |
| <4000 | 5.6±1.46 | 2.2±0.31 | 5.9±0.90 | 0.37±0.07 | 6.2±0.78 | 0.53±0.09 |
| 4000–4999 | 3.8±0.73 | 2.0±0.27 | 6.4±0.81 | 0.24±0.04 | 5.9±0.76 | 0.28±0.03 |
| 5000–5999 | 3.3±0.41 | 3.1±0.58 | 5.2±0.51 | 0.48±0.10 | 5.3±0.54 | 0.41±0.06 |
| 6000+ | 4.5±0.92 | 3.0±0.58 | 4.5±0.77 | 0.64±0.16 | 4.8±0.72 | 0.35±0.11 |

* Statistically significant trends, $p < 0.01$.

progressive diminution in the maximum slopes of dilatation and descent. These trends were rather clear-cut.

Thus, we have confirmation of the basic initial assertion that overdistention of the uterus is associated with prolongation and general slowing of progress in the active phase. At the same time, overdistention appears not to affect the latent phase in any discernibly adverse way. Indeed, the foreshortening of the latent phase in multiple pregnancies persists in all groups regardless of the degree of overdistention.

An explanation for this latter phenomenon was desired. Exploring the lead suggested by Eastman (1961), we examined our material with regard to the prelabor cervical dilatation that had been attained. We have already detailed the influence of initial cervical dilatation on the course of labor, particularly as it affects the duration of the latent phase (see Chapter 16). Among patients with multiple pregnancy, the distribution of initial dilatation was considerably different from that in singleton pregnancies. For example, 62.0 percent of nulliparas with single births start labor with dilatation of less than 2 cm; this contrasts sharply with 25.8 percent in twin pregnancies. At the other extreme, 7.2 percent of singleton labors begin with 3 cm of dilatation or more, compared with 39.4 percent in twin labors. Moreover, only 2.2 percent of singleton labors start with 4 cm of cervical dilatation or more, versus 19.7 percent in twin labors. Comparable findings were encountered among multiparas as well. The marked contrast was noteworthy and confirmed the need for fuller consideration of this factor.

The labor data were subdivided according to initial cervical dilatation so that the influence of this factor might be weighed more objectively. Analysis carried out in this way revealed interesting findings (Table 42). The apparent foreshortening of the latent phase that had been encountered in the composite twin group (see above) was completely erased when comparable subgroups were examined simultaneously. However, the effect did not carry

*Table 42. LATENT-PHASE DURATION BY PRELABOR CERVICAL DILATATION IN MULTIPLE PREGNANCY*

| *Initial Cervical Dilatation (cm)* | *Nulliparas* | | *Multiparas* | |
|---|---|---|---|---|
| | SINGLETON | MULTIPLE | SINGLETON | MULTIPLE |
| 1.0–1.9 | 8.6±0.29 | 7.3±1.53 | 5.3±0.20 | 7.1±1.73 |
| 2.0–2.9 | 6.6±0.64 | 6.4±2.00 | 4.0±0.42 | 3.8±0.67 |
| 3.0–3.9 | 4.9±0.60 | 7.4±1.73 | 4.2±0.28 | 3.9±0.75 |
| 4.0+ | 4.5±0.91 | 4.0±0.86 | 3.4±0.39 | 3.0±0.48 |

through into similar comparisons of data on the subsequent course of labor. Here, in every subgroup in both nulliparas and multiparas, the active-phase duration was longer than in comparable singleton pregnancies. The same observation applied to other differences that had previously been noted to exist, namely, in deceleration-phase and second-stage durations as well as in maximum slopes of dilatation and descent. Thus, we appear to be able to account for all the effects on latent phase by merely considering the factor of prelabor cervical dilatation in multiple pregnancies.

Earlier, we noted that the factors of heavy sedation and uterotonic stimulation may also have affected the course of labor in these patients. It was felt necessary to evaluate the potential influence of these factors, therefore. The usual technique for providing correction, involving idealization of the labor data (see Chapter 7), was inapplicable here because of the high incidence of prematurity and the unusual distribution of initial cervical dilatation. Accordingly, it was necessary to resort to use of matched pairs. Patients were matched by such factors as maternal age, parity, the presenting infant's birth weight, fetal position, use and degree of analgesia, uterotonic stimulation, and conduction anesthesia.

When this was accomplished, the labor data (Table 43) that were compiled revealed essentially the same changes that had been seen earlier (Table 40) among unmatched cases. These included significant foreshortening of the latent phase and prolongation of the deceleration phase and second stage, together with decreased maximum slope of descent. When still more critical matching was accomplished to take into account the factor of initial cervical dilatation, the labor data precisely paralleled the information shown

*Table 43. LABOR DATA FOR MATCHED MULTIPARAS WITH TWINS*

| *Pregnancy Group* | *Latent Phase (hr)* | *Active Phase (hr)* | *Maximum Dilatation (cm/hr)* | *Deceleration Phase (hr)* | *Maximum Descent (cm/hr)* | *Second Stage (hr)* |
|---|---|---|---|---|---|---|
| Singleton | 5.6±0.76 | 1.8±0.17 | 6.3±0.63 | 0.15±0.02 | 6.8±0.44 | 0.16±0.02 |
| Multiple | 2.7±0.39* | 1.8±0.17 | 6.6±0.76 | 0.26±0.04* | 5.0±0.54* | 0.31±0.04* |

* Statistically significant, $p < 0.01$.

in Table 43, except for the latent-phase duration. When corrected in this manner according to initial cervical dilatation, the latent-phase durations in singleton and multiple pregnancies were identical.

Dysfunctional labor patterns were encountered significantly more often among multiple pregnancies than expected in both nulliparas and multiparas. All aberrations were represented, including prolonged latent-phase, protraction, and arrest disorders. In nulliparas, one-third of gravidas with twin gestation presented some form of dysfunctional pattern in the active phase; one-sixth of the multiparas were similarly affected. The most noteworthy increase was seen in cases with protraction disorders; these included 21.2 percent of nulliparas and 10.2 percent of multiparas (4.8 and 0.3 percent expected among singleton pregnancies). This finding, together with the high rate of arrest disorders, strongly corroborated the postulation by Eastman (1961) that multiple gestation was commonly associated with disordered labor patterns.

These findings lead one inevitably to the conclusion that the labor pattern in association with multiple pregnancy is significantly altered. First, because of the high incidence of major degrees of prelabor cervical dilatation, one finds a clearly defined foreshortening of the latent phase. Second, the associated uterine overdistention appears to result in protraction of the course of the active phase; this is particularly noteworthy during the deceleration phase and is reflected in the slope of descent. The combination of both influences tends to maintain the total duration of labor within a relatively normal range.

## *HYDRAMNIOS*

It is generally agreed that labor is prolonged in association with the uterine overdistention of hydramnios. Caldeyro-Barcia et al (1957) were able to demonstrate objectively that the overstretched myometrium retained its ability to contract strongly. Nevertheless, the contractions were of low intensity. It was presumed on this basis that associated labors must necessarily progress more slowly than normal. Furthermore, it was asserted that correcting the overdistention by withdrawal of the excess fluid returned myometrial contractility toward normal, thereby producing labor acceleration. Whether or not this assumption is correct remains to be determined. It is mere conjecture to relate the observed diminution in peak uterine contractility directly to a probable slowing of the progress of labor. The dissociation that may exist between contractions and actual labor progression was seen in association with other conditions and may also be relevant here. Moreover, the demonstrated sustained increase in basal tonus might somehow be compensatory and contribute a normalizing influence.

In order to demonstrate whether or not the actual course of labor is affected by hydramnios, investigations were undertaken in depth (Friedman and Sachtleben, 1964b). The approach was the same as that utilized for defining the effects of multiple pregnancy on labor (see above). It was of interest that in 16.9 percent of our cases, hydramnios was concurrent with multiple pregnancy. This was considerably higher than the expected incidence of 5 to 7 percent twins in our gravid population at large, and reflected the recognized correlation between twinning and hydramnios.

Maternal age, race, and parity were comparable to the general hospital population, but the incidence of prematurity was very high (40.3 versus 5.2 percent). As a concomitant of prematurity, malpresentations occurred in excessive numbers, including 5.8 percent breech, 3.8 percent brow, and 1.9 percent transverse lie. As to factors that might affect the course of labor, both oxytocin infusion and heavy sedation were given in expected frequencies.

## *Labor Course*

The labor data compiled for this series of patients with hydramnios (Table 44) were interesting only insofar as they reflected no adverse effects. Even when we confined our observations to those gravidas with hydramnios giving birth to infants weighing 2500 g or more, thereby eliminating the factor of prematurity from consideration, we could uncover no deleterious influence from the hydramnios. Indeed, in nulliparas (Fig. 42) there was a definite foreshortening of the active- and deceleration-phase durations, but the maximum slopes of dilatation and descent were only slightly increased.

These findings are in sharp contrast to the widely accepted contention that hydramnios produces prolonged labors. No objective evidence that progress was delayed could be found. On the contrary, labors among nulliparas with hydramnios were actually shorter than the average total duration for normal nulliparas, although the differences were relatively small.

These results are also distinctly different from those encountered in labors associated with multiple pregnancy (see above). With twins, foreshortening of the latent phase was ascribed to the degree of prelabor cervical dilatation that had been attained; the apparent slowing of progress in the active phase was attributed to uterine overdistention. In view of these seemingly para-

*Table 44. LABOR DATA IN HYDRAMNIOS*

| *Pregnancy Group* | *Latent Phase (hr)* | *Active Phase (hr)* | *Maximum Dilatation (cm/hr)* | *Deceleration Phase (hr)* | *Maximum Descent (cm/hr)* | *Second Stage (hr)* |
|---|---|---|---|---|---|---|
| Nulliparas | | | | | | |
| Normal | 8.6±0.27 | 4.9±0.15 | 3.0±0.08 | 0.90±0 05 | 0.32±0.10 | 0.95±0.04 |
| Hydramnios | 8.4±2.11 | 3.1±0.64* | 4.3±0.87 | 0.50±0.12* | 0.36±0.72 | 0.92±0.31 |
| Hydramnios at term | 8.6±2.33 | 3.2±0.68 | 3.8±0.64 | 0.57±0.12* | 0.34±0.68 | 1.09±0.31 |
| Multiparas | | | | | | |
| Normal | 5.3±0.19 | 2.2±0.07 | 5.7±0.16 | 0.23±0.01 | 6.0 ±0.20 | 0.29±0.01 |
| Hydramnios | 5.2±0.75 | 2.2±0.23 | 6.1±0.47 | 0.40±0.11 | 6.3 ±0.40 | 0.27±0.06 |
| Hydramnios at term | 4.5±0.64 | 2.1±0.29 | 6.1±0.47 | 0.40±0.14 | 6.3 ±0.42 | 0.27±0.08 |

* Statistically significant, $p < 0.01$.

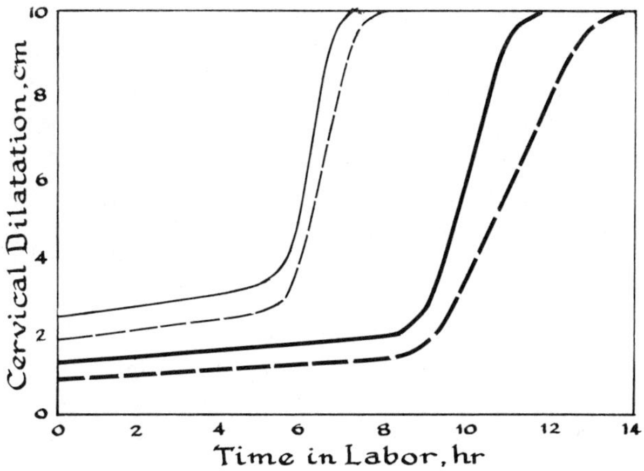


*Fig. 42.* Labor course in patients with hydramnios (*solid lines*) versus labor course in normal gravidas (*broken lines*), nulliparas (*heavy lines*), and multiparas (*light lines*) considered separately, demonstrating comparable latent-phase durations but foreshortened active phases as a consequence of the somewhat more rapid rates of dilatation that occur. A similar increase (not shown) in the slopes of descent is also encountered with hydramnios.

doxical results, reevaluation of these factors among patients with hydramnios was in order.

The distribution of initial cervical dilatation paralleled the distribution in gravidas with multiple pregnancy. Cervical dilatation of 3 cm or greater at the onset of labor was found in 25.0 percent of nulliparas with hydramnios and 45.0 percent of multiparas, both considerably in excess of expected frequencies (7.2 and 22.6 percent, respectively). On this basis alone, the latent phase in hydramnios should have been shortened. Since this was not the case, we must infer that there may be a relative slowing of progress of labor during the latent phase.

Closer examination on the basis of initial dilatation, however, clarifies this matter. We grouped women with hydramnios according to prelabor cervical dilatation that had been achieved. This yielded information on latent-phase duration, showing it to be entirely comparable in length to that expected in gravidas who had the same prelabor dilatation but without hydramnios. Thus, since the latent phase is actually not prolonged when this factor is taken into account, we are unable to implicate hydramnios as contributing to the slowing of progress here.

We might also presume that low infant weight could correct a potentially deleterious effect from overdistention due to hydramnios. Therefore, appropriate adjustments had to be made for this factor. Stratifying by birth weight so as to examine only those delivering term-sized babies (Table 44) yielded labor data showing unchanged patterns.

Myometrial suppression due to overdistention has been ameliorated by means of withdrawing excessive fluid (Caldeyro-Barcia et al, 1957). It was, therefore, felt essential to determine the effect, if any, of timely amniotomy. Our investigations showed that in two-thirds of patients with hydramnios, the membranes had not ruptured prior to the beginning of the active phase of dilatation and in one-third, the membranes remained intact well into the second stage. Patients were accordingly grouped by the time of membrane rupture: before or during the latent phase, during the active phase, or during the second stage. Labor data derived from these groups (Table 45) showed no significant differences among them. There was a slight but insignificant trend in the accumulated data toward lengthening of the latent phase in patients with membranes left intact until late in labor. At the same time, there was somewhat of an increase in the rates of active dilatation and descent. These were not reflected in consistent changes in the durations of active or deceleration phases.

*Table 45. LABOR DATA BY MEMBRANE STATUS IN HYDRAMNIOS*

| *Time of Rupture* | *Latent Phase (hr)* | *Active Phase (hr)* | *Maximum Dilatation (cm/hr)* | *Deceleration Phase (hr)* | *Maximum Descent (cm/hr)* | *Second Stage (hr)* |
|---|---|---|---|---|---|---|
| Latent phase | 5.2±1.12 | 2.2±0.41 | 5.3±0.74 | 0.36±0.09 | 5.5±0.80 | 0.37±0.07 |
| Active phase | 6.2±1.32 | 2.7±0.44 | 5.9±0.67 | 0.53±0.22 | 6.0±0.77 | 0.41±0.20 |
| Second stage | 6.6±1.52 | 2.3±0.27 | 6.0±0.75 | 0.37±0.08 | 6.2±0.79 | 0.49±0.16 |

At first, this was thought to represent a partial confirmation of the implication that the contractions of low intensity seen in hydramnios produce slowed labor. The latent-phase duration seemed especially to reflect this phenomenon. However, the rest of labor did not. In fact, the maximum slopes of dilatation and descent appeared to present contradictory information. Of course, paradoxical alterations in the latent phase may have been the result of influences quite distinct from those of uterine overdistention. This was indicated by the finding that one-third of the patients whose membranes had ruptured early in labor received uterotonic stimulation. Moreover, premature rupture of the membranes was a common finding in this group. It has been amply documented that latent-phase duration is expectedly foreshortened in association with premature spontaneous rupture of the membranes (see above). Thus, serious doubts are raised as to the real significance of the latent-phase data here. On the other hand, the findings with regard to maximum slopes of dilatation and descent take on somewhat greater significance.

Any possible effect that the factor of hydramnios had on labor may thus be masked in unpredictable ways by other factors, such as rupture of the membranes, sedation, or stimulation. In order to reduce such inherent analytic pitfalls, matched pairs of cases were examined. This was expected to allow us to compile groups in which many unrelated variables are maintained constant in order to assess more critically the true effect of the single factor under study. Patients with hydramnios were paired with normal gravidas according to such factors as age, parity, sedation, stimulation, anesthesia, analgesia, fetal weight and position, as well as pertinent items of time of rupture of the membranes and initial cervical dilatation. The labor data derived from these groups (Table 46) showed no important differences.

*Table 46. LABOR DATA IN HYDRAMNIOS BY MATCHED PAIRS*

| *Pregnancy Group* | *Latent Phase (hr)* | *Active Phase (hr)* | *Maximum Dilatation (cm/hr)* | *Deceleration Phase (hr)* | *Maximum Descent (cm/hr)* | *Second Stage (hr)* |
|---|---|---|---|---|---|---|
| Normal | 5.5±0.89 | 2.2±0.07 | 6.4±1.08 | 0.28±0.06 | 6.6±0.98 | 0.20±0.05 |
| Hydramnios | 4.7±0.75 | 2.0±0.30 | 6.7±0.64 | 0.21±0.05 | 6.8±0.78 | 0.13±0.05 |

These findings require some explanation. On the one hand, we may presume that the aforementioned suppression of myometrial activity does not actually slow the clinical course of labor. On the other hand, it is possible that measures utilized for the management of these labors succeed in correcting the myometrial dysfunction. Indeed, the high incidence of dysfunctional patterns (see below) found among them gives more support to this second possibility. In either event, the overall course of labor in association with hydramnios is rather normal.

Major disorders of labor occurred in 16.7 percent of nulliparas and 12.5 percent of multiparas with hydramnios. The exceedingly high incidence of protraction disorders found with multiple pregnancies was not duplicated here. There was fairly even distribution among prolonged latent phase, protraction disorders, and arrest disorders in the hydramnios series.

Objective findings tend to exculpate hydramnios as a primary contributor to the prolongation of labor. This is in contradiction to current popular belief. Even though dysfunctional labor frequently does occur in patients with hydramnios, the composite labor pattern falls within normal limits. Actually, labor tends to be somewhat shorter than in comparable normal cases, although the differences are small. We are consistently unable to demonstrate any objective evidence of delay in labor progression. In general, the dilatation and descent patterns in patients with hydramnios are normal. Good responses are seen either to nonintervention or to amniotomy among patients with disordered labors. These observations clearly illustrate the relatively inconsequential nature of any possible deleterious effect due to hydramnios, if any does exist, and the ease with which such an effect is corrected.

Our data do not refute the studies of Caldeyro-Barcia et al (1957) purporting to show myometrial suppression due to overdistention of the uterus. Our data merely question the assumption that progress in labor must directly mirror the amplitude and frequency of uterine contractions. It is possible that other factors are acting to compensate for the depression of myometrial function in hydramnios. We may conjecture, for example, that a prime compensatory mechanism is the increased basal tonus. It may serve to place a continuous stress of long duration in the form of circumferential forces acting to dilate the cervix. This feature of uterine contractility as a force acting to effect uterine work (in dilating the cervix, for example) is generally not taken into account in assessing myometrial function. When amniotic fluid is released, the basal tonus tends to be diminished and the intermittent myometrial contractions are augmented. It is conceivable that the mechanical forces acting to dilate the cervix may thus be more or less equivalent in their effects before and after amniotomy.

In dysfunctional labors, the force exerted by the increased basal tonus may be insufficient to produce normal dilatation and descent patterns. Following amniotomy good response may be expected and was occasionally seen. However, similar responses were encountered in some patients whose dysfunctional labor pattern was treated expectantly. In none was the result dramatic—that is, the established course of labor did not change significantly—although progress continued without abatement until delivery. Regardless of possible theoretical explanations, these findings seem to be representative of the clinical course of labor that should occur in association with hydramnios.

## *PLACENTAL SITE*

High implantation of the placenta has been proposed as possibly related to prolonged labor (Csapo, 1963a). Csapo's idea that the placenta releases its progesterone locally, thereby blocking the intrinsic spontaneous activity of the myometrium, especially in the region of the placenta, supports this contention (Csapo, 1956). Earlier onset of labor, averaging 4 days, was reported (Harris, 1975) in patients with placental implantation in the right upper quadrant of the uterus, as compared with left upper quadrant sites. This supported the concept that a pacemaker may exist at the right cornu. Csapo has presented evidence attempting to verify the association of prolonged labor with fundal implantation of the placenta (Csapo, 1959, 1963a, 1963b, 1970). In order to substantiate or refute this theory, additional objective data were sought (Little and Friedman, 1964). Our purpose was to try to elucidate the relationship between placental site and labor progress.

Placental location in the uterus was determined by measuring the shortest distance from the placental margin to the free edge of the chorioamniotic membranes. This method and its reliability were detailed (Little, 1964). The cases that were selected included gravidas who had single births with membranes complete. A large series, exceeding 10,000 patients, was analyzed.

The median placental distance from the membrane opening was 5 to 9 cm, encompassing 39 percent of all cases. Those cases in which the minimum membrane width was greater than 10 cm were considered to represent upper uterine segment implantations. Any errors due to the examination technique would tend to classify the placenta into cases with lower position in the uterus—that is, closer to the cervix by virtue of the shorter distance from placental edge to membrane edge as a result, say, of tearing of the membranes during the delivery. It was fully realized that some of the placentas assigned to the low group may actually have been located higher in the uterus.

There were no significant variations in the distributions of the placental site by maternal age or length of gestation. Despite the lack of variation by age, there was a slight yet significant tendency for the placentas of nulliparas to be located in the lower portions of the uterus. This finding was rather inconsistent with the generally accepted association of placenta previa with multiparity. The discrepancy could not be explained away on the basis of patients having been delivered by cesarean section for placenta previa.

There were also no relevant differences in the type of vaginal delivery, although there was a tendency (statistically insignificant) for breech presentation to be associated with high implantation. The lengths of the various stages of labor (Table 47) were essentially identical for all placental site groups. Since the most reliable measurements were expected to be found in the high implantation groups, these were carefully examined. There was no evidence of any association with prolonged labor.

*Table 47. PLACENTAL SITE DISTRIBUTION BY LABOR DURATION (percentages)*

| *Duration (hr)* | *Placental Site (cm)* | | | | | |
|---|---|---|---|---|---|---|
| | 0 | 1–4 | 5–9 | 10–14 | 15–19 | 19+ |
| First stage | | | | | | |
| <3 | 19.9 | 18.0 | 21.1 | 18.2 | 14.3 | 26.9 |
| 3–7 | 39.9 | 41.2 | 41.6 | 39.5 | 49.4 | 38.5 |
| 7–20 | 36.6 | 37.3 | 34.2 | 39.7 | 31.8 | 26.9 |
| 20+ | 3.6 | 3.5 | 3.1 | 2.6 | 4.5 | 7.7 |
| Second stage | | | | | | |
| <0.5 | 66.1 | 69.2 | 73.0 | 70.6 | 71.8 | 80.8 |
| 0.5–2 | 29.1 | 26.6 | 24.3 | 26.9 | 25.6 | 19.2 |
| 2+ | 4.8 | 4.2 | 2.7 | 2.5 | 2.6 | 0 |

Additional confirmation was seen in the absence of a relationship between the placental site and the incidence of clinical forms of disordered labor. More recent study of data obtained by graphic analytic means has confirmed these earlier results. Thus, our data suggest that placental site does not appear to have any demonstrable effect on the course of labor.

Csapo's studies (1970) of oxytocin-induced labors concluded that labors with high implantations were more likely to fail attempted induction or to require more stimulation for success. The magnitude of contractions needed, however, was unaltered. This was interpreted to mean that the unfavorable effect of placental site was mediated by changes in the character of the myometrial effort, perhaps in deranged propagation. Although the results of such studies appear to be at odds with ours, this may not be the case at all. We have repeatedly emphasized that discordance may exist between changes in contractility and the absence of corresponding change in dilatation or descent pattern. This may represent still another example of this paradoxical phenomenon.

## *PLACENTAL WEIGHT*

Along similar lines, the relationship between placental size and the course of labor deserves to be investigated. Analogous to considerations of the possible effect of placental site (see above), this bears on the issue of the blocking effect of the progesterone produced by the placenta on uterine activity, as set forth by Csapo (1955). It has been suggested by Hendricks (1966) that a correlation exists between placental weight and the length of labor. Data derived from graphic analysis of labor courses (Friedman and Sachtleben, 1969a) were felt to offer means for providing confirmation or refutation.

Labors were followed prospectively for purposes of constructing detailed dilatation and descent curves. Carefully weighed and examined placentas gave the information necessary for the ensuing analysis. Patients were grouped according to placental weight by 100-g increments. In this way, any relevant trends in the course of labor as affected by placental weight could be detected. Study was limited to gravidas delivering singleton infants weighing between 2500 and 4000 g in order to assure relative homogeneity in patient composition.

Distributions of maternal age and parity were comparable among the several subgroups. Similarly, there was relative uniformity with regard to fetal presentation, position, cephalopelvic disproportion, and the distribution of membrane rupture. There was likewise a high degree of uniformity in prelabor cervical dilatation and fetal station. The only exceptional distribution was in gravidas delivered of large placentas in whom sedatives and uterotonic stimulation were used in somewhat greater frequencies than expected.

It is well recognized that there is a close correlation between fetal size and placental size. The ratio between fetal and placental weights remains fairly constant under normal circumstances of fetoplacental development (Gruenwald and Minh, 1961; Hendricks, 1964b). This being the case, it was not unexpected to find a trend in infant weight with progressive placental weight, larger babies being associated with larger placentas. Fetal size in turn affects the course of labor (see Chapter 15). Thus, it becomes important to take the factor of birth weight into account here. Although the patient population was relatively uniform, factors of fetal size, sedation, and stimulation required special attention so that appropriate analytic corrections might be made. If not, conclusions based on the comparative labor data might otherwise be invalid.

## *Labor Course*

When patients were grouped according to parity and placental weight, the labor data proved to be comparable throughout (Table 48). There was a slight tendency for the latent- and active-phase durations in multiparas to be progressively longer with larger placentas. All other data were remarkably stable.

*Table 48. LABOR DATA BY PLACENTAL WEIGHT*

| *Placental Weight* (g) | *Latent Phase* (*hr*) | *Active Phase* (*hr*) | *Maximum Dilatation* (*cm/hr*) | *Deceleration Phase* (*hr*) | *Maximum Descent* (*cm/hr*) | *Second Stage* (*hr*) |
|---|---|---|---|---|---|---|
| Nullipara | | | | | | |
| <400 | 8.8±0.91 | 3.7±0.44 | 3.5±0.49 | 0.63±0.09 | 3.7±0.52 | 0.70±0.14 |
| 400–499 | 8.8±0.77 | 3.5±0.51 | 3.7±0.27 | 0.58±0.05 | 3.7±0.30 | 0.64±0.08 |
| 500–599 | 8.8±0.89 | 3.6±0.30 | 3.7±0.29 | 0.63±0.08 | 3.7±0.33 | 0.63±0.05 |
| 600+ | 9.2±1.38 | 3.5±0.34 | 3.2±0.37 | 0.56±0.06 | 3.4±0.40 | 0.71±0.10 |
| Multiparas | | | | | | |
| <400 | 5.9±0.80 | 1.8±0.18 | 5.4±0.47 | 0.24±0.04 | 5.5±0.51 | 0.24±0.08 |
| 400–499 | 6.6±0.71 | 2.1±0.19 | 5.8±0.39 | 0.27±0.02 | 5.8±0.42 | 0.24±0.03 |
| 500–599 | 6.0±0.67 | 2.1±0.14 | 6.0±0.41 | 0.28±0.03 | 5.8±0.44 | 0.26±0.03 |
| 600+ | 6.8±0.69 | 2.3±0.24 | 5.9±0.70 | 0.27±0.04 | 6.1±0.80 | 0.22±0.02 |

As mentioned earlier, there were some differences among these groups in fetal size, sedation, and stimulation. It was, therefore, necessary to consider the possibility that underlying trends may have been masked by these factors. Thus, the material was first reanalyzed after correcting for differences in analgesic and oxytocin usage. Newly derived data were essentially the same as the less refined data for nulliparas. In multiparas, however, the latent phase trend that was seen earlier no longer existed, whereas that for the active phase persisted without change. No new trends were uncovered by this approach.

Further breakdown of labor data according to both placental and infant weight was accomplished in order to attempt to distinguish between the relative influences of these separate factors on the course of labor. This was done for all measurable phases and slopes. Increasing fetal weight yielded progressive prolongation of all phases of labor in multiparas and of all phases except the latent phase in nulliparas. Parallel changes were not seen with increasing placental weight, however, when the fetal weight was simultaneously taken into account.

An example of this type of analysis is shown in Table 49 for active phase data in nulliparas. Horizontal tiers of data maintain a stable placental

*Table 49. LABOR DATA* BY PLACENTAL AND INFANT WEIGHT (grams)*

| Placental Weight | Infant Weight 2500–2999 | 3000–3499 | 3500–3999 |
|---|---|---|---|
| <400 | 3.5±0.48 | 3.8±0.98 | — |
| 400–499 | 3.3±0.67 | 3.5±0.44 | 3.9±0.94 |
| 500–599 | 3.0±0.37 | 3.6±0.39 | 3.9±0.85 |
| 600+ | 3.0±1.04 | 3.5±0.53 | 3.6±0.43 |

* For active-phase duration (hours) in nulliparas.

weight while indicating the trend for active-phase duration to increase with heavier infant weights. Vertical columns, on the other hand, yield essentially no trends with increasing placental weight when the infant weight is kept constant. If any tendency exists at all, it is for shorter active phases to be associated with larger placentas. This goes counter to the argument of an inhibitory effect accruing from a progesterone block. These data thus show that placental weight is unlikely to influence the course of labor; moreover, the effect of infant weight on the labor pattern is independent of any potential effect that placental weight might have.

As a critical test of whether placental weight affects labor progress, matched pairs of patients in the extreme placental weight groups (less than 400 g and more than 600 g) were examined. These patients were chosen to be comparable in as many ways as could be defined, including parity, age, sedation, stimulation, anesthesia, fetal presentation, position, and size, status of membranes, prelabor station, and dilatation. The labor data from these groups were identical, all previously encountered trends having been eliminated.

As final confirmation, each patient's labor record was examined carefully within the several placental weight subgroups to determine the incidence of disordered labor. The overall incidence was 8.4 percent, uniformly distributed in each of the groups. Thus, no relationship appeared to exist between placental weight and the frequency of dysfunctional labor, confirming our failure to verify any relationship between placental size and the course of labor.

## *LEIOMYOMATA UTERI*

There is a general clinical impression that myomas and other anatomic distortions of the uterus tend to increase the duration of labor and the frequency of abnormal labors. No studies are available to indicate whether or not this contention is true with regard to uterine anomalies, and our experience as yet has not been sufficiently large to warrant presenting detailed information here. Isolated case reports of normal labor progression serve as testimonials, however, to the probability that our impressions are incorrect.

As to labor with fibroids, this relationship has not been borne out by close scrutiny in the past. In one study of total labor duration in gravidas with fibroids, Grandin (1949) reported only 11.4 percent of labors lasting longer than 30 hours; simultaneously, there were 5.5 percent precipitate labors shorter than 3 hours in duration. Contrary but unconvincing evidence by Campbell (1933) suggests that as many as 26.2 percent have prolonged labors (not otherwise defined), while 54.1 percent have labors that are unusually short. It is clear that this matter deserves to be clarified by means of the objectivity available in the form of graphic analysis of relevant data.

Gravidas with fibroids, as expected, tend to be somewhat older than the general gravid population. Parity and gravidity are not dissimilar from that expected. However, there is a significant increase in the prematurity rate among these patients, almost twice the expected number delivering small babies. Both sedation and uterotonic stimulation were administered more often than to parturients without fibroids. The distribution of the time of membrane rupture was normal throughout. Prelabor cervical dilatation was likewise about as expected, but station at the onset of labor was relatively high, on the average. It was necessary, therefore, that these factors be taken into account in analyzing the labor course data obtained from them.

## *Labor Course*

Contrary to expectations based on clinical impression, the labor pattern (Table 50) in multiparas with fibroids was entirely normal. Moreover, in nulliparas, there was significant foreshortening of the latent, active, and deceleration phases. Comparable changes were not encountered in the maximum slopes of dilatation and descent or in the duration of the second stage.

In order to help verify and clarify these unanticipated findings, patients were grouped according to gross size of the fibroids. The only trends encoun-

*Table 50. LABOR DATA WITH LEIOMYOMATA*

| *Group* | *Latent Phase (hr)* | *Active Phase (hr)* | *Maximum Dilatation (cm/hr)* | *Deceleration Phase (hr)* | *Maximum Descent (cm/hr)* | *Second Stage (hr)* |
|---|---|---|---|---|---|---|
| Nulliparas | | | | | | |
| Normal | 8.6±0.27 | 4.9±0.15 | 3.0±0.08 | 0.90±0.05 | 3.2±0.10 | 0.95±0.04 |
| Fibroid | 6.3±0.51* | 3.9±0.28* | 3.1±0.20 | 0.56±0.07* | 3.3±0.24 | 0.83±0.12 |
| Multiparas | | | | | | |
| Normal | 5.3±0.19 | 2.2±0.07 | 5.7±0.16 | 0.23±0.01 | 6.0±0.20 | 0.24±0.01 |
| Fibroid | 5.1±0.45 | 2.2±0.13 | 5.9±0.39 | 0.24±0.03 | 6.1±0.42 | 0.20±0.03 |
| Matched Nulliparas | | | | | | |
| Normal | 7.3±0.82 | 4.1±0.49 | 2.9±0.25 | 0.64±0.08 | 3.2±0.22 | 1.06±0.18 |
| Fibroid | 6.9±0.88 | 4.0±0.47 | 3.2±0.30 | 0.67±0.14 | 3.3±0.31 | 0.98±0.12 |
| Matched Multiparas | | | | | | |
| Normal | 5.2±0.69 | 1.9±0.21 | 6.9±0.78 | 0.18±0.02 | 6.8±0.72 | 0.21±0.03 |
| Fibroids | 4.7±0.52 | 2.0±0.18 | 6.6±0.59 | 0.21±0.04 | 6.8±0.80 | 0.18±0.05 |

* Statistically significant, $p < 0.01$.

tered by this manipulation were those suggesting that increasing tumor size was associated with slight lengthening of the latent and deceleration phases as well as increasing maximum slope of dilatation. In multiparas, the same subclassification produced shortening of the latent phase and of the second stage. These trends were statistically insignificant but were relevant because they failed to provide consistent evidence that fibroids inhibit labor.

Special attention was directed to the location of the fibroids, particularly the intramural variety, which is felt to be most deleterious to efficient uterine action. Examining such patients showed no meaningful changes in the course of labor in nulliparas. In multiparas, there was a mere suggestion that the active-phase maximum slope was diminished somewhat, but the second stage was more rapid.

Disordered labors were not found in unusual numbers either. In nulliparas, there were 14.3 percent definable disorders; in multiparas, 10.9 percent. These were distributed among the several varieties of aberrant labors about as expected for gravidas in general.

In a final effort to ensure that factors known to inhibit or augment labor were not somehow masking an underlying effect by fibroids, matched pairs of cases were sought for purposes of critical comparison. The labor data (Table 50) from these patients clearly demonstrated that fibroids are entirely without specific influence on the course of labor.

We may conclude from these observations, therefore, that the labor that ensues in gravidas who have leiomyomata is normal in all characteristics unless acted upon by other factors present. Moreover, there is no evidence to suggest that other factors are any more likely to affect the labor adversely in these women than in normal parturients.

# Maternal Conditions

## CHAPTER 18

Multiparas with severe anemia may have slow labor progress; this is not the case in anemic nulliparas. Gravidas with febrile conditions fall into two groups: some are characterized by rapid labors, others by abnormally slow progress, apparently due to disparate conditions prevailing when labor was triggered to begin by the infection. Parturient cardiacs experience labors essentially comparable to those without heart disease. Labor in patients with neurologic disorders involving motor function is normal on the average, but the descent process may be delayed as a consequence of poor or absent expulsive efforts. The psychologic state of the gravida cannot yet be shown to affect the labor pattern.

Obstetrics is replete with dogmas and old-wives' tales about the course of labor generally expected to occur in association with various disease states. Generally unsupported except by clinical impression, these pronouncements deserve to be probed. In this chapter we will review available objective evidence on the labor patterns of gravidas with various conditions, including anemia, cardiopathy, infection, and neuromuscular and psychiatric problems.

### *MATERNAL ANEMIA*

It has been conjectured that the amount of circulating hemoglobin may be related to the myoglobin content of muscle, since both compete for available iron stores. Such stores may be severely limited in anemic patients. Since myoglobin is a fundamental element for uterine contraction, it is probable that the efficiency of labor is a function of its concentration in the myometrium. The hemoglobin level, therefore, may mirror myoglobin concentrations in the myometrium, and labor may vary accordingly.

Anemia may affect the course of labor in other ways as well. For example, it is generally recognized (Harrison and Ibeziako, 1973) that a significant correlation exists between uncorrected anemia and birth weight. Retarded fetal growth results from severe anemia. Small fetuses in turn are associated with altered labor patterns (see Chapter 15).

In order to determine whether maternal anemia alters the course of labor, a large series of gravidas was studied. The group consisted of 252 nulliparas and 257 multiparas. They were surveyed with regard to pertinent obstetric data, hemoglobin levels, and labor courses. While the distribution of hemoglobin values was normal, the modal value occurred at 11.0 g-percent and ranged from 6.5 to 18.0 g-percent. Blood levels referred specifically to those obtained just prior to or early in labor.

The average age was identical with comparable patients from our gravid population at large, but showed interesting trends in the several subgroups according to hemoglobin level. For example, among nulliparas, there was a distinctive tendency for younger patients to be more anemic. The same trend was encountered in multiparas, but the correlation was less clear. This confirms the tenet that young gravidas, especially teenagers, are less likely to have adequate preventive or corrective prenatal care. Along similar lines, our data confirmed the relationship between anemia and the birth of small babies, weighing less than 2500 g (Table 51). These resulted both from premature delivery and intrauterine growth retardation. This relationship is, of course, not unexpected. There is adequate documentation of increased prematurity rates among debilitated, undernourished, and indigent patients.

Distributions of factors such as fetal presentation and position, time of rupture of the membranes, cephalopelvic relationships, type and degree of sedation and stimulation were all uniform throughout the various hemoglobin subgroups. Conduction anesthesia was found to have been administered consistently more often in nulliparas with higher hemoglobin levels, perhaps reflecting the preference for this type of anesthesia among more affluent patients and their physicians. The distribution of parity was unusual among multiparas in that there was an obvious trend for the more anemic patients to have had more prior viable pregnancies. The association of anemia with grand multiparity is also well recognized.

*Table 51. AGE AND SMALL INFANT FREQUENCY BY HEMOGLOBIN LEVEL*

| *Hemoglobin* (g-%) | *Nulliparas* Age (yr.) | *Nulliparas* Infants <2500 g (%) | *Multiparas* Age (yr.) | *Multiparas* Infants <2500 g (%) |
|---|---|---|---|---|
| <10.0 | 22.9 | 15.2 | 27.9 | 9.6 |
| 10.0–10.9 | 23.5 | 13.4 | 27.3 | 4.6 |
| 11.0–11.9 | 24.0 | 3.1 | 28.4 | 1.4 |
| 12.0–12.9 | 24.9 | 5.1 | 28.7 | 7.5 |
| 13.0+ | 25.5 | 10.3 | 29.9 | 7.1 |

The labor data of the several subgroups stratified by hemoglobin level (Table 52) showed no startling trends in nulliparas, but an impressive alteration in the average labor course in multiparas. Among nulliparas, second-stage duration increased progressively with higher hemoglobin levels. This appeared to be related to the incidence of conduction anesthesia, which had been given much more often to patients with increased hemoglobin levels. Applying suitable corrections for this discrepancy entirely erased the trend in second-stage duration. In contrast, there was a very clear trend in multiparas characterized by slowing of progression in the active phase with diminishing hemoglobin levels. This applied to the active-phase duration as well as to the maximum slopes of dilatation and descent.

*Table 52. LABOR DATA BY HEMOGLOBIN LEVEL*

| *Hemoglobin* (g) | *Latent Phase* (hr) | *Active Phase* (hr) | *Maximum Dilatation* (cm/hr) | *Deceleration Phase* (hr) | *Maximum Descent* (cm/hr) | *Second Stage* (hr) |
|---|---|---|---|---|---|---|
| Nulliparas | | | | | | |
| <10.0 | 10.4±1.49 | 5.1±0.86 | 3.1±0.48 | 0.69±0.09 | 3.3±0.54 | 0.90±0.09 |
| 10.0–10.9 | 10.4±0.97 | 5.0±0.54 | 2.8±0.23 | 0.93±0.24 | 3.0±0.50 | 1.02±0.10 |
| 11.0–11.9 | 8.9±0.84 | 5.7±0.63 | 2.7±0.21 | 1.07±0.19 | 2.8±0.38 | 1.10±0.12 |
| 12.0–12.9 | 8.2±0.81 | 4.7±0.46 | 2.9±0.21 | 0.88±0.11 | 2.7±0.40 | 1.12±0.13 |
| 13.0+ | 9.7±1.05 | 4.5±0.36 | 2.9±0.28 | 0.77±0.14 | 2.8±0.42 | 1.26±0.22 |
| Matched Nulliparas | | | | | | |
| <10.0 | 7.7±1.29 | 4.9±1.02 | 3.4±1.10 | 0.72±0.14 | 3.6±0.86 | 1.02±0.18 |
| 13.0+ | 6.6±1.21 | 4.2±0.45 | 3.7±0.44 | 0.51±0.07 | 3.8±0.68 | 1.03±0.24 |
| Multiparas | | | | | | |
| <10.0 | 5.4±0.61 | 2.5±0.30 | 5.1±0.43 | 0.26±0.04 | 5.5±0.52 | 0.26±0.04 |
| 10.0–10.9 | 5.5±0.39 | 2.4±0.20 | 5.1±0.47 | 0.28±0.06 | 5.4±0.44 | 0.26±0.03 |
| 11.0–11.9 | 5.7±0.43 | 2.4±0.17 | 4.8±0.32 | 0.23±0.03 | 5.0±0.40 | 0.24±0.03 |
| 12.0–12.9 | 5.5±0.54 | 2.2±0.19 | 5.5±0.50 | 0.24±0.04 | 5.6±0.54 | 0.19±0.02 |
| 13.0+ | 4.4±0.51 | 1.8±0.19 | 6.5±0.54 | 0.26±0.06 | 6.0±0.60 | 0.25±0.03 |
| Matched Multiparas | | | | | | |
| <10.0 | 6.7±1.26 | 2.3±0.31 | 4.9±0.74 | 0.20±0.04 | 5.2±0.80 | 0.18+0.03 |
| 13.0+ | 5.6±0.45 | 1.6±0.27 | 6.3±0.63 | 0.16±0.03 | 5.9±0.71 | 0.22±0.04 |

It was assumed that unrecognized inhibitory or stimulatory factors might be acting to bring about these changes. Accordingly, we proceeded to develop an idealized series of patients for more critical comparison (see Chapter 7). The data derived in this manner revealed no consistent trends. The tendency among nulliparas for second-stage duration to increase with increasing hemoglobin was effectively negated. This approach, however, did not eliminate the active-phase trends previously described in multiparas. Because the numbers of cases were too small, statistical validity could not be established. Even if it had been possible, it is clear that the course of labor is so minimally influenced by maternal hemoglobin levels that this factor is not very pertinent in clinical terms.

The relative frequencies of disordered labors among these subgroups were essentially identical in nulliparas, regardless of hemoglobin level. In multipparas, on the other hand, we noted remarkable increases in the incidence of dysfunctional labor patterns with diminishing hemoglobin. There was an obvious trend (Table 53) from the total absence of abnormal labors among patients with hemoglobin levels of 13.0 g-percent or greater to an incidence of 13.4 percent in those with levels of less than 10.0 g-percent. The most commonly encountered aberration of labor among anemic multiparas was prolonged latent phase, constituting 9.5 percent (as compared with 0.4 percent expected among multiparas in general). In addition, there was an unusually large number of patients with protraction disorders; these conditions are found rather exceptionally in multiparas (3.9 percent versus 0.3 percent).

*Table 53. DYSFUNCTIONAL LABOR BY HEMOGLOBIN LEVEL*

| *Hemoglobin* (g-%) | *Nulliparas* (%) | *Multiparas* (%) |
|---|---|---|
| <10.0 | 13.6 | 13.4 |
| 10.0–10.9 | 11.8 | 6.2 |
| 11.0–11.9 | 12.1 | 6.2 |
| 12.0–12.9 | 9.9 | 5.0 |
| 13.0+ | 12.8 | 0.0 |

It thus became imperative to determine whether or not there were factors present in patients with documented anemia (other than the anemia itself) that resulted in abnormally slow progress in labor. Accordingly, the extreme tail groups (that is, those with very low hemoglobin and those with adequate levels) were more closely examined, with particular attention to the labor data. Suitable corrections were applied so that the two groups would be similar in all respects except the blood picture itself. Patients were matched by appropriate selection from each group. They were found not to differ significantly from each other as far as their labor courses were concerned (Table 52). Nulliparas presented nearly identical data.

The tendency was repeated for multiparas with good hemoglobin levels to progress more rapidly in the active phase than anemic gravidas, but the differences were not statistically significant. This relationship, therefore, could not clearly be denied. Although we have not been able to demonstrate it beyond reasonable doubt, our data point to the probability that severely anemic multiparas tend to have slower and more abnormal labors in general. This occurs even though such women tend to have higher parity and smaller fetuses.

## *MATERNAL INFECTION*

Almost no documentation exists on the relationship between obstetric infections and labor. There is a widely held clinical impression that prolonged labors frequently result in puerperal infections, especially in conjunction with prolonged rupture of the membranes. In studies of dysfunctional labor patterns, however, we were unable to verify this contention. Maternal morbidity in association with the several varieties of labor disorder was found to be essentially the same as in normal labors (Friedman and Sachtleben, 1961a, 1961b, 1962a).

However, it must be pointed out that these studies were not specifically designed for investigation of prolonged rupture of the membranes. On the contrary, within these study groups, the distribution of membrane rupture was approximately the same as in the normal population. The issue of rupture of the membranes as it affects the course of labor has been discussed elsewhere (see Chapter 17). Suffice it to say that we have no objective evidence to indicate that labor aberrations per se necessarily contribute to the development of intrapartum infection. Whether preexistent infection produces abnormal labor, on the other hand, is an issue that appears never to have been raised or resolved.

An analysis has been carried out to determine the effect of intrapartum infection on the course of labor (Friedman, 1973a). A group of patients with significant fever in labor was studied, including patients with amnionitis, respiratory and urinary tract infectons. While maternal age, race, and parity distributions were about as expected, the frequency of premature infants was almost twice that of the general gravid population. Similarly, almost three times as many as expected had premature rupture of the membranes. It was clear that these differences would have to be taken into account in analyzing the effects of infection on labor.

The labor data derived from these patients (Table 54) showed that all aspects of labor were prolonged for both nulliparas and multiparas. When subjected to statistical testing, only the durations of the latent phase and the second stage in nulliparas were found to be significant. Nonetheless, the trends are apparent and worthy of our attention. Because of the high inci-

*Table 54.* *EFFECT OF FEVER ON LABOR COURSE*

| *Group* | *Latent Phase (hr)* | *Active Phase (hr)* | *Maximum Dilatation (cm/hr)* | *Deceleration Phase (hr)* | *Maximum Descent (cm/hr)* | *Second Stage (hr)* |
|---|---|---|---|---|---|---|
| Nulliparas | | | | | | |
| Afebrile | 8.6±0.3 | 4.9±0.2 | 3.0±0.1 | 0.90±0.05 | 3.2±0.2 | 0.95±0.04 |
| Febrile | 14.1±1.4* | 5.4±0.5 | 2.7±0.3 | 1.31±0.25 | 2.8±0.3 | 1.46±0.26† |
| Febrile at term | 16.1±1.7* | 6.2±0.6† | 1.9±0.2* | 1.63±0.30† | 2.0±0.2* | 1.85±0.31* |
| Multiparas | | | | | | |
| Afebrile | 5.3±0.2 | 2.2±0.1 | 5.7±0.2 | 0.23±0.01 | 6.0±0.2 | 0.24±0.01 |
| Febrile | 5.8±0.7 | 2.7±0.5 | 5.2±0.5 | 0.30±0.07 | 5.4±0.6 | 0.32±0.08 |
| Febrile at term | 6.5±1.0 | 3.2±0.8 | 4.9±0.7 | 0.37±0.12 | 5.0±0.7 | 0.39±0.12 |
| Matched pairs | | | | | | |
| Afebrile | 11.4±1.2 | 5.0±0.5 | 3.2±0.4 | 1.14±0.22 | 3.5±0.5 | 1.22±0.23 |
| Febrile | 8.7±1.0 | 4.6±0.4 | 4.3±0.4 | 0.80±0.13 | 4.2±0.4 | 1.05±0.16 |

* Statistically significant, $p < 0.01$.
† Borderline significance, $0.05 > p > 0.01$.

dence of prematurity in this group, we examined those at term separately. This resulted in an exaggeration of the aforementioned trend toward prolonged labors. In nulliparas, this effect was statistically verifiable.

There is a generally accepted clinical impression that patients with extrauterine febrile diseases—pneumonia, for example—tend to have short, premature labors. We utilized our data to attempt to test this hypothesis. The results showed that nulliparas with extrauterine infections were found to have labors that were somewhat longer than patients with amnionitis, but the differences were negligible in terms of dilatation and descent patterns.

Another contention is that fever itself may initiate labor, perhaps before optimal conditions have been reached. Our material was further analyzed, therefore, to determine the influence of prelabor fever as contrasted with that arising during the course of labor. There was essentially no difference between the two groups, except that those with fever arising prior to onset of labor tended to have somewhat more prolonged labors. Unfortunately, the numbers of patients in this subgroup were too small to permit meaningful statistical evaluation.

In order to test these implications still further, we felt it necessary to eliminate all extraneous factors; that is, all factors other than the febrile disorder under surveillance. We had in mind such factors as amniotomy, analgesia, uterotonic stimulation, intrapartum anesthesia, and fetopelvic disproportion, any of which may influence the course of labor. Accordingly, we resorted to the statistical technique of matching pairs of cases for comparison.

Patients in the febrile series were matched individually with afebrile patients according to various factors, including those just listed and others of potential significance as well, such as maternal age, gestational duration, fetal presentation and position, pelvic type, parity, birth weight, and maternal disease. Furthermore, since it is conceivable that the infection may have initiated labor under less than ideal circumstances, prelabor preparation in the form of cervical dilatation and station of the fetal presenting part was also taken into account.

The data on the courses of the labors of these subjects (Table 54) duplicated the trends showing prolongation of the various phases of labor, but none of these was found to be statistically significant. Thus, it seems from these data that fever or infection per se has no major direct effect on the course of labor. The persistent trends we encountered appear to be explainable on the basis of other factors, agents, conditions, or influences that are coexistent or preexistent in these labors.

The overall incidence of disordered labor patterns as defined by the dilatation and descent tracings was very high, totaling 71 percent in nulliparas and 20 percent in multiparas. The very common occurrence of abnormal labor was rather unexpected in view of the labor data we have just presented. Much greater evidence of the influence of such abnormal labors should have been expected in terms of more extreme prolongation of the phase durations and slowing of the rates of dilatation and descent. Although some effect was indeed encountered, it was not considered to reflect the full force of the dysfunctional patterns.

It was necessary, therefore, to consider what might have caused this paradoxical situation to occur. Indeed, the observation that dysfunctional labors occur so frequently among febrile patients stands in sharp contradistinction to the data (Table 54) purporting that there is little or no influence of fever on the course of such labors. This important discrepancy suggests the possibility that we are dealing with a heterogeneous group of patients. It is conceivable that the very slow dysfunctional varieties are counterbalanced by a group of rapid labors.

In studies of preterm labors (Friedman and Sachtleben, 1969b) two dissimilar forms of labor were found to occur in association with the birth of small infants (see Chapter 15). On a bimodal distribution curve, the more rapid group of labors could be readily distinguished from the dysfunctional. These distinctive labor groups were considered to represent separate populations of patients who were undergoing labor under disparate conditions. The prelabor preparation was believed to be somehow related to the labor that evolved. The more rapid variety of labor was deemed likely to be associated with conditions that make rapid progress feasible, such as minimal resistance and efficient, strong myometrial contractions. Dysfunctional patterns, on the other hand, reflected less favorable prevailing conditions before and during the course of the labor.

The issue of prematurity has been discussed previously (Chapter 15). Correcting for this factor by examining term labors exclusively only partially resolves this question. To determine whether or not two distinct subpopulations exist here, it was necessary to examine the distribution by labor phases more closely. A representative distribution curve for the latent phase in nulliparas is shown in Figure 43. The bimodality of this distribution stands out clearly against the slightly skewed normal distribution for nulliparas in general. This confirms the likelihood that we are dealing with two separate and distinct populations.

To delve further, we subdivided our nulliparas into two groups according to latent-phase durations longer than and shorter than 10 hours, respectively. This cut-off point was selected on the basis of the bimodal distribution pattern. It was interesting to note that 36.8 percent of patients in the group with short latent phases delivered premature infants, as contrasted with 12.0 percent in those patients with long latent phases. In the former group, 52.6 percent had premature rupture of the membranes, whereas only 20.0 percent of the latter group began labor with membranes ruptured. Prelabor preparation of the cervix was also distinctively different: 69.2 percent with foreshortened latent phases showed initial cervical dilatation of 2.0 cm or greater, and 68.8 percent in the long-latent group had dilatation of less than 2.0 cm.

These observations indicate that there is little doubt we are indeed dealing with two different groups of patients, one initiating labor under optimal conditions of prelabor preparation of soft tissues, and the other quite unprepared in that various factors are unfavorable for rapid, uninterrupted progression. The presence of resistant, relatively inelastic and unyielding cervical and vaginal tissue is undoubtedly coupled with inefficient, weak, or even

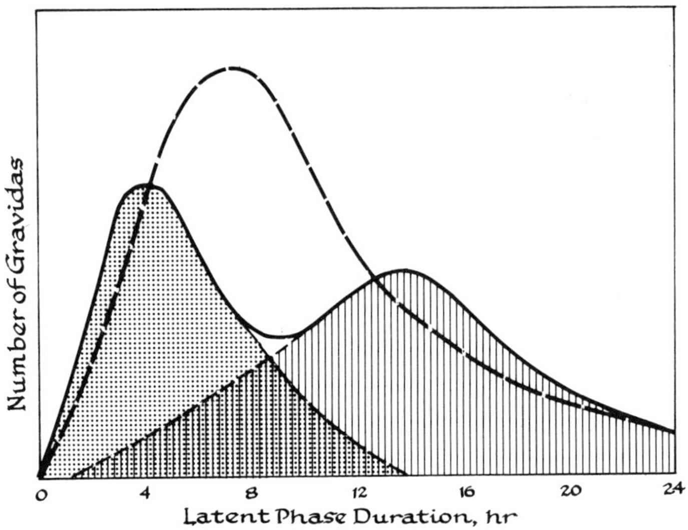


*Fig. 43.* Latent-phase duration in nulliparas, showing distribution curve for gravidas with intrapartum infection (*solid line*), contrasted with that for normal parturients (*broken line*). The bimodal distribution seen in association with infection supports the contention that they consist of two distinctly different population groups (see text).

(From Friedman EA: Obstetric infection in labor. In Charles D, Finland M (eds): Obstetric and Perinatal Infections. Philadelphia, Lea & Febiger, 1973).

dyskinetic uterine contractions in the latter group. Unfortunately, we have no documentation for this thesis.

It is reasonable, nevertheless, to conjecture that labor in the more favorable group was triggered to begin, perhaps by the febrile disorder, when everything was in readiness for the labor to begin. The ensuing labor evolved in a normal fashion. Patients with unfavorable factors, on the other hand, may be accounted for in two possible ways. First, the infection may be a secondary resultant of a long drawn-out, desultory labor. If this were frequently the case, our data comparing patients with postpartum fever and those in which the fever arose late in labor should be considerably different; instead, the differences between them are negligible.

A second and more plausible explanation invokes the consideration that the acute inflammatory process acts as a trigger mechanism for initiating labor in the fortuitous presence of conditions unfavorable for the labor to begin. There are no clear concepts today as to what factor or constellation of factors causes labor to begin under normal or abnormal circumstances. Nonetheless, we see here one group of patients in whom labor begins with conditions ideally suited for progression of normal labor patterns, and another contrasting group with quite unfavorable conditions that produce labors of poor quality or labors that are overtly abnormal.

## *CARDIOVASCULAR DISEASE*

There is a popular notion that women with cardiac disease have short, easy labors and generally deliver small babies. There is a growing body of information to confirm that cardiacs, especially those with cyanotic congenital heart disease, give birth to offspring much smaller than average size (Batson, 1974). As to whether or not they deliver prematurely, population studies suggest they do not (McGarry and Pearson, 1973), but there is no universal agreement in this regard.

Objective labor data are generally unavailable, but the investigation by McGarry and Pearson failed to show any difference in the total length of labor between women with cardiac disease and those without it. It seemed reasonable to attempt to resolve this issue by studying the labor patterns of such patients.

A total of 154 gravidas with documented rheumatic or congenital heart disease were observed in labor over a 7-year period of time, including 49 nulliparas and 105 multiparas. They tended to be somewhat younger than normal gravidas, but their prior obstetric experience was about as expected. The incidence of cephalopelvic disproportion in this group was very low, undoubtedly reflecting selection. As anticipated, there was an increased incidence of premature infants, 13.3 percent weighing less than 2500 g among nulliparas and 14.0 percent, among multiparas. The distribution of fetal presentations and positions was similar to that of the general gravid population. Similarly, the distribution of frequencies of membrane rupture was normal. Initial cervical dilatation and fetal station data were as expected also.

Differences did exist with regard to some exogenous factors known to influence labor. For example, conduction anesthesia was administered earlier and with greater frequency to many of these patients. The documented beneficial effect of this type of anesthesia for labor and delivery in cardiac gravidas is undoubtedly reflected by this practice. Sedative-analgesic agents were seldom used among these patients. By contrast, uterotonic agents were used more liberally than in normal patients.

From these data it can be seen that nearly all factors were acting to bring about a more expedient form of labor—that is, there was a relative absence of adverse influences and a relative preponderance of factors that have been documented to augment or enhance the course of labor progress. Specifically, pelvic problems were rare, there was an increased frequency of small babies, and use of sedation was diminished while oxytocin was given more frequently. It became apparent, therefore, that any evaluation of the course of labor must take these factors into account.

The labor data were studied in detail and compared with similar gravidas who did not have heart disease (Table 55). Clear-cut foreshortening of the deceleration phase and second stage was encountered in nulliparas, together with diminution in the slope of descent. In multiparas, only slight lengthening of the deceleration phase was encountered, and this was of bor-

*Table 55. LABOR DATA IN CARDIAC GRAVIDAS*

| Group | Latent Phase (hr) | Active Phase (hr) | Maximum Dilatation (cm/hr) | Deceleration Phase (hr) | Maximum Descent (cm/hr) | Second Stage (hr) |
|---|---|---|---|---|---|---|
| Nulliparas | | | | | | |
| Mean | 8.6±0.27 | 4.9±0.15 | 3.0±0.08 | 0.90±0.05 | 3.2±0.10 | 0.95±0.04 |
| Cardiacs | 7.8±0.92 | 4.3±0.31 | 3.2±0.43 | 0.62±0.06* | 2.6±0.21* | 0.72±0.07* |
| Class A | 7.3±0.99 | 4.4±0.38 | 3.1±0.63 | 0.65±0.07* | 2.7±0.16* | 0.66±0.09* |
| Class B and C | 8.6±1.29 | 4.1±0.56 | 3.3±0.51 | 0.58±0.10* | 2.4±0.24* | 0.83±0.11 |
| Matched pairs | | | | | | |
| Normal | 6.8±1.16 | 3.9±0.45 | 2.7±0.33 | 0.60±0.09 | 3.0±0.32 | 0.84±0.13 |
| Cardiacs | 8.7±1.30 | 4.5±0.60 | 3.0±0.54 | 0.62±0.07 | 2.6±0.40 | 0.73±0.14 |
| Multiparas | | | | | | |
| Mean | 5.3±0.19 | 2.2±0.07 | 5.7±0.16 | 0.23±0.01 | 6.0±0.20 | 0.24±0.01 |
| Cardiacs | 5.2±0.40 | 2.4±0.14 | 5.5±0.33 | 0.33±0.04† | 5.4±0.30 | 0.26±0.03 |
| Class A | 5.3±0.47 | 2.3±0.15 | 5.6±0.38 | 0.32±0.04† | 5.5±0.40 | 0.25±0.04 |
| Class B and C | 4.9±0.75 | 2.5±0.30 | 5.2±0.66 | 0.34±0.06 | 5.2±0.46 | 0.26±0.06 |
| Matched pairs | | | | | | |
| Normal | 4.7±0.81 | 1.9±0.24 | 6.6±1.03 | 0.18±0.03 | 6.4±0.82 | 0.27±0.04 |
| Cardiacs | 5.0±0.81 | 2.2±0.27 | 5.9±0.95 | 0.26±0.04 | 5.7±0.68 | 0.18±0.04 |

* Statistically significant difference, $p < 0.01$.
† Borderline significance, $0.01 < p < 0.05$.

derline significance. Aside from these negligible differences from normal, labor among cardiac patients was essentially the same as in normal parturients. When the material was further broken down according to functional cardiac classification, no additional trends were encountered.

Despite these findings, an increased incidence of dysfunctional labor patterns was seen, totaling 18.4 percent in nulliparas and 13.3 percent in multiparas. The disorders were distributed among all varieties of aberrations but concentrated somewhat in protraction and arrest problems. Conduction anesthesia could be incriminated in many of these cases as possibly etiologic because it had been given too early, to too high a level, or in conjunction with excessive sedative medication. However, it could not be determined whether or not the cardiac condition might also have been a contributing factor here. This is a particularly pertinent question in view of the beneficial factors that were acting to influence the course of labor in these cases.

Accordingly, it was necessary to examine this material by special statistical techniques. Pairs of cases were matched for a series of miscellaneous factors so that two groups of comparable patients could be examined to learn the real effects of cardiac disease on labor, if any. We found (Table 55) that the previously seen changes in labor pattern entirely vanished, except for persistently prolonged deceleration-phase duration in multiparas (not statistically significant). This finding was reminiscent of the prolongation in deceleration phase seen with conduction anesthesia (see Chapter 19).

Stratifying for the factor of peridural anesthesia, we determined that the deceleration phase of multiparous cardiacs was considerably longer with epidural anesthesia than without it, although the difference was only of borderline significance (0.38 ± 0.06 hour versus 0.24 ± 0.03 hour). It is interesting to note that peridural anesthesia in normal multiparas produced an essentially identical average deceleration phase (0.43 ± 0.05 hour). Since so many of the cardiac patients received conduction anesthesia during the deceleration phase, the resultant effect should not have been unexpected. We may conclude, therefore, that heart condition per se does not appear to influence the course of labor directly.

## *NEUROLOGIC DISEASE*

Almost nothing is known about the course of labor in association with major neuromuscular disorders. Isolated case reports and small anecdotal series describing pregnancies in patients with paraplegia or tetraplegia have been reported (Robertson and Guttmann, 1963; Rossier et al, 1969; Bakr and Robertson, 1973). Unsupported generalizations appear in a few obstetric textbooks to the effect that "The uterus is unaffected even if there is severe paraplegia, so that labor progresses normally up to the second stage. Expulsive efforts may be impeded because of abdominal wall involvement, and a forceps operation may become necessary" (Greenhill and Friedman, 1974). A similar excerpt referring to gravidas with paraplegia asserts that "labor often is easy and comparatively painless. The second stage may be prolonged by an inability to increase intraabdominal pressure, ie, bear down" (Pritchard and MacDonald, 1976). Most other textbooks in current use fail to mention the matter altogether.

Collective experience in any one institution is very limited indeed. The review by Bakr and Robertson (1973), although limited to 40 patients, is perhaps the most extensive one published to date. A difficult problem appears to be diagnosing the onset of labor. This is especially the case with spinal cord lesions above the tenth thoracic dermatome level. Here, there is no perception of pain during the course of labor. Frequent examinations are necessary in order to overcome the problem of recognizing when labor begins.

The situation is compounded still further should labor begin prematurely. Whereas premature labor may indeed be a hazard, it does not appear to occur very frequently. Nonetheless, it is recommended that such patients be admitted to the hospital at about 32 to 34 weeks' gestational age or even earlier if the cervix begins to efface. While this precaution may not reduce the risk of premature labor, it will ensure that the delivery takes place in the hospital setting.

It is of interest to note that some patients with spinal cord injury are able to recognize the onset of labor by the perspiration and piloerection associated with uterine contractions. These signs are undoubtedly mediated by reflex autonomic mechanisms. They may serve as useful and important signals for clinicians called upon to care for these patients. Autonomic hyperreflexia is particularly exaggerated in patients with spinal cord injuries above T-4 or T-5 and may also result in some paroxysmal hypertension, headache, bradycardia, and blockage of the nasal passages. Afferent stimuli arising in the pelvis appear to cause reflex vasoconstriction leading to hypertension (Rossier et al, 1969).

As to labor progression, the labors tend to be relatively short and uneventful. Inductions have been carried out mostly by amniotomy with good effect if timed correctly. Spontaneous deliveries can occur, particularly if the baby is small. However, forceps are often indicated because the patient cannot develop any expulsive force as a consequence of the paralysis of the accessory muscles. This tends to prolong the second stage overall.

Our own experience with such patients is also extremely limited. Dilatation and descent patterns are available for study in a relatively small number. Onset of labor, as indicated above, is impossible to time accurately. Therefore, the duration of latent phase can only be estimated and must be considered unreliable. The maximum slope of dilatation, on the other hand, is readily measurable. It is generally about as expected for comparable gravidas. Because analgesics and conduction anesthesia are not required in these gravidas, the rates of dilatation tend to approach the "ideal" labor pattern (see Chapter 7).

Descent, on the other hand, is often inhibited. This seems to result directly from the inability of these patients to bear down effectively. Not unexpectedly, the deceleration phase and second stage are likewise prolonged. This is not to imply that the delivery procedure is necessarily difficult. On the contrary, the deliveries tend to be rather easy because the fetus is small and the perineum is relaxed.

## *PSYCHOLOGIC FACTORS*

Observant obstetricians are aware of the effect that emotional factors have on the course of labor. A classic example is the cessation of uterine contractions that may occur when the obstetrician first enters the hospital room. It is postulated that this phenomenon may be mediated by neurohormonal mechanisms. They may act through endogenous secretion of epinephrine, a recognized inhibitor of uterine activity (see Chaper 19). It has become increasingly obvious that the psychologic status and emotional preparation of the gravida may be very important as far as labor progression is concerned.

Much enthusiasm has been generated for psychophysical training methods for relieving pain and anxiety during labor and delivery. Proponents assert that ideal conditions of painless childbirth can be achieved, and there are many testimonials supporting this contention. Despite extensive discourses and reviews on the subject of psychoprophylactic preparation of the pregnant patients (Buxton, 1962; Chertok, 1967; Lamaze, 1958; Read, 1959), objective evaluation has been slow in coming. The current widespread popularity of these approaches clearly supports the claim that many gravidas who participate achieve substantive subjective benefits. However, objective alterations have not as yet been confirmed by clinical investigation.

The problem of providing experimental proof is compounded by the lack of suitable controls. It is recognized that patients preferentially select themselves for prepared childbirth programs (Leonard, 1973). They tend to be older, more educated, and less indigent than gravidas who do not participate in such programs. At the same time, however, they do not seem to manifest significant differences in terms of anxiety or psychologic makeup.

Because they tend to differ from the general gravid population, it is essential that appropriate controls be devised for assuring that data will be interpretable. Most studies can be criticized because control samples are either poorly defined or absent, or because statistical analysis has not been undertaken or has been inadequately reported. There is general agreement among them, nevertheless, that such patients use less analgesics and anesthetics and have higher frequencies of spontaneous deliveries.

Some reports have suggested that labor is shortened (Van Auken and Tomlinson, 1953; Thoms and Karlovsky, 1954), but more recent and better controlled studies show no differences (Davis and Morrone, 1962; Davis and Curi, 1968; Laird and Hogan, 1956; Scott and Rose, 1976; Zax et al, 1975). Since these studies involved comparisons of average lengths of labor only, it is conceivable that significant differences could easily be missed (Barnes, 1976). This is especially pertinent in view of the large number of known factors that can influence the labor pattern; it is clear that these must be taken into account here.

Other study methods have been used to assess the effects of psychologic factors on labor. Kapp et al (1963), for example, compared psychologic attitudes and personality characteristics of gravidas with disordered labor against similar traits in women with normal labor. The labor abnormality in this investigation was characterized by inefficient uterine action in that no progress in dilatation or effacement occurred in the absence of cephalopelvic disproportion. It is difficult to know from the report whether these were specifically patients with arrest of dilatation or merely gravidas in the latent phase (or even in false labor). Nonetheless, they were found to be rather different from normal gravidas in their attitudes to motherhood, sex, and marriage, their adjustments to pregnancy, and their anxieties. The shortcomings of this approach are similar to those mentioned earlier. However, the observations may be relevant and, if verified, meaningful for clinicians.

Labor was also studied by objective graphic techniques in a small group of women (Friedman, 1955a). These patients had been prepared for childbirth by formal classwork through a series of lectures, demonstrations, and exercises. Their labor courses were compared with those of corresponding unprepared patients. The study patients were unselected in that inclusion in the classes was not specifically solicited. Nevertheless, self-selection was apparent and will be referred to again (see below).

Extensive evaluation of dilatation and descent patterns (Table 56) indicated that mean labors of prepared patients were essentially identical with those of comparable unprepared patients. Except that they were generally somewhat less heavily sedated, they constituted a cross-section sampling of

*Table 56.* LABOR DATA BY PSYCHOLOGIC PREPARATION

| Patient Group | Latent Phase (hr) | Active Phase (hr) | Maximum Dilatation (cm/hr) | Deceleration Phase (hr) | Maximum Descent (cm/hr) | Second Stage (hr) |
|---|---|---|---|---|---|---|
| "Prepared" | 8.4±0.80 | 5.0±0.92 | 2.6±0.27 | 0.89±0.13 | 2.9±0.22 | 1.04±0.14 |
| Ward Service | 8.8±0.30 | 5.1±0.19 | 3.1±0.09 | 0.92±0.06 | 3.2±0.10 | 0.97±0.05 |
| Private Service | 7.1±0.45* | 4.0±0.22* | 2.9±0.16 | 0.72±0.08 | 2.9±0.18 | 0.79±0.07 |

* Statistically significant, $p < 0.01$.

the gravid population. Sedation had been administered to these patients rather infrequently, and this was especially apparent early in labor. This reflected the kind of support these patients received.

In an effort to investigate the matter of psychologic preparation by examining a larger cohort of patients, we compared private and ward service patients. The preparation among these groups was felt to be quite different because of financial, nutritional, intellectual, and emotional factors, as well as by the confidence exhibited by them and the reassurance and personalized attention that they received from their obstetricians.

It was interesting, therefore, that private patients demonstrated a significant shortening of both the latent and active phases (Fig. 44). Neither the deceleration phase nor the maximum slope of dilatation was altered, suggesting that foreshortening of the active phase primarily reflected a significant decrease in the duration of the acceleration phase. The close relationship between latent and acceleration phases is now well recognized. Second-stage duration and maximum slope of descent were also unaffected.

Management of these patient groups was essentially identical. It was conceivable, therefore, that the differences in labor patterns could be attributed to differences in psychologic preparation. However, other factors were undoubtedly also at play here, differences in nutritional status being the most obvious.

One could conjecture at length as to whether or not psychologic preparation can influence the course of labor. It is clear that no study has yet given the final answer. The basic problem is our inability to be truly objective in determining the degree of psychologic preparation achieved by any particular patient. Classes in psychophysical preparation may attract many individuals who possess underlying anxieties and deep-seated fears.

If the psychologic state of the gravida does influence the course of labor—perhaps through the inhibition of uterine contractility by anxiety—then those gravidas with disturbed attitudes should have disturbed labors. Including such patients in the prepared groups will necessarily alter the outcome data adversely. They will effectively erase any potentially beneficial effect on labor that the preparation might have had in more normal individuals. Such courses may have value in correcting the theoretically detrimental effect

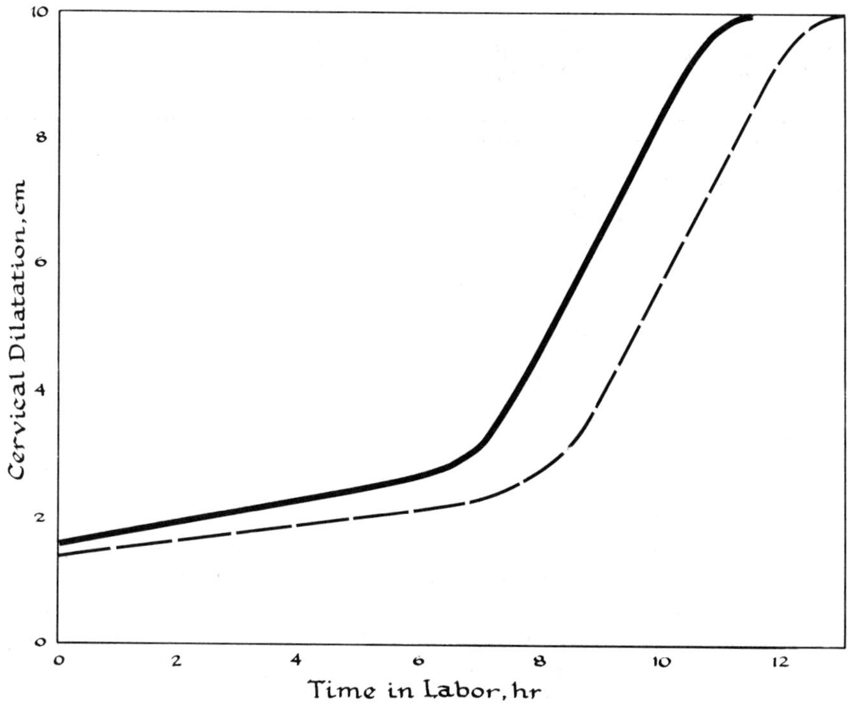


*Fig. 44.* Effect of patient status (and indirectly, perhaps psychologic preparation) on the dilatation pattern in nulliparas, showing significant foreshortening of the latent and acceleration phases in private patients (*solid line*), as contrasted with nonprivate ones (*broken line*). The remainder of the dilatation curve and the entire descent curve are unaffected.

that anxiety has on labor; moreover, these may have an ameliorating effect on normal gravidas.

We are unable to ascertain whether such benefits occur without some method for adjudging and measuring the emotional state of the participants in advance. Since the classes tend to be self-selecting (Leonard, 1973), satisfactory statistical analyses for investigating true effects cannot be designed. It is necessary, therefore, to await the development of a means whereby psychologic status and preparation may be objectively indexed. Since psychologic testing at this time is still imperfect, the question of the relationship between formal preparation for childbirth and the subsequent course of labor remains unanswered.

# Exogenous Factors

## CHAPTER 19

Information is presented on the documented effects of the gamut of pharmacologic agents on the course of labor. The discrepancy between the effects of drugs on contractility and their influence on the progression of dilatation and descent is stressed. It is clear that reliable and unassailable verification of specific effects is rarely available.

It is obvious that many pharmacologic agents given to the woman in labor may affect her fetus. There is a growing field of fetal pharmacology concerned with the burgeoning knowledge currently being evolved in this important subject area. Much less is known concerning the effects of drugs on uterine activity and the course of labor. In this chapter we will concentrate on the potential effects that various exogenously administered agents may have on the labor process.

Unfortunately, the obstetric literature contains contradictory reports on specific drug actions. There appears to be such marked variability and acknowledged subjectivity of evaluation that diametrically opposed responses may be recorded for a given agent. Moreover, in vivo investigations are often at variance with those carried out in vitro, and animal studies sometimes differ from one another and from observations in humans. Species specificity has been invoked to explain some of these discrepancies, but it is clear that many are more likely due to the inconsistencies in experimental conditions and control.

While there is a great deal of basic information available to us for review, total integration and rationalization of conflicting evidence cannot yet be accomplished. Our objective here will be to present documented effects and to delineate controversial issues concerning those medications that are likely to be used in pregnancy and during labor.

## *ANALGESICS AND SEDATIVES*

### *Narcotic Agents*

Morphine and meperidine (pethidine, Demerol) have been showed to have a variable effect on both the isolated and intact myometrium, as well as on the course of labor. Uterine contractions have been reported to be inhibited (Campbell et al, 1961), unaffected (Eskes, 1962), and even enhanced (DeVoe et al, 1969b). Experimental design in some studies made comparisons difficult, but even among those with similar experimental approaches, contradictory results were sometimes seen. This variation has been explained without supporting evidence (Snyder, 1949) as likely to be the result of exposing a deficiency in expulsive uterine forces by the drug. Analogously, one could postulate that the drug corrects some underlying deficiency; it is possible that this is its mechanism of action when used to correct prolonged latent phase disorders (Chapter 9). Alternatively, it is conceivable that the alleviation of pain and anxiety will diminish the release of epinephrine from the adrenal medulla (Filler et al, 1967). Epinephrine inhibits uterine activity (see below).

Notwithstanding the discrepant experimental evidence, the overall clinical impression is that both morphine and meperidine diminish uterine activity and labor progress. Testifying to this effect are the significantly altered dilatation and descent patterns that are encountered in heavily sedated patients. This is especially evident when the sedation is administered early in the first stage, prior to active dilatation (see below). There is a clear difference in the response of the uterus to sedation according to the phase of labor in which the sedation is administered. The latent phase, for example, is most sensitive and is readily inhibited. The normal active phase, on the other hand, is least responsive, although subtle changes can sometimes be demonstrated, especially with sophisticated devices for measuring progressive dilatation objectively (see Chapter 4). Moreover, the abnormally progressive active phase—particularly one characterized by a protraction disorder—tends to be almost as sensitive as the latent phase (Chapter 10).

These differences may offer partial explanations for some of the variable results that have been reported in experimental studies. It is reasonable to expect major inhibition of uterine contractility when the narcotic agent is given in the latent phase, whereas no effect at all may be detectable from the same dosage of medication given during the active phase or second stage. Unless the researcher is aware of such differences in sensitivity, the results will be difficult to interpret.

The problem of studying sedative effect in the clinical setting was readily resolved by grouping each patient on the basis of the degree of sedation achieved, rather than on the type or amount of drug used (Friedman, 1955a, 1956b). Labors that are uncomplicated except for the sedation effect achieved may readily be compared with each other and with an "ideal" series of like patients (see Chapter 7).

*Table 57.* LABOR DATA BY SEDATIVE EFFECT

| Sedation Group | Latent Phase (hr) | Active Phase (hr) | Maximum Dilatation (cm/hr) | Deceleration Phase (hr) | Maximum Descent (cm/hr) | Second Stage (hr) |
|---|---|---|---|---|---|---|
| Nulliparas | | | | | | |
| Unmedicated | 7.4±0.49 | 3.5±0.54 | 3.4±0.20 | 0.42±0.05* | 3.6±0.18 | 0.77±0.08 |
| Light | 7.7±0.37 | 3.7±0.22* | 3.3±0.13 | 0.72±0.08 | 3.4±0.14 | 0.80±0.06 |
| Moderate | 8.6±0.30 | 4.9±0.18 | 3.0±0.10 | 0.90±0.06 | 3.2±0.12 | 0.95±0.05 |
| Heavy | 9.8±0.48 | 6.3±0.34* | 2.4±0.11* | 1.03±0.07 | 2.5±0.14* | 1.02±0.06 |
| Multiparas | | | | | | |
| Unmedicated | 4.4±0.45 | 1.8±0.16 | 6.2±0.31 | 0.18±0.10 | 6.6±0.32 | 0.24±0.04 |
| Light | 5.0±0.24 | 2.0±0.10 | 5.9±0.20 | 0.21±0.08 | 6.4±0.30 | 0.27±0.02 |
| Moderate | 5.3±0.21 | 2.2±0.08 | 5.7±0.18 | 0.23±0.01 | 6.0±0.22 | 0.29±0.02 |
| Heavy | 5.8±0.22 | 2.8±0.08* | 5.1±0.38 | 0.36±0.06* | 5.0±0.44 | 0.20±0.02 |

* Statistically significant, $p < 0.01$, when compared with data from moderately sedated group.

The average phase durations of unmedicated nulliparas (Table 57) were almost identical with the ideal labor pattern, except for abbreviation of the deceleration phase. Comparison with sedated patients, however, showed that all phases except the second stage were markedly foreshortened and all slopes, sharply steepened. Although there were very few cases classified as precipitate (Chapter 13), there were also no dysfunctional labors, and none required uterotonic stimulation.

Lightly medicated nulliparas demonstrated somewhat less impressive labors; they were better than the overall mean, but not quite so good as the ideal labor mean. The only deviation here was the short active phase. Dysfunctional labor occurred among these nulliparas rather rarely (2.9 percent). Interestingly, all of these were associated with peridural anesthesia and had occiput posterior positions. Oxytocin was utilized in 8.8 percent; in two-thirds of these, the oxytocin was used to attempt to correct a dysfunctional pattern.

Heavily sedated patients in the nulliparous group averaged significantly prolonged active-phase durations and low maximum slopes of dilatation and descent, as compared with the total series. Figure 45 graphically contrasts the mean curves of the lightly and heavily medicated patients. Disordered labors were significantly more frequent among heavily sedated patients (13.6 percent), mostly characterized by arrest disorders. Oxytocin was used in 24.0 percent; in nearly one-half of these, it was used for correcting the labor disorder (failing in about one-third).

The complicating factors that were represented in the heavily sedated group suggested the possibility that the slowed progress might reflect the complications rather than the medication. It is possible, for example, that a patient who is undergoing a disordered labor may be more deeply sedated by a standard dosage of drug. Similarly, a prolonged labor may require more frequent and, therefore, apparently heavier medication. A significant bias may have been unwittingly introduced.

Accordingly, the groups were made more alike by selecting only those

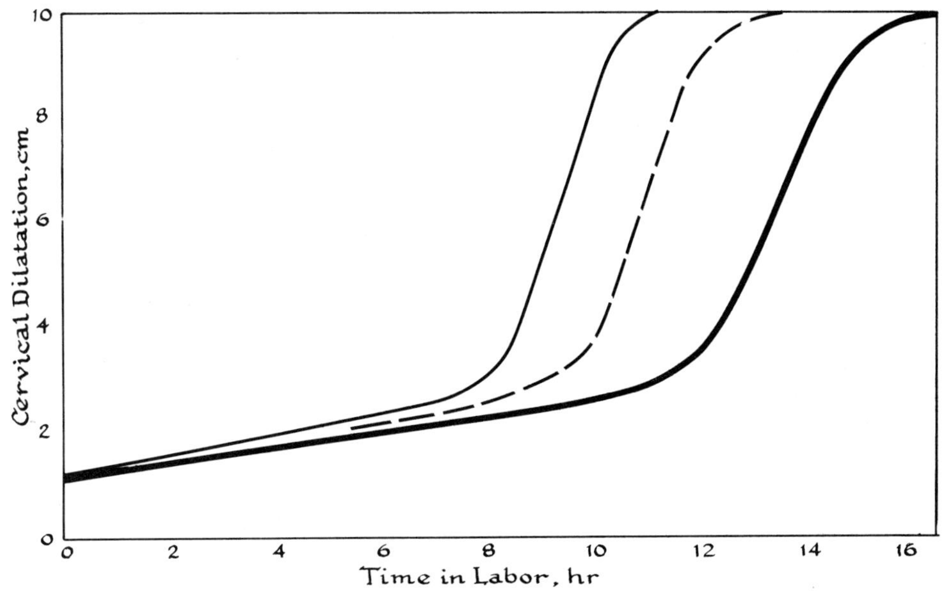


*Fig. 45.* Effect of sedation on the course of labor in nulliparas, as shown by the contrast between the dilatation curves traced by patients who are heavily sedated (*heavy line*) and those traced by lightly sedated or wholly unsedated patients (*light line*). The mean pattern for all nulliparas considered collectively (*broken line*) falls in between. Large amounts of sedation can prolong the latent and active phases while also diminishing the slopes of dilatation and descent (the last not shown).

patients with completely uncomplicated labors (except for the variable of medication, of course) and comparing them with each other. Analysis demonstrated significant prolongation of the latent (9.6 ± 0.67 hours) and active (4.9 ± 0.20 hours) phases, together with flattening of the maximum slopes of dilatation and descent (2.7 ± 0.16 and 2.9 ± 0.25 cm/hr) among heavily medicated patients. These findings verify those encountered in the uncorrected group of heavily sedated patients.

These data from nulliparas should convince us that sedation does indeed have a profound influence on the course of labor. Heavy sedative-analgesic medication slows cervical dilatation and is associated with a high incidence of dysfunctional labor. This in turn necessitates stimulation by uterotonic agents and results in more frequent operative deliveries.

It may be argued that many of these patients were heavily sedated in efforts to rest them temporarily because they were not progressing well. Careful observation of our data demonstrated that sedation under these circumstances had been given before the abnormal labor pattern was recognized; in most instances, the abnormal pattern was a secondary occurrence.

To verify this contention, patients were selected who had been excessively sedated during the latent phase only. These labors were examined and found to be normal in all respects except for latent-phase prolongation ($14.9 \pm 1.2$ hours). This value alone was statistically significant, being 6.3 hours longer than the expected mean (Fig. 46). Among these patients, no other inhibitory factor was noted to occur with significant frequency.

Among multiparas studied in the same manner, unmedicated patients demonstrated no significant deviations in their labor courses from the average multiparous pattern, although progress tended to be more rapid overall. Lightly medicated gravidas likewise exhibited normal labor curves, but also showed a tendency toward foreshortening of the various phases and steepening of the slopes of dilatation and descent. By contrast, those who were heavily sedated averaged significantly prolonged active and deceleration phases; flattened maximum slopes of dilatation and descent were only of borderline statistical significance. These findings confirmed those in nulliparas, except that the duration of the second stage was rather abbreviated. The short second stages suggested that sedative-analgesic agents are primarily inhibitory in the latent phase, less so in the active phase, and least during the second stage. In fact, it does not appear to impede progress in the second stage at all in multiparas.

This material cogently demonstrates that excessive sedation given during the latent phase will prolong the latent phase significantly. It is clear that the latent phase is remarkably sensitive to narcotic-analgesic-sedative medication. Sedation is likewise implicated in slowing the rate of cervical dilatation in the active phase, but not to the degree seen in the latent phase. The same applies for its ability to inhibit fetal descent. It appears that labor, once it is established by having entered the active phase, is not easily de-

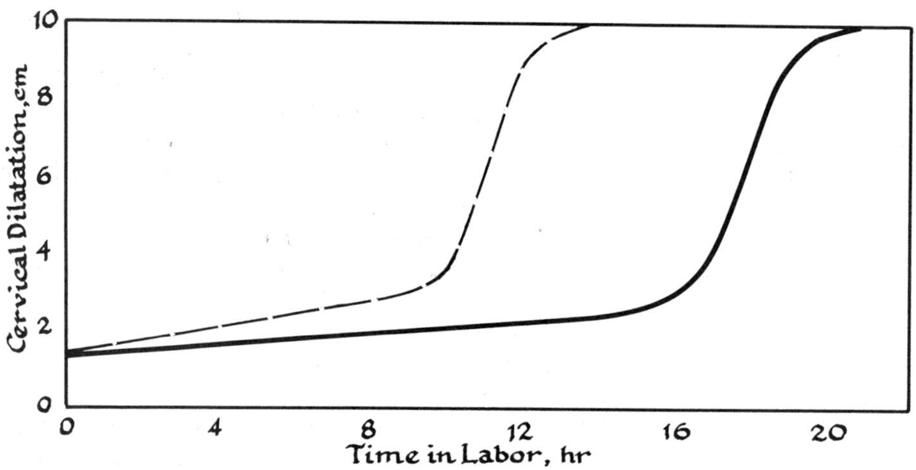


*Fig. 46.* Sedative-analgesic agents given during the latent phase significantly prolonged the latent phase only, illustrated here in nulliparas (*solid line*), compared with the average nulliparous dilatation curve (*broken line*). Neither the descent curve nor the rest of the dilatation pattern is adversely affected.

terred from its course. Nevertheless, the active phase can be slowed somewhat by large doses of analgesic medication. This is particularly the case if the rate of dilatation or descent is already abnormal. Protraction disorders (see Chapter 10) are readily compounded by the administration of sedation, which leads to the development of arrest problems.

The objective here is not to denigrate the use of sedation in parturition. Instead, we have merely demonstrated that objective investigatory methods can be employed to study the effects of drugs on labor and the comparative effects among drugs. Although adequate laboratory control of drug levels is lacking and experimental design is imperfect, the conclusions are probably valid. The specific action has also been clearly demonstrated through the use of objective measurements of the dilatation course (see Chapter 4).

The effects of various other narcotic-analgesic agents on myometrial function and the course of labor have been dealt with in various reports. It should be emphasized again, however, that the published results are not necessarily definitive. The clinical pharmacology in most instances fails to take into account differences in responses that may be expected according to the phase of labor in which the drug was given. Without clearly defined specifications of the means used for controlling such important variables, the observations tend to be unreliable.

Heroin was shown to have no appreciable effect on labor (Snyder, 1949). Methadone, on the other hand, diminished uterine tone somewhat when studied by various objective means (DiFrancesco, 1963). The course of labor was shortened in uncontrolled clinical studies of oxymorphone (Simeckova et al, 1960; Snow and Sattenspiel, 1962). Alphaprodine (Nisentil) was shown to have a variable action similar to meperidine in objective experiments (DiFrancesco, 1963). The same variability was encountered among patients given phenazocine (Prinadol) during labor when they were studied on the basis of the duration of labor (Corbit and First, 1961; Olson and Riva, 1964; Sadove et al, 1960). Pentazocine (Fortral, Talwin) appears to be somewhat less inhibitory than meperidine (Duncan et al, 1969).

### *Barbiturates*

Uniform opinion holds that large doses of barbiturates may seriously inhibit uterine contractility and slow the progress of clinical labor (Alfonsi and Massi, 1963; Campbell et al, 1961). Diminished myometrial function appears to be closely related to the dosage administered. No effect is seen with minimal doses, but diminished frequency and duration of contractions occur with larger doses. Complete cessation of uterine activity takes place with anesthetic doses of barbiturates (Snyder, 1949). This has been shown with use of pentobarbital (Nembutal) sodium (Campbell et al, 1961; Talbert et al, 1958) and thiopental (Pentothal) sodium (Alfonsi and Massi, 1963; Snyder, 1949). No inhibitory effect is seen with phenobarbital (Luminal) when used in vitro to study its effect on isolated human uterine muscle (Talbert et al, 1958). External hysterography (Dodek, 1934) failed to show any effect from amobarbital (Amytal) administered in labor.

### *Other Analgesics*

Tribromoethanol (Avertin) has been shown to prolong the interval between contractions as well as to delay labor even in low doses; moreover, it can produce marked uterine atony in larger doses (Dodek, 1934). Paraldehyde appears to be capable of prolonging labor by decreasing uterine activity, particularly after amnesic doses (Greenhill, 1962). The earlier it is given, the longer and more persistent its effect and the more difficult it is to overcome the myometrial inhibition that has been produced (Snyder, 1949).

Neuroleptanalgesia has also been used in labor (Ovadia and Halbrecht, 1967). The agent used was Innovar (a mixture of Droperidol and Fentanyl). While effective in reducing discomfort and improving patient cooperation, it did diminish the duration and frequency of contractions so that oxytocin infusion and instrumental delivery were often found to be necessary. Controlled studies have not as yet been reported.

### *Narcotic Antagonists*

The narcotic antagonists, N-allylnormorphine (Nalorphine, Nalline) and levallorphan (Lorfan), have been shown to act upon the uterus in a variable manner. In general, its effect is simliar to that of meperidine, but at a diminished level (DiFrancesco, 1963). These agents have not been shown to be capable of counteracting the depressive effect of narcotic-analgesic drugs on the uterus. No extensive experience has as yet been reported with the newer agent, naloxone hydrochloride (Narcan); however, it is likely to have no uterine effect since it appears to be devoid of a depressant effect on the neonate.

## *TRANQUILIZERS*

### *Promazine*

Reports dealing with the effects of various psychoactive agents on uterine contractility and the course of labor are largely unsubstantiated and conflicting. There are very few controlled objective studies and these tend to be inundated by the deluge of clinical reports consisting mostly of series of testimonials. The clinical action of promazine (Sparine) has been shown to range from inhibition (Pollock et al, 1960), to no effect (Matthews, 1963), and even to stimulation (Stewart, 1961). Objective measurements of intrauterine pressure were also inconsistent. One study showed no effect (Caldeyro-Barcia, 1958), while another demonstrated in vitro depression of spontaneous action in proportion to the concentration, and in vivo diminution in amplitude and frequency of contractions (Zourlas, 1964). During the 2-hour interval in which the drug was active, labor progress was completely stopped.

### *Chlorpromazine*

Chlorpromazine (Thorazine) prolonged labor in some clinical studies (Carrol and Hudson, 1955; Savage, 1955) ; others showed it to have no effect on labor (Hershenson et al, 1954; Norton et al, 1956) ; still others found it capable of shortening labor (Christhilf et al, 1960; Harer, 1956) . Intraamniotic pressure recordings yielded no demonstrable effect (Alfonsi and Massi, 1963; Caldeyro-Barcia et al, 1958) as well as a contradictory depressant effect (DiFrancesco, 1963; Vanden Driessche et al, 1954) with diminished basal tonus and intensity. This latter was associated with progressive loss of contractile coordination.

Unfortunately, these studies presented a spectrum of patient populations and management principles, including concurrent administration of other sedative-analgesic medications. The issue was confused. Examining the data carefully could lead one to infer that concomitant diminution in the amount of sedative necessary for pain relief might result in improved contractility. Thus, labor progression may indeed have been enhanced as a secondary effect of the use of these agents, but the agents themselves could not be considered to be uterotonic in the sense of having stimulated the uterus to contract more effectively.

### *Promethazine*

Interpretation of clinical data was particularly difficult for promethazine (Phenergan) administered in labor. When this agent was used in conjunction with other analgesic medications, it was concluded that the labor was definitely foreshortened (Eckerling et al, 1959; Stewart, 1961) . There was clear documentation that the requirements for analgesia were diminished. The resultant labors were shorter than comparable labors in which the patients had been given greater quantities of analgesic-sedative drugs.

The sensitivity of the uterus to sedation, particularly during the latent phase of the first stage, is now well documented (see above) . There can be little doubt, therefore, that the shortening of labor resulting from the use of promethazine was not necessarily due to its uterotonic activity, but was rather a secondary benefit due to the lesser amount of narcotic required for pain relief. Objective study using intrauterine amniotic fluid pressure-catheter recording has produced contrary information (Zourlas, 1964) . Promethazine characteristically inhibits both the amplitude and frequency of uterine contractions without apparently influencing the resting tonus.

### *Perphenazine*

Variable results have also been reported for perphenazine (Trilafon) . No objective studies have been published to date, however. In clinical investigations that measured only total duration of labor and did not adjust for analgesic agents given simultaneously, perphenazine showed a range of effects from none (Gready et al, 1959), to inhibition (Phillips et al, 1960), and even to enhancement (Harer, 1958; Stewart, 1961).

### *Prochlorperazine*

No real effect on labor could be determined for prochlorperazine (Compazine) in uncontrolled clinical studies (Kappelman, 1962; Stewart, 1961). An unusually well-controlled, objective investigation (Vasicka and Kretchmer, 1959) showed that prochlorperazine delayed the patient's subjective awareness of uterine contractions, but had no apparent direct effect on uterine contractility, with regard to either the mechanism of labor or its duration.

### *Chlordiazepoxide*

Evaluations of small pharmacologic doses of chlordiazepoxide (Librium) showed no response tocographically (Soiva et al, 1964). At higher levels, there was marked relaxation that did not appear to affect the rhythmical contractility; at still higher concentrations, relaxation increased to the point of diminishing the frequency of the contractions or even stopping them (Berger, 1961). In another study that utilized both internal and external tocography (DiFrancesco, 1963), there were no demonstrated changes at low doses, increased tone and incoordination of the contractions at moderate doses, and diminished resting tonus with inhibited spontaneous contractility at high doses. Since the conditions imposed by these several experiments differed somewhat, the responses obtained were dissimilar.

### *Dimenhydrinate*

Dimenhydrinate (Dramamine) is an antihistaminic with both antiemetic and ataractic effects. It was found to shorten labor (Rotter et al, 1958; Scott et al, 1963). No corrections, however, were made for the possible effects of the drug on analgesic potentiation; acceleration of labor occurred primarily in those patients who required and received less analgesia. A well-designed, double-blind, clinical study of dimenhydrinate demonstrated antihistaminic, atropine-like, local anesthetic and soporific effects, but no change in labor duration (Harkins et al, 1964).

### *Diazepam*

As to the effects on labor of the psychotropic drug diazepem (Valium), the experimental findings are variable. Labors are reported to be shortened (Baumgarten, 1963; Rouchy et al, 1966) or unaffected (Lee, 1968; Nisbet et al, 1967). Again, the shorter labors in some reports may have been the result of the smaller amounts of narcotics required to achieve comparable analgesic effects. This possible source of confusion has been avoided by controlled, double-blind studies showing no demonstrable effect on labor duration. Indeed, a relaxing effect on myometrium has been found in vitro (Landesman and Wilson, 1965). This suggests that the enhancing action reported to exist clinically may be erroneous.

Objective studies of labor progression using the dilatation and descent patterns were undertaken in order to resolve this issue (Friedman et al, 1969d). Patients were assigned to receive diazepam or placebo on the basis of random coding. Despite the randomization, control and double-blind design, the index and control groups were not identical. Whereas they were comparable with regard to age, station and cervical dilatation at the onset of labor, and infant weight, they were dissimilar in other important factors. For example, the use of supplementary analgesia was considerably diminished in those receiving diazepam (Niswander, 1969). Equilibrating such disparities was essential.

Uncorrected dilatation and descent data demonstrated no statistically significant differences, but some trends were encountered. Gravidas receiving the placebo showed consistently slower dilatation and descent patterns, with prolonged latent, active, and deceleration phases; the second-stage durations, on the other hand, tended to be shorter.

When the two series were examined by studying only those patients receiving comparable analgesic medications, with particular attention paid to the dosage and the time in labor when given, these trends vanished. Patients receiving diazepam showed essentially the same labor courses as those given the placebo in regard to active- and deceleration-phase durations. The maximum slopes and second stage differences persisted, however. Moreover, the latent phase was somewhat lengthened overall in gravidas receiving diazepam.

In an attempt to eliminate the potential influence of other extraneous factors, the technique of matching pairs of patients for purposes of critical evaluation was undertaken. Patients from the diazepam and placebo groups were matched carefully according to comparable parity, maternal age, fetal position, initial station and cervical dilatation, supplementary analgesia, uterotonic stimulation, and infant weight. The labor data from these groups (Table 58) once again revealed a slight increase in the dilatation and de-

*Table 58. LABOR DATA WITH DIAZEPAM TRANQUILIZATION*

| *Group* | *Latent Phase (hr)* | *Active Phase (hr)* | *Maximum Dilatation (cm/hr)* | *Deceleration Phase (hr)* | *Maximum Descent (cm/hr)* | *Second Stage (hr)* |
|---|---|---|---|---|---|---|
| Matched nulliparas | | | | | | |
| Untreated | 7.0±1.21 | 3.7±0.35 | 2.6±0.28 | 0.78±0.09 | 2.8±0.32 | 0.73±0.08 |
| Treated | 6.3±1.23 | 3.1±0.36 | 3.4±0.43 | 0.69±0.10 | 3.5±0.44 | 0.75±0.11 |
| Matched multiparas | | | | | | |
| Untreated | 7.5±1.17 | 1.9±0.17 | 5.0±0.51 | 0.30±0.04 | 5.4±0.58 | 0.24±0.04 |
| Treated | 7.0±1.21 | 1.7±0.16 | 5.5±0.58 | 0.22±0.05 | 5.8±0.62 | 0.19±0.03 |

scent rates among those receiving diazepam. In addition, all phases were slightly shorter, although none of these findings were statistically significant.

We were thus able to show that patients receiving pharmacologic doses of this ataractic agent progressed uneventfully during labor at almost precisely the expected pace as appropriately matched patients to whom it had not been given. From this we may conclude that diazepam does not adversely affect the course of labor. Moreover, it does not appear to stimulate or augment labor either. Of course, these patients received significantly less supplementary analgesia; this in turn appears to permit the labors to proceed unencumbered by the relative inhibitory effects of analgesics (see above).

### *Other Ataractic Agents*

A variety of related substances have been studied to determine their effects on labor. Hydroxydione (Viadril) is a corticosterone derivative with hypnotic and basal anesthetic actions; it appears to produce no appreciable change in intrauterine pressure patterns in the usual pharmacologic doses (Alfonsi and Massi, 1963). After prolonged use, however, it yields diminished resting tonus, lower contractile amplitude, and increasing irregularity. Hydroxyzine hydrochloride (Atarax, Vistaril) does not affect the course of labor progression in the first stage (Inmon, 1963).

Methotrimeprazine (levomepromazine) has pharmacologic effects similar to chlorpromazine and appears to depress uterine activity in a manner analogous to meperidine. This was shown in a well-designed clinical study (De Kornfeld et al, 1964). No effect on the course of labor or on the use of analgesic medication was found with the antidepressant monoamine oxidase inhibitor, nialamide (Niamid), in a double-blind clinical study (Stein and Paxson, 1963). Ethchlorvynol (Placidyl) was shown to have little effect on tocographic patterns, but resulted in shorter labors when compared with patients who were given other narcotic analgesics primarily for pain relief (Boros and Priver, 1964).

## *INHALATION ANESTHETIC AGENTS*

The effects of many inhalation anesthetics on the myometrium is dose-related. Moreover, there is a wide range of action, from the inconsequential effects of nitrous oxide to the markedly inhibitory effects of halothane. There is general agreement that nitrous oxide does not influence myometrial contractility. This is based on both clinical and experimental studies in vivo (Alfonsi and Massi, 1963; Caldeyro-Barcia, 1958). However, a depressant effect has been demonstrated in isolated human uterine muscle (Talbert et al, 1958). Ethylene also exhibits little or no influence on the course of labor (Greenhill, 1962; Snyder, 1949). Trichlorethylene is similarly without effect in the laboratory or the clinical setting (Alfonsi and Massi, 1963; Talbert et al, 1958). Flowers (1953), however, showed that prolonged use of trichlorethylene reduced uterine contractility somewhat.

### *Ether*

Diethyl ether and divinyl ether anesthesia inhibits labor; this has been well documented experimentally and clinically. Ether diminishes tonus, amplitude, and frequency of uterine contractions, whether the contractions are spontaneous or induced by oxytocin (Alfonsi and Massi, 1963; Van Liere et al, 1964). Its effect appears to be the result of direct action on uterine muscle. Contractions are abolished in the lower first and upper second plane of anesthesia (Vasicka and Kretchmer, 1959). Ether anesthesia produces an arrest of labor progression that is resistant to the influence of uterotonic stimulation (Alfonsi and Massi, 1963).

Comparable inhibition of uterine activity has been shown with use of chloroform in both clinical and laboratory experiments (Duncan et al, 1956; Lindgren and Smyth, 1961; Moya, 1960). Chloroform depresses uterine contractility in analgesic doses and in the first plane of anesthesia. There is significant diminution in amplitude and frequency of contractions. With increasing depth of anesthesia, this leads ultimately to complete relaxation. Here, too, the effect is likely to be the result of direct myometrial action.

### *Cyclopropane*

The effects of cyclopropane on isolated uterine muscle strips are difficult to interpret; this agent has been reported to depress myometrial function (Talbert et al, 1958) as well as to increase the basal tonus (Munson et al, 1969). However, in subanesthetic or light first-plane anesthetic levels, it appears to have no effect on the intact uterus (Alfonsi and Massi, 1963; Moya, 1960). Deeper levels of cyclopropane anesthesia, on the other hand, result in progressively decreasing frequency of uterine contractions without significantly influencing the tonus or amplitude.

Cyclopropane tends to be somewhat less effective in inhibiting myometrial function than other inhalation agents (Bosomworth et al, 1962). Therefore, it is of relatively little clinical value when complete uterine relaxation is required as, for example, when intrauterine obstetric manipulations are to be done (Moya, 1960).

### *Halothane and Halogenated Ethers*

Halothane (Fluothane) is a strong inhibitor of myometrial function (Munson et al, 1969) in vitro. In clinical use it is effective even at light anesthetic levels. Contractility will be rapidly and markedly diminished from the inhalation of as little as 0.5 percent halothane mixture (Crawford, 1962). In concentrations of 0.8 percent it can produce prolonged uterine relaxation (Moir, 1970). In objective studies of uterine contractility, halothane markedly reduces the intensity of uterine contractions with first-plane anesthesia and practically abolishes them with second-plane anesthesia (Vasicka and Kretchmer, 1961). The effect is seen within 2 minutes of administration (Miller and Stoelting, 1965). During the administration of halothane anesthesia, the uterus becomes unresponsive to uterotonic stimulation with oxytocin (Alfonsi and Massi, 1963). Contractility returns to normal when tissue concentrations are significantly reduced; this usually takes about 5 minutes after the agent has been discontinued (Miller et al, 1966).

Because uterine relaxation is so prompt and complete, halothane has been recommended as the agent of choice for treatment of tetanic uterine contractions or for use whenever uterine relaxation is needed for purposes of obstetric manipulations (Moya, 1963). It must be emphasized, however, that severe postpartum atony with hemorrhage may result (Stoelting, 1964).

Other halogenated ether compounds also depress uterine muscle function markedly. These include methoxyflurane (Penthrane), fluroxene (Fluoromar), enflurane (Ethrane) and isoflurane (Forane). They are especially inhibitory in high concentrations (Munson, 1974).

## *REGIONAL ANESTHESIA*

### *Local Anesthetic Agents*

Isolated human myometrium can be directly inhibited by high concentrations of various local anesthetic agents, including procaine, tetracaine (Pontocaine), lidocaine (Xylocaine), chloroprocaine (Nesacaine), dibucaine (Nupercaine), hexylcaine (Cyclaine), and propoxycaine (Blockain), as shown by McGaughey et al (1962). Concentrations of lidocaine well in excess of those used clinically, for example, will decrease uterine frequency and amplitude while increasing the baseline tonus. At still higher concentrations, it further reduces contraction amplitudes, but there are concomitant increases in the frequency and resting tone. When administered intravenously (Evans et al, 1969), lidocaine first produced an increase in uterine activity, followed by substantial diminution in contractility. Decreased contractility—with and without preceding transient hypercontractility—occurred after paracervical injection of both lidocaine and mepivacaine (Carbocaine) (Vasicka et al, 1971).

Thus, if high concentrations of local anesthetic agents reach the myometrium, they may be stimulatory. This perhaps occurs when the drug is administered inadvertently by the intravenous route or directly into the myometrium. Under normal circumstances, however, low blood levels of drug appear to have only a slight depressant effect on uterine contractility, or none at all (Munson, 1974). Nevertheless, there appear to be variations in the effect on labor according to the method by which these agents are administered. It is clear that the type of conduction block technique must be taken into account.

### *Spinal Anesthesia*

The effect of spinal anesthesia on labor has been studied extensively, but the reports are sometimes contradictory. In well-established labors, no consistent effect is seen with spinal anesthesia to the second thoracic level (Alvarez et al, 1959). Even anesthesias to the sixth cervical level are said to be without effect (Vasicka and Kretchmer, 1961), provided hypotension is avoided (Vasicka et al, 1964). However, there have been reports of disruption of rate, rhythm, strength, and gradient of contractility with anesthetic levels above the tenth thoracic dermatome (Browne and Browne, 1964; Reynolds et al, 1954). External hysterography showed a significant rise in basal tonus at still lower anesthetic levels (Dodek, 1934); it resulted in diminished frequency and amplitude of contractions lasting about 30 minutes after the anesthetic was given. Contractility subsequently returned to normal even though the anesthesia was maintained.

To confound the relationship between spinal anesthesia and its effect on labor, striking improvement in incoordinate uterine dysfunction has been reported following the administration of spinal anesthesia (Caldeyro-Barcia, 1958). Such reports may be open to question because factors other than the anesthesia are undoubtedly at play. The type of labor pattern, for example, is important. We have shown that spinal anesthesia given prior to the onset of the phase of dilatation in the first stage will impede progress of the latent phase, forestalling the normal progressive changes of late labor (Friedman and Sachtleben, 1961a). Moreover, regional block will inhibit a labor that is progressing abnormally, most particularly one characterized by a protraction disorder (see Chapter 10). In general, however, spinal block given to the patient during the course of a normally progressing active phase—and to a level not exceeding that necessary for uterine pain relief, namely, the tenth thoracic dermatome—should not influence the labor course.

### *Peridural Anesthesia*

There is a general impression that caudal and epidural anesthesia has a negligible effect on the course of labor, unless misused. Most clinical studies are in agreement that well-established labor is not retarded (Bromage, 1961; Vasicka et al, 1964; Sala et al, 1970; Epstein et al, 1970). Not all are in agreement, however. Some have found that anesthetic levels above the tenth thoracic dermatome disrupted the contractility pattern (Browne and Browne, 1964) and actually impaired labor progress (Friedman and Sachtleben, 1959). Protraction and even arrest of labor in the second stage is especially common with this form of anesthesia (Potter and MacDonald, 1971). Inefficient flexion and rotation of the fetal presenting part are undoubtedly the result of diminished voluntary expulsive efforts. The reduced effectiveness of the abdominal and diaphragmatic muscles, in turn, is a consequence of anesthetic abolition of the perineal reflex. Thus, myometrial contractility is uninvolved.

The effect of peridural anesthesia on labor has been evaluated by objective graphic means (Friedman and Sachtleben, 1959; Friedman, 1965c). A large series of patients given caudal anesthesia early in labor was investigated. They were found to be somewhat dissimilar from the general gravid population due to diminished numbers of patients with fetopelvic disproportion, malpositions, and abnormal labors prior to the administration of the anesthesia. It was important, therefore, to be sure that appropriate comparisons would be made with similar patients who had not received the anesthesia. It was interesting to note that when compared with the overall nulliparous labor data, nulliparas who labored under caudal anesthesia illustrated no deviations in either direction. Even when we deleted all complicated cases so as to create an "ideal" caudal group for comparison with the ideal group of nulliparas discussed in Chapter 7, we found that the labor patterns were essentially unaltered (Table 59).

*Table 59. LABOR DATA WITH CONDUCTION ANESTHESIA*

| *Anesthesia Group* | *Latent Phase (hr)* | *Active Phase (hr)* | *Maximum Dilatation (cm/hr)* | *Deceleration Phase (hr)* | *Maximum Descent (cm/hr)* | *Second Stage (hr)* |
|---|---|---|---|---|---|---|
| Nulliparas | | | | | | |
| No anesthesia | 8.3±0.32 | 4.6±0.20 | 3.0±0.12 | 0.88±0.05 | 3.2±0.16 | 0.92±0.04 |
| Caudal | 7.6±0.46 | 4.4±0.26 | 2.9±0.20 | 0.97±0.12 | 3.0±0.24 | 1.00±0.08 |
| Epidural | 8.7±0.64 | 4.7±0.44 | 2.6±0.34 | 1.08±0.05* | 2.7±0.39 | 1.37±0.15* |
| Multiparas | | | | | | |
| No anesthesia | 5.0±0.22 | 2.2±0.07 | 5.7±0.18 | 0.23±0.02 | 6.1±0.22 | 0.24±0.02 |
| Caudal | 5.5±0.28 | 2.4±0.11 | 5.2±0.25 | 0.43±0.05* | 5.3±0.26 | 0.33±0.02* |
| Epidural | 5.8±0.36 | 2.6±0.35 | 5.3±0.47 | 0.40±0.06* | 5.1±0.30* | 0.32±0.02* |

* Statistically significant, $p < 0.01$.

The multiparas who were given caudal anesthesia were found to be more representative of a cross-section sampling of the hospital multiparous population. Contrasting the labor data from these two groups yielded information showing that the only significant variations from normal were prolongation of the deceleration phase and second stage, together with reduction in the maximum rate of descent, among those who labored with caudal anesthesia.

Stratification of the data was pursued for the purpose of determining those factors that yielded adverse results when present concurrently with peridural anesthesia. Whereas the analyses were unable to provide definitive results due to inadequate numbers of relevant cases, certain inferences were possible. We have seen that both cephalopelvic disproportion (Chapter 16) and excessive sedation (see above) will act to inhibit the dilatation and descent patterns of labor, whether anesthesia is given or not. Although not definitively verifiable, these changes appear to be enhanced in association with conduction anesthesia. Thus, factors known to slow the various portions of the labor curve can be expected to have these alterations augmented in the presence of peridural anesthesia.

Analogously, the same may be said about factors known to have a potentially beneficial effect on labor progress. Oxytocin, for example, is effective in speeding the rates of dilatation and descent in otherwise normal labor (see below); the effect is essentially identical among gravidas who receive such uterotonic stimulation with and without anesthesia. It is clear that even in the presence of conduction anesthesia, oxytocin affects the course of labor by producing an overall speeding of dilatation and descent. The only exception is a perceptibly diminished effect on the deceleration-phase duration.

We learned that in many instances the possible deleterious effects of anesthesia may have been masked or compensated for by the stimulatory effect of oxytocin. When this interaction of opposing forces was assessed analytically, we were able to define the influence of anesthesia on the course of labor more precisely. In general, conduction anesthesia in nulliparas yielded an essentially normal dilatation pattern and a terminally inhibited descent pattern. In multiparas, dilatation was characterized by marked prolongation of the deceleration phase, as well as slight lengthening of the active phase and second stage; the descent curve was affected to the same degree as in nulliparas with terminal reduction in slope.

More importantly, factors that were known to alter the labor curves adversely—such as cephalopelvic disproportion, fetal malposition, and excessive sedative-analgesic medication—were found to act qualitatively in precisely the same way in association with peridural anesthesia. Indeed, these effects were quantitatively much exaggerated.

We had earlier seen (Chapter 9) that the administration of conduction anesthesia during the latent phase readily inhibited progress and prolonged the latent phase. When we studied conduction anesthesia and its effects on labor, however, this anticipated result could not be reconfirmed. Slowing of cervical dilatation by the premature application of conduction anesthesia was certainly observed frequently. However, the overall data did not reflect this fact. This was eventually explained by the common practice of allowing the effective level of anesthesia to abate temporarily when it was apparent that the clinical labor had slowed or stopped. Alternatively, oxytocin stimulation had been used. The resultant effect could thus be reversed easily if recognized promptly.

Membranous dystocia from unruptured chorioamniotic membranes occurred quite rarely in association with conduction anesthesia. It was characterized by arrest of descent in the second stage, unaccompanied by any evidence of bony or positional dystocia. Because it took place so late in labor, the foregoing labor pattern was in general not significantly altered. As expected, amniotomy promptly corrected any untoward effect with regard to terminal descent.

Epidural anesthesia has also recently been studied by the same approach. Heretofore unpublished data from appropriately comparable patients (Table 59) show that patients receiving adequate levels of lumbar epidural anesthesia have significantly prolonged deceleration phase and second stage; this applies both to nulliparas and multiparas. Additionally, there are clear trends toward slowing of the rates of dilatation and especially of descent. The data for mean slopes of descent attain statistical significance.

On the basis of these objective studies, we were able to formulate criteria for limiting the use of conduction anesthesia. Proper administration entails withholding it until the active phase of labor has been entered. Moreover, it should not be preceded with an excess of analgesic-sedative drugs. Conduction anesthesia should be avoided in cases presenting documented or suspected cephalopelvic disproportion or those with diagnosed fetal malpositions. The untoward effects on the course of labor may be readily reversed in most instances by allowing the anesthesia to wear off or by administering uterotonic stimulation in the form of oxytocin infusion.

### *Paracervical Block*

The affect on labor of paracervical block is paradoxical. It has been shown to produce a transient reduction in uterine contractility (Sandmire and Austin, 1964; Bonica, 1970; Jenssen, 1973). Others have found variable tocographic effects in objective studies of contractions (Cooper and Moir, 1963). At the same time, it is alleged to enhance cervical dilatation (Davis et al, 1962; Jenssen, 1973). It is conceivable that the latter merely represents the rapid advancement that one anticipates will normally occur as labor progresses. It is likely that the expected acceleration in dilatation that occurs as labor enters the active phase is mistakenly attributed to the agent or technique immediately preceding this natural event.

### *Pudendal Nerve Block*

The commonly used pudendal nerve block anesthesia does not appear to interfere with myometrial function (Greenhill, 1962). Some retardation of second stage progress, however, has been reported (Lee, 1959). Paradoxically, combined paracervical and pudendal nerve block has been alleged to speed cervical dilatation in an uncontrolled anecdotal report (Kobak and Sadove, 1961). Inconsistent results have also been obtained with the use of uterosacral block anesthesia (Pitkin and Goddard, 1963).

### *Paravertebral Block*

Paravertebral lumbar sympathetic block appears to promote uterine contractility, as shown by increasing resting tonus and contractile amplitude (Reich, 1951, 1953). Studies based on intraamniotic pressure and external tocography have shown that bilateral lumbar paravertebral sympathetic block may accelerate the course of labor (Hunter, 1963). Normal uterine contractions appear to be improved by this approach; abnormal contractility may even be corrected. The same potential shortcomings, as noted earlier with regard to evaluation of the effect of paracervical block (see above), may apply here as well. Because no attempt was made to take into account the expected labor progression at the time the block was instituted, it is difficult in retrospect to ascribe the changes that occurred to the anesthesia that had been given. More appropriately designed investigations are needed to determine whether or not such measures do actually augment labor progress.

### *Neuromuscular Blocking Agents*

There is almost total agreement that uterine function is unaffected by skeletal muscle relaxants such as *d*-tubocurarine (Tubarine), gallamine (Flaxedil), decamethonium (Syncurine), or suxamethonium (succinylcholine, Anectine) (Tunstall, 1963; Healy, 1971). Isolated reports to the contrary have appeared, however, suggesting that labor may be shortened (French, 1958) or, contrariwise, that the frequency and strength of contractions may be depressed by profound curarization (Pittinger et al, 1953; Felton and Goddard, 1966). In vitro study has shown that myometrial strips are unaffected by concentrations of these agents in massive doses (Reier and Moster, 1970).

Despite these findings, other investigators have reported diminished intensity of uterine contraction with succinylcholine (Alver et al, 1962; DiFrancesco, 1963). Nevertheless, essentially all clinical studies have shown that labor progression, with regard to both dilatation and descent as well as uterine contractility, is unaffected; similarly, the response of the uterus to uterotonic agents is unaltered (DiFrancesco et al, 1962).

## *UTEROTONIC AGENTS*

Various agents are in wide clinical use for purposes of inducing or augmenting labor, or both. The wealth of clinical experience attests to their efficacy. Undoubtedly, the most widely used is oxytocin, currently available commercially as the synthetic products Syntocinon and Pitocin.

Sparteine sulfate (Tocosamine, Spartocin) enjoyed brief popularity (Plentl et al, 1961; Plentl and Friedman, 1963), but its use has waned considerably in recent years on the basis of isolated reports of adverse effects, including tetanic contractions (Bedrosian and Gamble, 1963) and uterine rupture (Boysen, 1963). Since response to sparteine can be variable and unpredictable, it must be used with caution, even though the incidence of complications is small (Greenhill and Friedman, 1974). There is clear need for constant attendance and supervision during its use (DeVoe et al, 1969a).

Prostaglandins, although not yet formally approved for clinical usage in late pregnancy in the United States, have been shown to be useful for inducing and stimulating labor. They are available abroad. It is likely that approval for commercial distribution will be forthcoming here soon. Accordingly, we will confine our discussion to the effects on labor of oxytocin and prostaglandins.

## *Oxytocin*

The identification and synthesis of the oxytocic fraction of the pituitary gland secretion by du Vigneaud et al (1953a, b, 1954) and Tuppy (1953) was a milestone in the annals of biochemistry. The pharmacologic similarity between natural and synthetic oxytocin has been demonstrated (du Vigneaud et al, 1954; Konzett et al, 1956). Response of the gravid myometrium to this agent has been clearly demonstrated under well-controlled laboratory and clinical conditions.

Moreover, critical evaluation of its physiologic effect on the gravid uterus in vivo as it relates to labor progression was also accomplished (Friedman, 1957b). This involved extensive analysis of dilatation and descent patterns in gravidas to whom oxytocin was administered as an intrapartum uterotonic stimulant.

It was determined that the drug is—within the narrow limitations of its use and when applied with appropriate caution—a safe, effective agent for clinical use. It is inappropriate for us to dwell on the prerequisites, precautions, and techniques relevant to its administration; all standard obstetric textbooks detail these extensively. Our interest here lies instead in our ability to quantitate its effect on labor progression.

When administered by standard infusion technique, using either dilute solution by intravenous drip or delicately controlled infusion pump, clinically normal labor can be simulated. Patients subjected to these measures represented a cross-section sampling of the gravid population.

The labor patterns were examined with specific reference to the effect that may have been produced by oxytocin. The durations and slopes of the several phases were measured to compile information on those aspects of labor that followed the use of the oxytocin (Table 60). These data were compared with comparable material obtained from similar unselected spontaneous labors. The differences were felt to represent the drug effect.

*Table 60. LABOR DATA WITH OXYTOCIN STIMULATION*

| *Group* | *Latent Phase (hr)* | *Active Phase (hr)* | *Maximum Dilatation (cm/hr)* | *Deceleration Phase (hr)* | *Maximum Descent (cm/hr)* | *Second Stage (hr)* |
|---|---|---|---|---|---|---|
| Nulliparas | | | | | | |
| Unstimulated | 8.6±0.27 | 4.9±0.15 | 3.0±0.08 | 0.90±0.05 | 3.2±0.10 | 0.95±0.04 |
| Oxytocin | 3.6±0.63* | 3.1±0.24 | 3.8±0.32* | 0.57±0.07* | 4.0±0.28* | 0.80±0.07 |
| Multiparas | | | | | | |
| Unstimulated | 5.3±0.19 | 2.2±0.07 | 5.7±0.16 | 0.23±0 01 | 6.0±0.20 | 0.24±0.01 |
| Oxytocin | 3.2±0.21* | 1.9±0.10* | 7.0±0.50* | 0.20±0.04 | 7.4±0.48* | 0.17±0.03* |

* Statistically significant, $p < 0.01$.

Subjecting the differences to statistical analysis permitted us to determine relative significance.

It was found that all phases of labor, when acted upon by oxytocin, are significantly foreshortened or accelerated in both nulliparas and multiparas, with the exception of the deceleration phase in multiparas and the second stage in nulliparas. The maximum slopes of both dilatation and descent were significantly more steeply inclined while oxytocin was being given (Fig. 47).

It may or may not be appropriate to consider whether the results of stimulation are desirable. Nonetheless, it is apparent that oxytocin is an effective uterotonic agent in labor. If comparison is made with labor data derived from "ideal" nulliparas (see Chapter 7), it can be seen that labors enhanced by oxytocin approach this allegedly ideal pattern. Statistically, the values are identical, except for the significantly foreshortened latent phase associated with the use of oxytocin. This last observation strongly suggests that oxytocin stimulation markedly speeds up the process of softening and effacement of the cervix that occurs during the latent phase.

When we stratify our data to examine only those subjects whose labors were induced, we obtained confirmatory evidence. Among nulliparas, this subgroup showed that all phases of labor were abbreviated and that the slopes of dilatation and descent were steepened significantly. Oxytocin inductions in multiparas again showed significantly shortened average latent-phase and second-stage durations, but the average intervals of active and

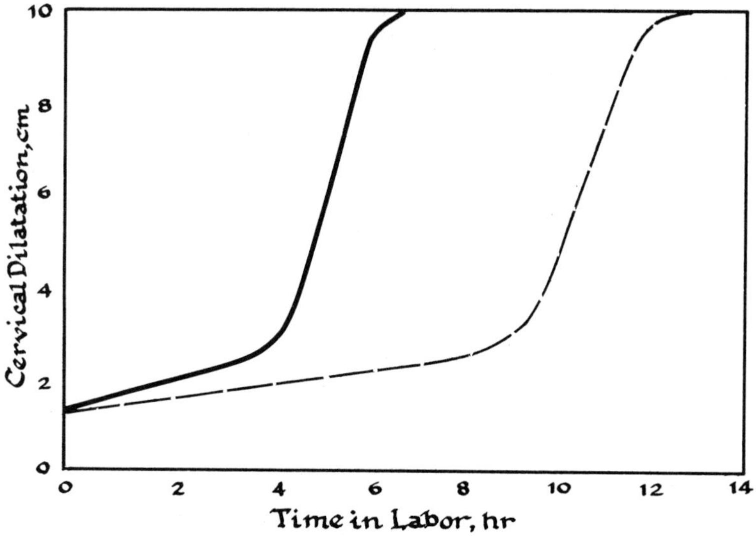


*Fig. 47.* Influence of uterotonic stimulation with oxytocin infusion on the dilatation pattern of otherwise normal nulliparas (*solid line*), as compared with unstimulated spontaneous labors in similar patients (*broken line*). The labor process is clearly speeded by this means, including significant shortening of the latent and active-phase durations and increasing of the maximum slopes of dilatation and descent (not shown).

deceleration phases were not significantly altered (although reduced in length somewhat). The slopes of dilatation and descent remained significantly increased in multiparas.

Thus, we have determined that oxytocin produces a significant foreshortening of all phases of the first stage of labor in nulliparas; additionally, there is an apparent though insignificant diminution in the duration of the second stage. In multiparas, the drug causes reduction in duration of all phases except the deceleration phase. The maximum slopes of dilatation and descent are correspondingly greater in both nulliparas and multiparas under the influence of oxytocin stimulation.

One may question whether the effects that we note here are desirable. It is incontrovertible that oxytocin possesses therapeutic efficacy for changing many desultory or even arrested labors (see Chapter 11) into normal patterns. As to its use for inducing labor or for stimulating otherwise normal labor in progress, we observed no untoward side effects, but it should be emphasized that oxytocin had been administered in a most cautious manner throughout. The rate of administration had been regulated by the uterine response that was elicited so that excessive and potentially harmful stimulation could be avoided.

The overall effect of speeding the normal pattern of labor progress has been equated with a theoretical ideal in all its components except the latent phase. It is conceivable that the abbreviation of the latent phase by oxytocin may cause some harm, but this has not as yet been demonstrated. The theoretical hazards of fetal damage, cervical laceration, hemorrhage, or other reported consequences of overstimulation were not encountered. Again, it must be stressed that these perils are real, however, and can be avoided only by critically vigilant administration.

Concern over the differences between spontaneous and oxytocin-stimulated labor is made all the more meaningful by the objective demonstration that the contractions produced are not the same (Johnson et al, 1970). This is further compounded by the demonstration that the fetus may be adversely affected by such contractions; the incidence of abnormal fetal heart rate patterns, for example, was determined to be significantly increased during oxytocin infusion, especially if given in association with peridural anesthesia (Schifrin, 1972). The issue of elective use of oxytocin for purposes of speeding the course of labor, therefore, remains unresolved.

## *Prostaglandins*

The clinical use of prostaglandins $E_2$ and $F_{2\alpha}$ ($PGE_2$ and $PGF_{2\alpha}$) in obstetrics has burgeoned in recent years. They are currently accepted for their efficacy in terminating midtrimester pregnancies. Extensive clinical research has also shown them to be effective for inducing labor at term. As stated above, they have not yet been approved for use in labor or for commercial distribution for this purpose in this country, but they are available abroad and continue to be used widely.

The pioneering work of Karim et al (1968, 1969) with $PGF_{2\alpha}$ given by intravenous infusion at rates of 0.05 μg per kilogram per minute confirmed its value as a clinically useful uterotonic agent. Later well-controlled, double-blind clinical investigations have likewise verified its efficacy (Anderson et al, 1972). Potentially serious hypertonus of the uterus is occasionally seen with its use, however (Spellacy and Gall, 1972), suggesting that this agent may not be particularly advantageous over oxytocin. The contractility patterns produced by $PGF_{2\alpha}$ appear to be identical with those of oxytocin (Anderson and Schooley, 1975).

$PGE_2$, when administered intravenously, provides no special advantages over $PGF_{2\alpha}$ (Beazley and Gillespie, 1971). However, oral administration of $PGE_2$ appears to offer a new dimension (Karim, 1971; Karim and Sharma, 1972). Specific information concerning the type of labor progression produced by oral administration of $PGE_2$ was made available on the basis of the analysis of dilatation and descent patterns (Friedman and Sachtleben, 1974; Friedman et al, 1975b).

Dose-finding investigations were undertaken in sequential series of patients. Unacceptably high frequencies of side effects, including nausea, vomiting, and diarrhea were encountered with the highest dosage regimen. This involved administering incremental doses from 0.5 mg to 3.0 mg, increasing by 0.5 mg every half hour for the first 3 hours, followed by maintenance doses of 0.5 mg half-hourly during the next 7 hours. Because of the undesirable side effects, this regimen was deemed to be unacceptable, particularly since there was no justification for its continued use in the form of counterbalancing benefit.

Lower dosage regimens were found to be useful for inducing labor. These consisted of administering either 0.5 mg or 1.0 mg hourly for 10 doses. Side effects for both regimens were relatively infrequent. Vomiting and diarrhea, for example, occurred in 26 and 32 percent, respectively. However, these manifestations tended to be more severe in the higher dosage group. In addition, instances of uterine hypercontractility were encountered more frequently in the latter group. Abnormal fetal heart rate patterns were also seen, but these were generally unassociated with hypercontractility and tended to be innocuous. There were no apparent ill effects to either mother or fetus from the hypercontractility or fetal heart rate abnormalities.

Labor was successfully induced in 76 percent of patients given low dosage $PGE_2$ orally and in 78 percent of those given high dosage. Discounting those subjects in whom the induction failed technically on the basis of discontinuation for side effects, we derived success rates of 79 and 83 percent, respectively.

The dilatation and descent patterns from these patients were compared with a matched series of comparable gravidas whose labors had been unstimulated. The factors taken into account for matching included maternal age, parity, the prelabor Bishop Score—an objective measure of inducibility (Bishop, 1964)—as well as fetal position, status of the membranes, sedation, and anesthesia. The Bishop Score is detailed in Chapter 22 with regard to its usefulness in labor induction.

It was found (Table 61) that the high dosage regimen consistently yielded

*Table 61. LABOR DATA WITH ORAL PROSTAGLANDIN $E_2$ INDUCTION*

| *Matched Groups* | *Latent Phase (hr)* | *Active Phase (hr)* | *Maximum Dilatation (cm/hr)* | *Deceleration Phase (hr)* | *Maximum Descent (cm/hr)* | *Second Stage (hr)* |
|---|---|---|---|---|---|---|
| Unstimulated | 5.3±0.22 | 2.5±0.16 | 4.6±0.33 | 0.34±0.04 | 4.1±0.36 | 0.46±0.05 |
| Low dosage (0.5 mg qh) | 4.3±0.49 | 2.5±0.24 | 5.1±0.43 | 0.32±0.04 | 4.5±0.91 | 0.42±0.06 |
| High dosage (1.0 mg qh) | 3.7±0.49* | 2.2±0.21 | 6.1±0.66† | 0.29±0.04 | 5.2±0.78 | 0.48±0.13 |

* Statistically significant, $p < 0.01$.
† Borderline significance, $0.05 > p > 0.01$.

labors characterized by shorter phases and more steeply inclined slopes than labors on the low dosage schedule. None of these differences was statistically significant, however. Comparison with the unstimulated control labors did show significant foreshortening of the latent phase with high dosage $PGE_2$ and somewhat less foreshortening (not statistically significant) with the low dosage regimen. The high dosage data showed much more rapid progress, except for second-stage duration, throughout the rest of labor when compared with the unstimulated matched control subjects. This was not duplicated for the low dosage subgroup data. The latter were found to be essentially identical with that of the comparable unstimulated group once the active phase had been entered.

These findings demonstrated little difference between the two dosage regimens with regard to their ability to induce labor. Needless to say, the more suitable the candidate for induction, the more likely for the induction to be successful by either dosage regimen. Moreover, the labor that results from such uterotonic stimulation—although more rapid in the higher dosage group—is at least as actively progressive as normal unstimulated labor. In addition, its latent phase is likely to be foreshortened as well. The low dosage regimen has a clear advantage in the lower intensity of side effects associated with its use. Thus, the balance between therapeutic efficacy and adverse effects leans favorably toward the low dosage regimen. On this basis, 0.5 mg of $PGE_2$ administered hourly can be recommended for clinical use.

## *UTERINE-INHIBITING AGENTS*

It is well beyond our scope to discuss the growing list of pharmacologic agents employed for purposes of attempting to arrest premature labor. Various antispasmodic smooth muscle depressants and myovascular relaxant agents have variable suppressing effects on uterine contractility. In general, they appear to work best when labor is early and not well established. This observation suggests that some of the patients in whom such agents have been most successful may not have been in labor at all.

Among the drugs that have been reported to be most useful in this regard are intravenous alcohol (Fuchs et al, 1967; Zlatnick and Fuchs, 1972), pregnenolone (Scommegna et al, 1970; Bieniarz et al, 1971), and a group of $\beta$-adrenergic agents. Some of the last are selective $\beta_2$-receptor stimulants which act to relax smooth muscle of the uterus, bronchi, and vessels of the skeletal musculature. They have fewer cardiovascular effects than other comparable agents, such as isoproterenol. Those currently under intensive investigation include salbutamol (Ventolin) (Liggins and Vaughn, 1973; Korda et al, 1974), ritodrine (Premar) (Landesman et al, 1971; Barden, 1972; Renaud et al, 1974), and orciprenaline (metaproterenol, Alupent, Metaprel) (Baillie et al, 1970; Belizan et al, 1975). The $\beta$-mimetic effect of these agents often inhibits uterine contractility effectively in clinical use. This has been shown by objective in vitro studies as well. Unfortunately, the doses required to obtain a clinical effect are so large that side effects become limiting.

Another $\beta$-stimulant that has been examined for its uterine inhibiting effect is isoxsuprine (Vasodilan) (Hendricks, 1964a). Unlike the selective $\beta_2$-receptor stimulants, it produces major cardiovascular side effects, including tachycardia and diastolic hypotension. An unrelated drug, diazoxide (Hyperstat) (Landesman et al, 1969), is an effective diuretic, but it also inhibits uterine function. Although use of these drugs is promising, their clinical applicability has not yet been fully verified.

Ethyl alcohol solution given intravenously was shown to slow or stop normal spontaneous labor and to relax the tetanically contracted uterus (Fetchko, 1951). However, it does not affect oxytocin-induced labor (White, 1955). Fuchs et al (1967) described use of alcohol in a therapeutic program that appears to be effective in arresting premature labor. Beginning with a loading dose of 7.5 ml per kilogram body weight of a 9.5 percent solution, one may often forestall labor; a maintenance dosage of 1.5 ml per kilogram per hour is usually needed for up to 10 hours. A controlled study has recently verified the effectiveness of this regimen (Zlatnick and Fuchs, 1972).

Studies on isolated human myometrium (Johnson et al, 1963) have also shown that other antispasmodic agents depress the gravid uterine muscle. These include such widely diversified agents as adiphenine (Trasentine), dicyclomine (Bentyl), valethamate (Murel), thiphenamil (Trocinate), and methylisooctenylamine (Octanil, Isometheptene). Still others, such as amyl nitrite and nitroglycerin, have no consistent effect in clinical usage (Jeffcoate et al, 1952). Indeed, amyl nitrite was once advocated for purposes of reducing uterine hypertonicity during tetanic contractions. In actuality, it may lower uterine tonus in only about one-half the cases in which it is used, probably mediating its action by way of uterine vasodilatation (Kumar et al, 1965).

Drugs that inhibit the synthesis of prostaglandins from arachadonic acid may also prove useful in preventing premature labor (Zuckerman et al, 1974). Indomethacin has been shown to be effective in this regard in limited clinical situations. Much work remains to be done in the assessment of these potentially useful agents.

## *STEROID AND RELATED HORMONES*

### *Estrogens*

It is generally agreed that estrogens stimulate uterine contractions. Indeed, the capacity of the gravid uterus to contract becomes manifest only if it has been primed with estrogenic substances (Caldeyro-Barcia, 1959). Animal and human experiments support this contention by showing increased spontaneous uterine activity, manifested by more frequent contractions of greater amplitude (Pinto et al, 1964a, b; Reynolds, 1965). The contractions produced by estradiol are not the same as those of oxytocin; they are shorter, of lower intensity, more frequent, less coordinated, and generally painless. Moreover, estrogens appear to reduce the threshold of myometrial responsiveness to oxytocin. Some investigators have not been able to verify this last effect (Jeffcoate et al, 1952; Kobak and Sadove, 1961), and in one in vitro study using rat myometrium, estrogens actually blocked contractile response to oxytocin (Barnafi and Croxatto, 1963).

Shabanah et al (1964a, b) proposed the concept that estrogens control actomyosin synthesis in the uterine myofibrils while assisting the synthesis of high energy phosphates (ATP) to provide the energy for actomyosin contraction. At the same time, estrogens control synthesis and activation of acetylcholine and the resulting myometrial response. Furthermore, acetylcholine and compounds with acetylcholine-like activity stimulate the release of oxytocin; the action of oxytocin on the myometrium is in turn only manifest in the presence of acetylcholine. Estrogens also control the synthesis of the catecholamines (see below). The response by myometrium to the sympathetic neurohormonal transmitters is influenced by the level of progesterone. If these concepts are substantiated, the physiology of myometrial function will be greatly clarified.

### *Progesterone*

The response of myometrium to progesterone is not well understood. Most animal experimentation shows that progesterone can inhibit uterine contractility, diminish spontaneous contractions, and overcome the ability of the uterus to respond to uterotonic agents (Bengtsson, 1957; Caldeyro-Barcia, 1959; Csapo, 1963b; Fuchs, 1964, 1971; Kroc et al, 1959; Reynolds 1965). The evidence in man, however, is contradictory. Progestational agents are capable of preventing uterine activity as a consequence of hypertonic saline-induced abortion (Bengtsson, 1962); they inhibit spontaneous contractility of human myometrium in vitro (Bygdeman and Eliasson, 1964; Kumar et al, 1962); they sometimes reduce uterine activity in premature labor (DiFrancesco, 1963) and even diminish spontaneous contractions at term (Hendricks et al, 1961). Nonetheless, the clinical effects are inconsistent and tend not to be verifiable (Kelly, 1961; Kumar et al, 1963a; Reynolds, 1965; Taubert and Haskins, 1963; Wood et al, 1963). Discrepancies can be explained by variations in technique and instrumentation in the study of myometrial function.

### *Other Hormones*

Gonadotrophins may inactivate the rabbit myometrium, but the evidence is indirect and inconclusive (Reynolds, 1965). Aldosterone has an antiprogesterone effect; it has been shown to accentuate spontaneous uterine activity when administered intravenously (DiFrancesco, 1963).

The water-soluble ovarian extract, relaxin, has not been completely characterized as to its effect on myometrial function. It has been shown to relax the symphysis pubis and soften the cervix in lower animals, but clinical reports on its effect on uterine activity are conflicting. It is alleged to inhibit uterine contractions, thus slowing or stopping premature labor (Eichner et al, 1956); in contrast, it may speed cervical dilatation (Birnberg and Abitbol, 1957) and shorten the first stage of labor (Rothman et al, 1959). These actions have not been verified objectively. Indeed, in vitro experiments utilizing isolated human uterine muscle showed no effects whatsoever (McGaughey et al, 1958). Likewise, no consistent inhibition or stimulation of uterine contractility has been demonstrated either in controlled clinical studies or objective physiologic investigations (Israel and Groeber, 1960; Kelly and Posse, 1956; Poseiro et al, 1959; Slate and Mengert, 1960; Ware and Haynes, 1962).

## *AUTONOMIC BLOCKING AGENTS*

The most commonly utilized postganglionic cholinergic blocking agents in obstetrics are atropine and scopolamine. They are generally supposed not to have any effect on uterine activity (Snyder, 1949) and to exert no significant influence on the course of normal labors (Shaaban and Youssef, 1959). However, they do appear to have some antispasmodic action. Intraamniotic pressure studies show that both drugs relax the lower uterine segment and diminish basal uterine tonus as well as contraction frequency. In addition, in some incoordinate states, uterine activity has been regulated. In the excised uterus, the circular muscular fibers (but not the longitudinal ones) are relaxed by atropine. In clinical usage these effects appear to be negligible, however.

Of the adrenergic blocking agents, perhaps the most widely used in obstetrics are the ergot alkaloids and their derivatives. In practice today, their use is limited to the postpartum period because they produce unphysiologic and intensive contractions if given during labor. The amine alkaloids, ergonovine and the semisynthetic methylergonovine, are effective uterotonic agents, with rapid onset of action and negligible adrenergic activity. They are effective orally as well as parenterally.

The dihydrogenated alkaloids, on the other hand, tend to have far less effect on uterine contractility but have greater adrenergic effects than the naturally occurring amino acid alkaloids from which they are derived. Dihydroergotamine is said to raise the basal tonus of the uterus (DiFrancesco, 1963) ; alternatively, it is reported to have no effect on the uterus (Goldfarb, 1954) ; it may also increase the tonus and frequency of contractions but reduce their intensity (Caldeyro-Barcia, 1960) ; it may even lead to uterine atony in the third stage of labor (Friedman, 1957b) .

No direct effect on uterine muscle has been demonstrated from large doses of the more potent adrenergic blocking agents, dibenamine and dibenzyline. The imidazolines, tolazoline (Priscoline) and phentolamine (Regitine) , on the other hand, appear to stimulate the uterus directly both in vivo and in vitro in many species. Although these agents should be expected to act in the same way in humans, the effect on uterotonic activity has not as yet been reported. Similarly, the benzodioxans, piperoxan and prosympal, stimulate the smooth muscle of the uterus directly.

Of all the ganglionic blocking agents, nicotine is perhaps the most widely prevalent. Aside from the documentation of the association between smoking and low infant body weight, uterine stimulation has been seen in vivo but not in vitro (Kumar and Zourlas, 1963) . Whether this effect is due to direct stimulation or to the release of oxytocin by a nicotinic effect on the neurohypophysis, as shown in rats (Bisset and Walker, 1957) , has not yet been clarified in humans.

Nicotinic properties have been ascribed to the quaternary ammonium compounds, notably the tetraethylammonium ion. Although this substance has been almost entirely replaced by hexamethonium as a therapeutic autonomic ganglionic blocking agent, it has been shown to be mildly uterotonic. It appears to improve contractility in some incoordinate dysfunctional labors (Jeffcoate et al, 1952) .

Of the parasympathomimetic agents in current clinical use, the choline ester, acetylcholine, is of little interest because of its pharmacologic instability. Nonetheless, acetylcholine in large doses does produce good uterine response in the intact gravid uterus (Shabanah et al, 1964b) . No such effect is seen after administration of smaller doses (Embrey, 1958; Shaaban and Youssef, 1959) . Myometrial responsiveness to oxytocin is said to become manifest only in the presence of acetylcholine (Shabanah et al, 1964b) . The synthetic choline derivative, carbachol, has been shown to have the same effect as acetylcholine.

The cholinesterase inhibitors, which prevent the destruction of acetylcholine, should be expected to yield an effect upon the uterus that is similar to acetylcholine. Nevertheless, the uterus is apparently unaffected by physostigmine, except in high concentrations. It is postulated that this comes about because of the lack of continuous release of acetylcholine by the uterus. Thus, the myometrium will not be stimulated by a drug that acts through inhibition of cholinesterase.

Similarly, neostigmine does not stimulate the pregnant uterus, except at term. At one time, neostigmine was used to correct delayed anovulatory menstruation; as such, it has been stigmatized erroneously as an abortifacient. In actuality, it is very unlikely to induce abortion. Among the cholinergic alkaloids, pilocarpine produces uterine contractions in the uterus that has been primed by estrogens (Reynolds, 1965).

Paradoxical effects have been obtained with the sympathomimetic agents. It is generally stated that epinephrine inhibits contractility of the pregnant uterus, while norepinephrine stimulates contractions. This has now been verified experimentally, using purified active principles. Both in vitro and in vivo studies demonstrate that epinephrine diminishes the frequency and amplitude of contractions, but does not appear to affect the basal tonus (Zuspan et al, 1962). Rebound of uterine activity often follows, but this is not invariable (Pose et al, 1962). Such action is recognized to affect both spontaneous and oxytocin-induced uterine contractions.

Norepinephrine, on the other hand, initiates spontaneous contractions and augments uterine activity by increasing the frequency and amplitude of contractions (Cibils et al, 1962). In many instances, however, the contractions produced by norepinephrine are not well coordinated. They differ from contractions produced by oxytocin both qualitatively and quantitatively (Cibils and Spackman, 1962).

Other vasopressor amines have also been evaluated (Senties et al, 1970). Methoxamine (Vasoxyl) and mephentermine (Wyamine), for example, consistently showed a stimulating effect on the gravid uterus. The response was primarily manifested by increased frequency of contractions proportional to the dose, and by increased basal tonus at high dosage levels. Stimulation was occasionally seen even in response to doses too small to produce blood pressure changes. It suggested that the uterus at term may sometimes be more sensitive to these agents than the vasculature.

Reynolds (1965) has attempted to integrate the many paradoxical effects that drugs appear to have on uterine activity. Some may exert their action directly, while others may indirectly excite the uterus by cholinergic nervous activity, even though they may not themselves be adrenergic. Consequently, a sympathomimetic effect on the uterus is obtained indirectly. Such observations may be valid, but our current state of limited knowledge on the interrelationships of neural and hormonal function with the control of myometrial activity does not permit us to verify them.

## *OTHER DRUGS*

Magnesium sulfate inhibits the spontaneous contractility of isolated myometrium (Kumar et al, 1963b; Talbert et al, 1958). It diminishes intensity, frequency, and basal tonus. Clinical studies of its effect on the gravid uterus showed that the magnesium ion is capable of depressing uterine activity in proportion to blood levels. Suppression of myometrial function is most often manifest in decreasing contraction frequency (Kumar et al, 1963b); in addition, the intensity and resting tonus are variably inhibited (Hutchinson et al, 1964), and the duration of labor is somewhat prolonged (Hall et al, 1959).

Histamine stimulates the uterine muscle by direct action in vitro, but it has not been shown to have uterotonic effect when used in low dosage during pregnancy (McElin and Horton, 1949). The antihistamines, on the other hand, are often mildly spasmogenic, enhancing myometrial contractility. The controversial aspects of this type of response to antihistamines and the possible interpretation of this response has been discussed earlier (see above) in association with the use of dimenhydrinate, which was included among the tranquilizing agents.

Myometrial function has been augmented in both animal and human investigations from digoxin. It appears to cause an increase in the frequency of contractions associated with some degree of hypertonus between contractions (Norris, 1961). Similar results were obtained with the use of ouabain and strophanthin G in a clinical setting. Labor progress, however, was unaffected.

Bradykinin exerts an inconsistent uterotonic effect on isolated rat myometrium (Elliot et al, 1960), but no effect on the intact human uterus (Berde and Saameli, 1961). It does effectively relax smooth muscle in vitro, however, blocking both spontaneous and oxytocin-induced contractions of human uterine muscle strips and decreasing their frequency and amplitude (Landesman et al, 1963). The degree of relaxation is apparently proportional to the dose administered.

This general review of the effects of commonly used drugs on uterine contractility and labor progression has not provided clear-cut answers to questions that might be raised for application to clinical practice. Our understanding of physiology is still very limited, and clinical pharmacology has not always been helpful in this regard. The controversies we have touched on still await resolution by more sophisticated and better-designed experiments. As more critical approaches to the investigation of the complex labor phenomena are developed and applied, we are hopeful that the physiology of the pregnant uterus will be elucidated, and the true pharmacologic effects of the various exogenous agents will be more definitively demonstrated.

# Clinical Applications

# PART IV

# Diagnostic Approaches

## CHAPTER 20

Early diagnosis of disordered labor requires ongoing assessment of every labor in progress by graphic means. Various useful graph formats are reviewed, including those devoid of arithmetical calculation. Sources of error and means for identifying and correcting for them are detailed. Specifics are provided for evaluating the patterns as they evolve. The method of interpreting graphs dynamically in a stepwise fashion is proffered. This leads to a logical diagnostic sequence for clinical practice.

While we were evolving means for detecting, evaluating, and managing patients with abnormal labor in the foregoing chapters, we elaborated many details that may or may not be useful to the obstetric attendant. To this point, we have delved broadly, seeking answers to relevant and tangential clinical issues. It is now important to synthesize all the foregoing information for the purpose of providing practical programs of management. Such programs can be formulated on the basis of objective observations. These observations represent the epitome of the material we have reviewed thus far in digested, sorted, and ordered sequence.

Recommendations for clinical care are meant neither to challenge established dogma—although they frequently do so inadvertently—nor to replace authoritative pronouncements with equally unfounded tenets. Instead, they are offered as composite empirical reflections; they are the quintessence of a large experiential store of knowledge. Without exception, they are believed to be logical deductions based on confirmed relationships. Nothing is knowingly presented merely on opinion, faith, or preconception. By the same token, no concept is so firmly held that it could not be replaced by substitute recommendations based on newly derived and reliably objective data, whenever such data become available.

When applicable, we have tried to use the flow sheet (algorithm) approach in order to illustrate recommended programs succinctly. In this way, we hope that they will serve as useful references for the practitioner. While these effectively summarize management recommendations (Chapter 24), the reader is urged to study the detailed material on diagnostic aids (see below), problems in differential diagnosis and evaluation for etiologic and contributory factors (Chapter 21), issues relating to therapy (Chapter 22), and findings relating to the prognosis for the fetus and the surviving infant (Chapter 23).

By acquiring a working familiarity with the fundamental principles of the management programs, the attendant will develop his or her clinical proficiency considerably. The difficult diagnostic and management problems that laboring patients present to us will be much more readily resolved as a consequence. This applies equally to the physician in practice, the resident in training, the nurse or nurse-midwife, and the medical student—indeed it applies to anyone who is called upon to care for the obstetric patient in labor.

## *EARLY DIAGNOSIS*

Prompt and proper diagnosis is the keystone to sound clinical management. This medical maxim applies to many disciplines, but seldom is it more critical than in labor disorders. Moreover, early diagnosis is especially difficult to achieve here. Normal labor presents such marked variations in clinical appearance that many valuable hours may be lost before it is clear that the situation has become abnormal.

There is no firm conception as to when an abnormal labor condition may be said to exist. Our available clinical approaches tend to be very nebulous. In the past, we were all too often deluded into believing that any progress in the intensity, frequency, or duration of contractions, or in cervical dilatation or effacement, or in the descent of the fetal presenting part was probably adequate. This often held no matter what the price was in time and effort.

Hindsight enlightenment frequently came too late to avoid a potentially dangerous situation or to allow one to make corrections before irreversible damage had occurred. It is fortunate that most labors do progress normally. Only in the few abnormal instances does our diagnostic deficiency become critical. We need not belabor the point that our ability to diagnose abnormal labor is severely limited. This matter has been reviewed in much detail earlier (see Chapter 3).

The key to early diagnosis is the detection of disorders in labor progression—specifically, the expected evolution of the characteristic patterns of cervical dilatation and fetal descent. Only by following patients carefully, critically, and continually throughout the course of their labors will it be possible to trace these patterns accurately and diagnose disorders as they arise.

Continuous reevaluation is mandatory if abnormal progression is to be recognized. Our obligations to the laboring patient are clear. We cannot delegate our responsibilities to unskilled or untutored subordinates, except under unusual and exigent circumstances. Early recognition of the major labor disorders is essential if we are to be able to institute proper management expediently, thereby achieving our ultimate objectives of reducing fetal and maternal risks. Such early recognition cannot be accomplished without ongoing evaluations.

## *CHART FORMS*

### *Standard Graph*

The benefits of visual interpretation make the use of simple graphic forms particularly helpful. Any kind of square-ruled graph paper will do. Graphs are often incorporated as a permanent part of the patient's hospital record for future reference or study. One popular form currently in use (Fig. 48)

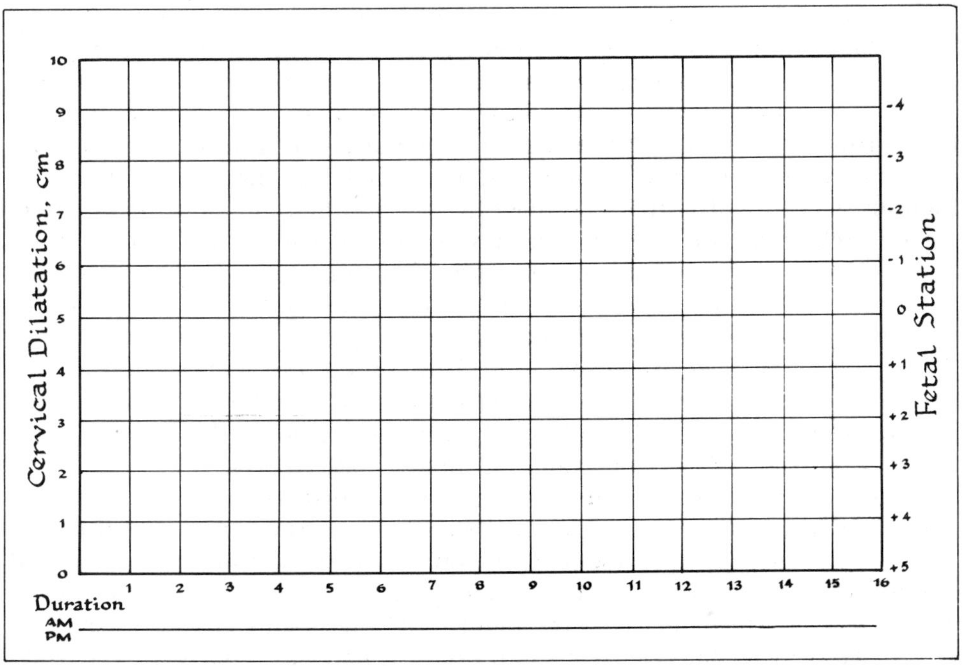


*Fig. 48.* A simple standardized graphic form that can be incorporated into the gravida's permanent hospital chart for purposes of recording the dilatation and descent patterns as they evolve during the course of her labor. The horizontal time scale refers to the number of hours that have elapsed from the time the patient first perceived the beginning of regular and unremitting uterine contractions. This form is currently in wide use.

provides a horizontal scale of elapsed time in labor, and two vertical scales representing cervical dilatation and fetal station, respectively. Such graphs are not meant to replace the narrative type of notations in hospital records, depicting events and observations and detailing diagnostic and therapeutic considerations. Instead, they serve to supplement these notes and to provide concise and utilitarian summations of the course of events.

A reasonable degree of accuracy and consistency is needed for estimating cervical dilatation and fetal station in order for the patterns to become meaningful. However, very little experience is necessary to achieve these ends. Inexperienced and even incompletely knowledgeable medical students and nurses are frequently quite capable of following labors and producing meaningful graphic representations of the dilatation and descent patterns after minimal instruction.

The single most common fault in constructing these graphs is inattention to uniformity in the baseline. It is important that the time scale be uniform throughout. Each subdivision of the graph should represent a given and constant unit of time. The easiest scale to use is 1 hour per division. If the scale is irregular or otherwise inconsistent, one cannot intelligently interpret the pattern that is traced.

One should begin the graph at the left margin with the onset of labor. Thus, the left side of the graph will represent the point in time when regular uterine contractions began. Since we have no objective way to pinpoint when labor actually begins in any given case, we need not agonize over the precise timing of onset of labor. Instead, we merely have to utilize the time reported by the patient when she first perceived the onset of regular contractions. Occasionally, this may have to be modified at some future time, when it is clear that the contractions have spontaneously ceased. We are then awakened to the realization that the foregoing episode actually represented an interval of false labor. Until then, however, we could not make the distinction.

The first entry of estimates of cervical dilatation and fetal station are recorded a certain number of divisions to the right of the left margin; the number of divisions is equivalent to the number of hours that have elapsed from the onset of labor. For example, for the patient who is first seen and examined 4 hours after the onset of perceived contractions, the observation of 2 cm of cervical dilatation should be entered on the fourth vertical line from the left margin (representing 4 hours of elapsed time in labor) and two divisions up from the lower border (representing 2 cm of dilatation). For convenience in identifying the determination, open circles (○) are generally used to designate cervical dilatation estimates as obtained by vaginal examination, and closed circles (●), for those obtained by rectal examinations. By contrast, the symbol x is usually used for station estimates.

Each subsequent point is entered in its appropriate place on the graph according to the amount of time that has elapsed from the previous entry. It is convenient to maintain two matched time scales simultaneously, one representing elapsed time in labor, the other, the actual clock time. If these scales are set forth at the time of the initial examination, no further difficulty should be encountered thereafter. New points can then be entered according to the clock time when they were obtained, and elapsed durations can be read directly from the corresponding scale as well.

### *Alert and Action Lines*

The graphic forms have been adapted for special needs. Numerous minor variants have been reported (Schulman and Ledger, 1964; Ledger, 1969; Beazley, 1972b; Notelovitz, 1973; Johansen, 1973; Margolis, 1974). Of particular importance was the modification made by Philpott and Castle (1972a). Their objective was to fulfill the special needs of paramedical personnel caring for maternity patients in Rhodesia. They sought a means for automatically signaling the presence of labor abnormalities. The magnitude of the problem they confronted can be appreciated because most of the deliveries were being carried out by midwives and maternity assistants. There was a clear need to establish simple and accurate guiding principles.

Based on the original cervical dilatation pattern, they constructed an Alert Line that would serve to flag those patients at risk. When a patient's dilatation pattern crossed this Alert Line, arrangements could be made for transferring her from the outlying periphery to a centrally located intensive obstetric unit. They used the working premise that active management should be effectively instituted within 4 hours of the time that the Alert Line had been crossed. This was believed by them to be sufficient time to allow safe transfer of the patient to the central unit for treatment.

The graph proposed by Philpott and Castle (1972a) (Fig 49) is a standard square-ruled graph upon which the Alert Line is drawn. This Alert Line represents the minimally acceptable rate of dilatation for nulliparas at the rate of 1 cm per hour. It is constructed by joining points representing 1 cm of cervical dilatation at zero time (taken as the time of admission, not the onset of labor) and full cervical dilatation at 10 cm 9 hours later. This single straight Alert Line was considered to be suitable for use in all nulliparas arriving at their institution with cervical dilatation of 3 cm or greater.

Observations of dilatation can be plotted on this graphic form in exactly the same way as previously described (see above). Active-phase progression can be observed as the pattern is traced. Should the pattern cross the Alert Line, the attendant is alerted to the possibility that an abnormal situation exists. Consultation should be obtained or the patient transferred promptly to another institution where more sophisticated monitoring, evaluation, and aggressive management may be undertaken. The Action Line is placed parallel to the Alert Line but removed by four hours; it indicates the time considered by Philpott and Castle (1972b) to represent when definitive action will be required.

Philpott and Castle have made an important and significant contribution to the practice of obstetrics in this way—especially as it is practiced in underdeveloped areas or wherever personnel are limited in number, sophistica-

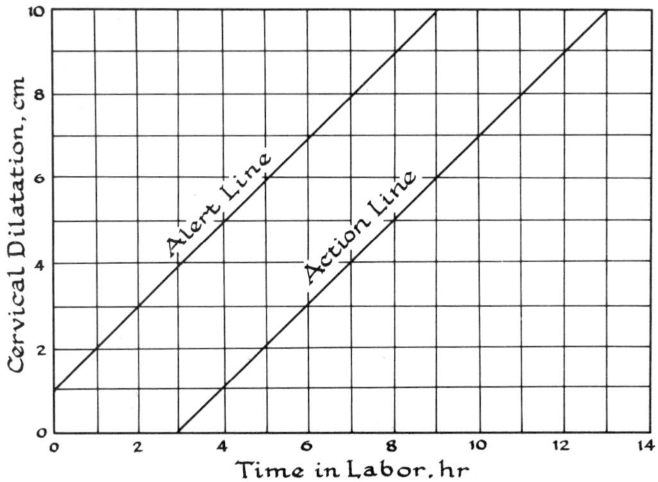


*Fig. 49.* A graphic guide for assessing labors in progress by plotting cervical dilatation against time, without taking into account the expected latent phase and assuming all patients have already entered the active phase of dilatation when first seen. If the dilatation curve crosses the Alert Line, it signals a potential problem in that the course may be either arrested or abnormally slow. Definitive diagnosis and therapy are expected by the time the curve crosses the Action Line placed 4 hours to the right of the Alert Line.
(From Philpott RH, Castle WM: J Obstet Gynaecol Br Commonw 79:595, 1972)

tion, or skills. Arbitrary critical limits of total duration of labor or nebulous concepts of uterine inertia, both of which are difficult to use and limited in value even in expert hands, have here given way to a very efficient and simple technique for plotting cervical dilatation against time on a standard graph. As the curve evolves, the abnormal labor pattern will cross the Alert Line to indicate to the observer that a problem is likely to exist.

This was shown to occur in 22 percent of nulliparas studied. Exactly one-half of these continued in labor to develop truly abnormal progression and crossed the Action Line, as indicated above. Clear evidence has been presented that labors crossing the Action Line are commonly associated with cephalopelvic disproportion; they frequently require operative delivery.

Two major drawbacks appear to limit the usefulness of this method somewhat. First, it does not take into account the latent phase or its normal extension. Philpott and Castle acknowledged this problem, but accepted this limitation because they were unable to define the beginning of labor in most of their cases. This appears to be a special problem inherent in underdeveloped areas. Nevertheless, it is probable that many of the patients who cross the Alert Line are actually in the latent phase. This would account for the large proportion of patients—amounting to 50 percent in their series—

who underwent active dilatation of the cervix and subsequently delivered without complication, all without ever crossing the Action Line. On this basis, the Alert Line concept is too sensitive because it designates so many normal labors as abnormal. The second drawback is that this approach does not consider progressive descent at the same time. Thus, disordered descent patterns are unrecognized.

By not taking cognizance of the contributions of the latent phase, one can expect a high frequency of false positive cases that comprise patients with perfectly normal labors who are considered to be abnormal merely on the basis of their having crossed the Alert Line. On the other hand, by ignoring descent, we will necessarily miss some very serious labor aberrations.

It is important to add here that despite these deficiencies, all due credit must be given to Philpott and Castle for having adapted the graphic method of labor analysis so effectively to a very difficult clinical situation. Their approach has resulted in wide application of this method throughout the world. It already has had a salutary effect on the practice of obstetrics everywhere it has been introduced.

## *Nonarithmetical Forms*

In order to improve the value of this graphic approach further, some slight additional modifications may be justified. These should include some means for recognizing and allowing for the evolution of the normal latent phase, and for simultaneously observing the development of the descent pattern for purposes of detecting its aberrations. This has been accomplished (Friedman et al, 1975) by utilizing the separate dilatation and descent forms shown in Figure 50. Comparable forms are available for use in nulliparas and multiparas. Those for nulliparas are designed with a series of parallel inclined dilatation-limit lines set at 1.2 cm per hour and comparable descent-limit lines at 1 cm per hour. The forms for multiparas provide dilatation limits of 1.5 cm per hour and descent limits of 2 cm per hour. The choice of these limits is based on the empirical observations analyzed and detailed in Chapters 7 and 8. Vertical indicators for the approximate maximally acceptable duration of latent phase are set at 20 hours for nulliparas and 14 hours for multiparas.

Use of this type of graph has provided a means for achieving nearly perfect diagnostic capability without requiring any form of mathematical computation of the rates of dilatation or of descent. The limits of normal latent-phase duration are provided for purposes of defining the disorder of prolonged latent phase. The expected rates of maximum dilatation and descent below which the abnormalities of protracted active-phase dilatation and protracted descent may be diagnosed are also presented. The inclined limit lines also provide means for assessing when arrest of dilatation and descent is occurring.

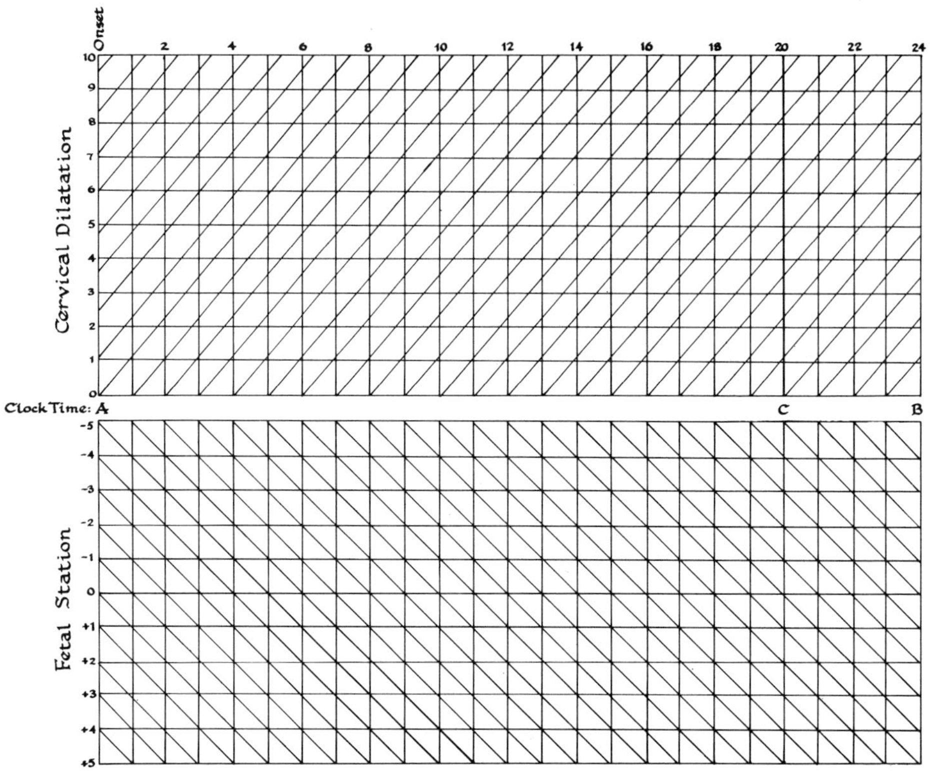


*Fig. 50.* A graphic form that permits obstetric personnel to plot and interpret both dilatation and descent curves in labor without the need for any arithmetical calculations. This form is designed specifically for use with nulliparas in that it provides inclined slope lines of 1.2 cm/hr for dilatation and 1.0 cm/hr for descent. A comparable form for multiparas (see Fig. 51) contains inclined lines of 1.5 and 2.0 cm/hr, respectively. The inclined lines represent acceptable minimal rates of normal dilatation *(upper form)* and descent *(lower form)*. As soon as the dilatation curve turns up (or the descent curve turns down), the very next inclined line is marked to serve as a guide for the diagnosis of abnormal progress. After the onset of labor (A) is determined, one completes the clock time scale (A to B), designating each division as 1 hour. Vertical line (C) at 20 hours represents the upper limit of the normal latent phase.

The following sequence, illustrated in Figure 51, should serve as a useful guide for implementing these labor forms:

1. Ascertain the patient's parity and select the proper form for nulliparas or for multiparas.
2. Determine the time of onset of labor and insert this time at the left margin of the time scale *(point A)*.

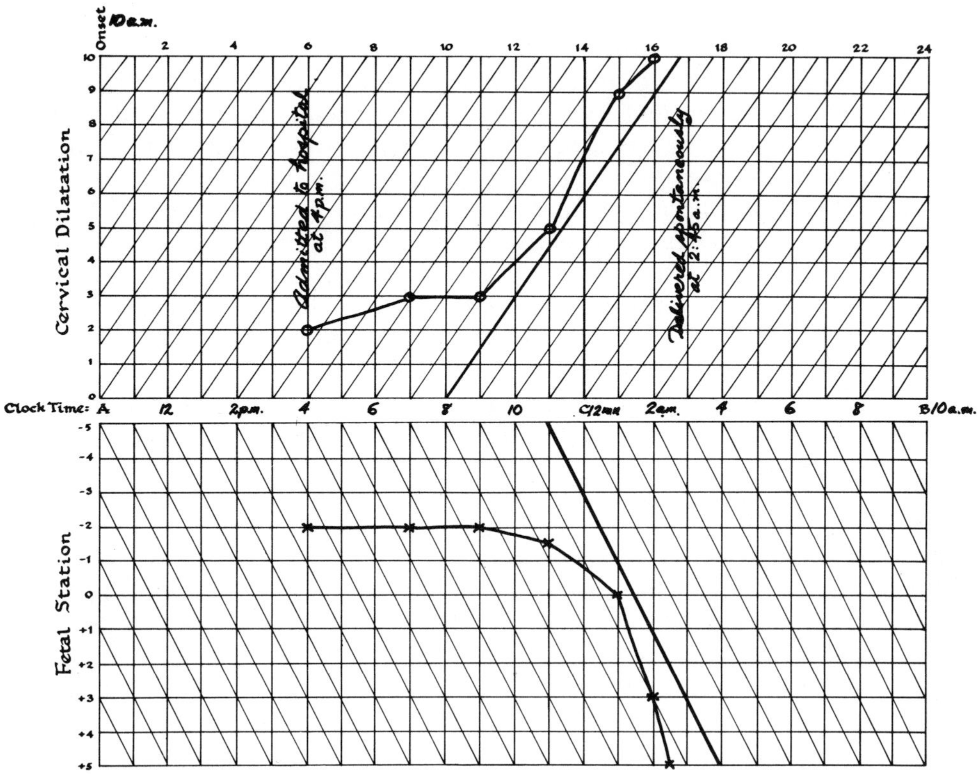


*Fig. 51.* Example of a multipara's dilatation and descent patterns, traced during the course of her labor as it unfolded. First entry was made when this patient was first seen at 4:00 P.M., 6 hours after labor began. The clock time scale was completed at that time, and the findings at each subsequent examination were entered. When the dilatation curve turned up at 13 hours (11:00 P.M.), the next inclined line was darkened. The same operation was carried out for descent at 15 hours (1:00 A.M.). The labor course bettered the minimum guideline set for this parturient and could therefore be considered entirely normal. Had the labor pattern crossed the inclined lines at any time, a specific abnormality could have been diagnosed at once (see text).

3. Complete the time line (*Clock Time*) by inserting a sequence of hours, using one division per hour up to the right-hand margin of the time scale (*point B*).
4. Mark the time of admission on the time line, inserting a vertical arrow at the correct point.
5. Insert the estimates of cervical dilatation (*upper graph*) and of fetal station (*lower graph*) at the appropriate points on the graph at the time of admission.
6. Insert each subsequent determination of cervical dilatation and fetal station at the proper times, as designated on the time scale.

7. Join each new point with the previous point by a straight line to evolve the patterns of cervical dilatation and fetal descent.
8. When the dilatation line turns upward, the active phase of labor has been entered. The next inclined line to the right should be darkened. This line represents the acceptable normal lowest limit of the rate of active-phase dilatation.
9. When the descent pattern turns down, darken the next inclined line to the right to indicate the acceptable lowest limit of the rate of descent.
10. If the dilatation line crosses the heavy vertical line at 20 hours in nulliparas (or 14 hours in multiparas) while still in the latent phase—that is, the pattern has not taken an upswing—the abnormality of *prolonged latent phase* exists.
11. If the active phase has been entered (recognized by the observation that the upswing has taken place) and the tracing crosses the inclined limit line that has previously been darkened, the diagnosis of *protracted active-phase dilatation* is made, provided progressive dilatation is continuing. If there is no further progress for 2 hours, however, the diagnosis is *secondary arrest of dilatation.*
12. After active descent has begun, if the descent line crosses the inclined limit line that has been darkened, diagnose *protracted descent* if progressive descent is continuing. Diagnose *arrest of descent* if there has been no further progress for 1 hour.
13. If the active phase dilatation line crosses the darkened inclined limit line above 8 cm of cervical dilatation, the deceleration phase has been entered. If this progresses for longer than 3 hours in nulliparas (or 1 hour in multiparas) without attaining full dilatation, diagnose *prolonged deceleration phase.*
14. If active descent has not begun by the time the deceleration phase of dilatation is entered, diagnose *failure of descent.*

In a consecutive series of labor studied by means of these modified graphic forms (Friedman et al, 1975), the diagnosis of the specific abnormality was made in every instance among the 11.3 percent dysfunctional patterns that occurred. Thus, there were no false negative diagnoses. Among the remaining graphically normal labors, a total of 1.4 percent misdiagnoses or false positive diagnoses were made. In each of these erroneous cases, the misdiagnosis was caused by the dilatation curve crossing the designated limit line during the acceleration phase. In every instance, the curve reached its maximum slope within another hour and either continued to progress in parallel with the inclined limit line or actually crossed back to the left of this line to reach full cervical dilatation quickly. The error, therefore, was promptly corrected. Discounting these left no incorrect diagnosis. Based on such experience, this graphic format appears to afford the practitioner an exceptionally insightful diagnostic capability. Moreover, this is accomplished without the need for developing even a minimal sophistication in mathematical calculations.

There are some difficulties, however, still persisting. Among them is the problem of accurately defining when the dilatation curve slopes upward and the active phase is entered. The difficulty especially pertains when there is some degree of change in cervical dilatation during the course of the latent phase. Although not wholly reliable, we may offer the following as a utilitarian aid. The uppermost rate of latent-phase dilatation, even when contractions are particularly vigorous and cervical resistance is negligible, rarely exceeds 0.6 cm per hour. By the same token, active-phase dilatation, except under the most unusual circumstances, is rarely less than this rate.

A rate of cervical dilatation slower than 0.6 cm per hour will usually, but not always, indicate that the patient is still in the latent phase. It is reflected on the nulliparous graphic form (Fig. 50) by a dilatation pattern that crosses two or more inclined limit lines for each centimeter of cervical dilatation that takes place. If fewer than two lines are crossed per centimeter, the rate of dilatation exceeds 0.6 cm per hour, and the patient is more likely to be in the active phase. This being the case, the next line to the right should then be designated to indicate the acceptable limit for the rate of dilatation in the active phase.

A word of caution is in order here. This "rule" should not be overinterpreted; it is meant merely as a guideline. When it is clear that there has been documentation of a perceptible change in the slope of dilatation, the active phase should be considered in progress—even if the new slope is less than 0.6 cm per hour. Of course, it is an abnormally protracted active phase. Nevertheless, the upswing defines the end of the latent phase and the beginning of the active phase, regardless of the dilatory course that the labor may be taking.

### *Labor Stencils*

Still another modification involves the construction of stencils for the purpose of forecasting the expected pattern of progression according to the degree of dilatation that has been achieved by the time the patient is admitted in labor (Studd and Duignan, 1972; Studd, 1973; Studd et al, 1975). Again, because of the confusion surrounding the time of onset of labor, these graphs were begun using the time of admission in labor as the starting point. Curves showing the average course of cervical dilatation were constructed for varying degrees of dilatation on admission. These composite data were then etched onto a stencil for use in conjunction with the aforementioned graphic records. The stencils were designed to provide a means to identify patients with disordered labor.

In practice, five separate patterns (Fig. 52) representing normal labor progression were compiled from groups of patients admitted at five different levels of cervical dilatation. The curves transcribed onto acrylic stencils are available for use as follows. When the patient is admitted in labor, the cervical dilatation is assessed. The appropriate stencil line is drawn according to the cervical dilatation completed up to that time. This line designates the expected progress for that patient.

Studd (1973) asserts that the labor pattern straying 2 hours or more to the

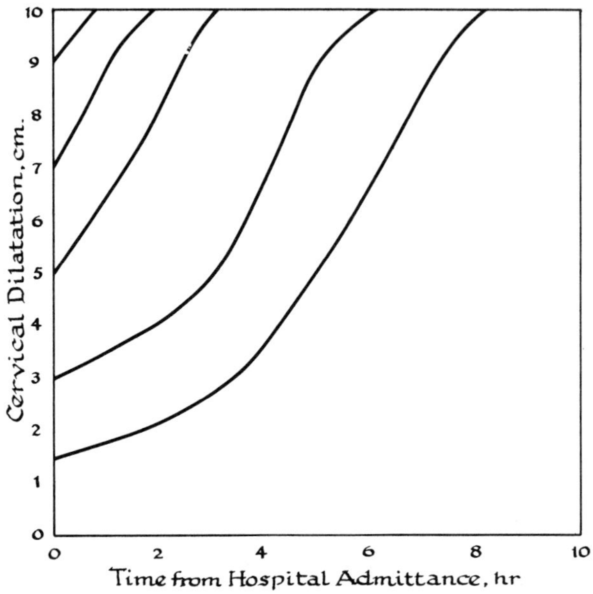


*Fig. 52.* Progressive courses of cervical dilatation in a series of nulliparas according to the degree of dilatation achieved up to the time of admission to the hospital. These curves were used to create stencils for the purpose of designating expected progression in a given gravida on the basis of the admission dilatation (compare with Fig. 32). (From Studd J: Br Med J 4:451, 1973).

right of the projected line may be considered abnormal and will require uterotonic stimulation. While issue may be taken with the recommendation for stimulation without a clearer idea of the type of disorder present and its causation (see Chapter 23), it is still commendable that this approach provides a very direct and simple means for identifying labors that are likely to be abnormal.

It should be noted that more than one-third (36 percent) of nulliparas and 13 percent of multiparas were deemed to be abnormal on this basis. This suggests that the technique is overly sensitive, designating many normal labors as dysfunctional. Indeed, both normal and abnormal latent phases will be flagged as seriously abnormal. This technique especially mislabels all those gravidas whose cervix may have reached 3 cm or more of dilatation while still in the latent phase (or even in false labor). These patients are uniformly declared disordered and categorically subjected to uterotonic stimulation to achieve the acceleration of progress that is expected of them. This routinized aggressive regimen can hardly be considered rational for all such cases. Quite the contrary: these patients tend to do well if their labors are allowed to evolve spontaneously or are deliberately rested by use of narcotic analgesics (Chapter 9).

While this approach is unlikely to overlook an abnormality of dilatation, it cannot distinguish protraction from arrest. It manages both of these groups of conditions automatically with uterotonic stimulation and without attempting to uncover those with prevailing fetopelvic disproportion. Moreover, unfortunately, it ignores the very serious descent problems entirely (see Chapters 10 and 11).

Studd (1973) uncritically uses a definition of disordered labor that stipulates a labor transgressing 2 or more hours from the mean labor curve. Note the use of the average pattern of progression. This does not take into account any measure of variance—that is, it ignores expected deviations of the normal population from the mean. The 2-hour designation is arbitrary at best. Data are presented to show that fewer operative deliveries occur after labors that progress more rapidly than the mean, as compared with those progressing more slowly. However, other factors may be at play to cause this difference. It is possible, for example, that the higher incidence of operative delivery among the slower labors reflects the aggressive attitude of the obstetrician (impatient to effect delivery, perhaps) rather than a consequence of the labor itself.

It has been suggested (Friedman, 1975a) that the appropriate cut-off be objectively determined by assessing outcomes according to the degree of delay patients exhibit (in a stepwise manner on the time scale). In this way a really meaningful definition of labor abnormality can be provided. It will be based on anticipated hazards to mother and fetus. Once this has been done, the stencil could be redesigned to yield the newly defined and much more critical limit patterns. These would serve to illustrate meaningful expectations in place of these average curves for normal labors.

## *SOURCES OF ERROR*

Certain minimum information is necessary in order to permit us to construct meaningful dilatation and descent curves for any given laboring patient. The prerequisites have been detailed earlier (see Chapter 7), including known time of onset of labor and at least two documented and "nonregressive" points along the active phase portion of the curves. Our ability to pinpoint when labor begins is admittedly limited (Chapter 3). Nevertheless, it is usually possible to ascertain from the patient when she first perceived regular uterine contractions. In our society, it is seldom the case that the patient cannot provide useful information in this regard. There are gravidas, of course, who are poor historians or who are so unobservant that they cannot be more precise. Moreover, there are areas where clock time is just unavailable; the African experience reported by Philpott and Castle (see above) attests to the modifications that are needed to adjust for this feature. For more highly developed areas, however, this is not a real problem, and it should be possible to define onset of labor with reasonable accuracy.

Graphs constructed by entering the first observation (usually obtained at the time of hospital admission) at the left margin of the form essentially ignore all the foregoing elapsed time from onset of labor. The graphs often give erroneous impressions of the evolution of labor to the attendant personnel. Thus, a serious source of error is the practice of beginning the labor curve at an inappropriate place on the graphic form. To do so, for example, might fail to provide a ready means for detecting when the latent phase is abnormally prolonged beyond the critical upper limits established for the latent-phase duration (Chapter 9).

Determinations of cervical dilatation and fetal station contain inherent errors analogous to the errors of any physical measurement. The magnitude of such error has been studied (see Chapter 3). An overall error of 3 percent in the measurement of cervical dilatation was found, with greatest accuracy at less than 3 cm and at more than 7 cm. Thus, between 3 and 7 cm, when progressive dilatation is occurring at its most rapid rate, accuracy of the measurement is poorest (although still rather good). Of course, since relative change is most important, the observation that rapid changes are taking place counterbalances the error factor. The accuracy of determinations of fetal station appears to increase with progressive descent, and the inherent error of these determinations is of the same order of magnitude as cervical dilatation. Again, since progressive descent is more important than its absolute measurement, comparable sequential determinations can be considered sufficiently accurate for our purposes.

Nevertheless, errors may be introduced into serial determinations by not ensuring that observations are made in a uniform manner. Interobserver variations exist. Individuals tend to err rather consistently—that is, a given individual will often overestimate (or underestimate) cervical dilatation or fetal station by a constant amount in a predictable manner. This consistency makes it possible for such an individual to create perfectly acceptable labor patterns provided he or she alone makes all the examinations. Thus, interobserver variations are minimized by reducing the number of observers as much as possible.

In practical terms, this might mean limiting examinations of a given patient to a single obstetric attendant. More realistically, it is often necessary for several people to be involved in patient care. Discrepancies in estimates of dilatation and descent can be minimized under these circumstances, if necessary, by constructing simultaneous curves based on the observations of each individual separately. Thus, the dilatation curve produced by one physician or nurse would be constructed only on the basis of those observations that he or she actually made, essentially ignoring all others. The tendency for some labor patterns to have "regressive" points (see Chapter 7) is almost entirely eliminated by this technique.

While the training, background, and experience of the observer appears to have little bearing on the accuracy of his or her estimates of dilatation and station, certain biases and expectations may. From time to time, labor patterns are seen to evolve in such a way as to suggest that the attendant is interpreting rather than measuring. The dilatation pattern, for example, may incorrectly show that the active phase has been entered, as evidenced by increasing cervical dilatation; similarly, the deceleration phase may appear to end in the second stage with full cervical dilatation and retraction. In such instances, subsequent observations (often by someone else who perhaps does not share the first observer's wishful expectations) show less by way of progression. Needless to say, such overenthusiastic optimism (or alternatively, undue pessimism) should be avoided. The labor patterns should reflect objective determinations and each recording should represent the most accurate information that can be obtained.

Examinations should be undertaken with uniform conditions whenever possible. Estimates made at the height of a uterine contraction will necessarily be different from those obtained during the quiescent intercontractile interval. Since a true estimate of cervical dilatation is at best difficult to achieve with a flaccid, elastic cervix, it is probably best to measure dilatation during contractions at all times. The same applies for estimating fetal descent, especially if the fetal head is not deeply fixed in the pelvis. While this may prove to be somewhat more uncomfortable for the patient, the benefits in useful information may make it acceptable, especially in those cases in which problems in labor progression occur.

Estimates of dilatation obtained by means of rectal examination tend to be somewhat smaller than those by vaginal examination. This is undoubtedly the consequence of the apparent inclusion of the thickness of the rectovaginal septum in the cervical os. The rectovaginal wall, of course, is usually soft and easily compressed, permitting one to discern anatomic landmarks readily. However, it may be difficult to be certain about cervical dilatation after the cervix has been completely effaced. Thus, vaginal examination is usually more accurate overall for the purpose of estimating cervical dilatation.

In contrast, the ischial spines are generally felt much more easily by rectal than by vaginal examination. This makes estimation of fetal station somewhat more accurate by the rectal route. The hazard, however, of estimating station rectally is that misinterpretation is more likely under certain circumstances. Since the examining finger is inserted rectally into the posterior aspect of the pelvis, it is conceivable that one may mistakenly assume a lower station for a fetal head that is occupying the hollow of the sacrum, especially in an occiput posterior position. The curve of the pelvis must always be borne in mind when estimating fetal station.

While the relative advantages of vaginal versus rectal examinations are debatable, there has been a general tendency toward using the vaginal approach exclusively. There is no evidence to support the contention that rectal examinations are safer than vaginal examinations (Peterson and Richey, 1962). Vaginal examinations are usually more comfortable for the patient, and the information obtained by this route is generally more reliable.

Potentially serious errors may result from misreading cranial molding as descent. The novice may mistakenly accept the formation of caput succedaneum as progressive descent, but this error is readily correctable by simple instruction. It takes considerably more sophistication to recognize that a fetal head fixed in the maternal pelvis is undergoing the process of molding, so that its forward leading edge appears to advance even though true descent is not occurring. The serious nature of this error is best understood when it is realized that one can wrongly diagnose protracted descent in a patient who has actually already experienced the more perilous disorder of arrest of descent. The implications of the differential diagnosis are discussed further in Chapter 21.

Here, proficiency and accuracy in estimating fetal station by vaginal examination is not necessarily helpful. It is more important to ascertain that true descent has taken place by means of abdominal examination (see Chapter 6). Periodic suprapubic palpation permits one to assess and confirm the true level of the fetal head according to its advancement into the pelvic inlet. This method ensures that descent as perceived by vaginal examination is not merely a reflection of molding of the fetal skull.

## *EVALUATING THE CURVES*

Some of the difficulties inherent in defining onset of labor have already been discussed (see above). The approach to recognizing the beginning of the active phase has also been reviewed in detail. Emphasis should be directed at recognizing the change in the rate of progression as the upswing of the dilatation curve (or the downswing of the descent curve) takes place. For some reason, this concept is sometimes difficult for the novice to grasp. As the pattern of the labor curves unfolds, the linear aspect of the latent phase can be seen to give way to the more steeply inclined slope of the active phase. The change is critical.

Moreover, calculating the slope between two consecutive points does not necessarily always provide a true overview of the evolution of the labor. This is particularly the case when the inherent errors in the estimates of dilatation or descent are ignored. While major changes in slope are generally obvious and easily appreciated, small changes tend to be either magnified or overlooked. Dismissing minor changes as insignificant is appropriate in most instances because these changes usually result from errors in measurement and therefore need not be considered as representing real change. However, such minor changes are sometimes very important, particularly in protraction disorders. When progression is occurring so slowly that the increment between observations is of about the same magnitude as the error of the measurement itself, it may take many hours before the situation is clarified.

A useful practice involves comparing the most recent observation with those made earlier in the sequence. Whereas the last and the next-to-last measurements may be similar in dimension to each other (the most recent perhaps 0.5 cm or less larger than the preceding one), earlier measurements may be much smaller, so that they more realistically reflect the progression that the patient has made in the course of her labor.

The absolute amount of dilatation or level of station is not entirely reliable as a milestone in the labor process. The majority of patients enter the active phase of dilatation with cervical dilatation of 2.5 cm or more. It does not follow, however, that those with dilatation exceeding 2.5 cm are necessarily in the active phase. It is well recognized that prelabor cervical dilatation occurs commonly, particularly in multiparas. Therefore, it is conceivable, for example, for gravidas to begin labor with cervical dilatation of 4 or 5 cm; prelabor dilatation far in excess of this—even to as much as full cervical dilatation—has been observed, although infrequently.

The duration of the latent phase in such labors tends to be short, reflecting the prelabor soft-tissue preparation that has occurred earlier (see Chapter 16). Nevertheless, some finite interval of latent phase is almost always documentable in these cases. This is not merely an academic exercise; it has important clinical relevance. For example, the additional slow dilatation that is likely to take place during the latent phase in these instances can be mistaken for protracted active-phase dilatation pattern, when in actuality the situation is nothing more than a normal latent phase. Differentiating these two conditions is of obvious clinical importance (see Chapter 21).

When the active phase begins, a change in the slope of dilatation is apparent at once. However, we should stress here that most gravidas do not attain their maximum rates of dilatation immediately. There is usually some period of time (which we have designated the acceleration phase) during which the dilatation pattern is speeding up to reach its maximum. If by chance one or more observations are made during the course of the acceleration phase, one may perceive this changing slope. It is not unusual, for example, for a patient to be diagnosed as having protracted active-phase dilatation pattern early in the active phase, only later to be found progressing quite normally, without any intervening event having occurred or uterotonic stimulation having been evoked.

Indeed, one of the serious pitfalls of automatized computer assessment systems is the unacceptable overdiagnosis of protraction disorders. Among nulliparas in one such series (Sokol et al, 1977), 26 percent had protracted active-phase dilatation and 10 percent, protracted descent (among their multiparas, 16 and 5 percent, respectively). Undoubtedly, the reason for this unusually high frequency is misdiagnosis based on blind calculation of the slopes of dilatation and descent between every two readings, without accounting specifically for the maximum slope attainable in a given case.

That the slope of dilatation or descent early in the active phase is abnormally protracted is not necessarily irrefutable evidence that a protraction disorder actually exists. While it is appropriate to suspect that the labor is actually abnormal when abnormal slopes are encountered, the diagnosis must be considered tentative until the curve of dilatation or descent reaches its maximum rate of progression (phase of maximum slope). It is this linear portion of the active phase that will serve best as a measure of normality.

Several methods are available for purposes of measuring the maximum slopes of dilatation and descent. Use of nonmathematical graph forms (see above) have reduced the need for arithmetical computation of the slopes. Nonetheless, it is important for the practitioner not to fear the minimum efforts involved here. The most difficult calculation involves nothing more than dividing the change in dilatation (or station) by the time interval for that change to occur. For example,

Onset of labor in a nullipara: 8:00 P.M.
Examination A at 2:15 A.M.: 2.5 cm and station 0
Examination B at 4:30 A.M.: 4.0 cm and station 0

Dilatation has changed from 2.5 cm to 4.0 cm, an increment of 1.5 cm, over an interval of 2 hours and 15 minutes (2.25 hours) ; dividing 1.5 by 2.25 yields a rate of dilatation of 0.7 cm/hr. The situation is unclear. If the patient is in latent phase, the degree of dilatation is uncommonly good; if in active phase, it is possible that she exhibits a protraction disorder. More likely than either of these is the possibility that she has just entered the active phase and is still accelerating. Time should clarify these issues.

Examination C at 6:00 A.M.: 7.0 cm and station +1

There has been a 3.0-cm change in dilatation over an interval of 1.5 hr; the slope of dilatation is now 2.0 cm/hr (derived by dividing 3.0 by 1.5) . The patient is now clearly in the active phase of the dilatation curve. Looking back, we may say the latent phase lasted until about 2:15 A.M., or 6.3 hours in duration. Although she may not as yet have reached her maximum rate of dilatation, progression is now quite normal. At the same time, descent appears to have begun. The fetal presenting part has descended 1 cm in 1.5 hours, a slope of 0.7 cm/hr. This may or may not be abnormal, according to the events that evolve subsequently.

Examination D at 7:15 A.M.: 9.5 cm and station +2

Dilatation has now progressed an additional 2.5 cm over a period of 1.25 hours, demonstrating a slope of 2.0 cm/hr. This verifies her maximum slope of dilatation. Meanwhile, further descent has taken place at a rate of 0.8 cm/hr (1 cm of descent in 1.25 hours) , suggesting the abnormality of protracted descent. Again, it is possible that the maximum rate of descent has not as yet been attained. This, too, should be clarified with the passage of more time.

Examination E at 8:45 A.M.: cervix fully dilated and fetal station +4

During the intervening 1.5 hours, the cervix has dilated the additional 0.5 cm and is now fully retracted in the second stage. Station has advanced 2 cm for a slope of 1.3 cm/hr (2 cm divided by 1.5 hours) , a normal rate of descent for this nullipara. We can see how easy it would have been to misdiagnose protraction disorders in this case, as discussed above. Equally important, we have illustrated how simple the calculations are for measuring the slopes of dilatation and descent.

If the arithmetic should still prove to be too difficult or threatening, simple devices are available to help provide the necessary information. One can create useful instruments for purposes of reading the slope directly from the graph on which it is being traced. Three examples are shown in the accompanying illustration (Fig. 53). By aligning the bottom edge along any horizontal coordinate of the graph, the inclination of the slope is immediately available, as shown. This can take the form of an etched plastic triangle, protractor, or rectangle. No calculations are required to obtain fairly accurate measurements of the rates of dilatation and descent.

Guide rules of this kind can be devised with stipulated limits of normal already inscribed (at 1.2 and 1.5 cm/hr for dilatation and at 1.0 and 2.0 cm/hr for descent). Although they are not as yet commercially available, it should be a relatively simple matter to produce one for personal use. The prototypes shown in Figure 53 may aid in this regard.

Measurement errors should be considered as an integral part of one's analysis of labor progression. Since it is so important to recognize when the slopes of dilatation and descent are abnormal, we should make every effort to identify those cases that are obviously abnormal as well as those that might possibly be so. This involves two kinds of manipulations. The first is the practice of discounting "regressive" points (see Chapter 7). These are observations that can be considered to have been in error because later estimates of dilatation and station show retrograde progress. The points in Figure 54A trace an irregular dilatation curve. However, when the regressive observations are deleted (Figure 54B), the sigmoid curve of normal dilatation emerges.

The second corrective maneuver involves smoothing or averaging the irregular curve or, alternatively, expressing the range of possibilities based on the inherent error of the measurements themselves. The inconsistencies in the dilatation pattern shown in Figure 55A fade quickly by this averaging process. It can be accomplished by statistical means (a "best fit" regression equation based on the method of least squares) or, more practically, by eye fit. This is an acceptable approach only if the variations from the smoothed curve are minimal.

Because the error of a given measurement rarely exceeds 0.5 cm, depicting these limits may prove useful in offering a means for assessing the extremes of the slope for any given pair of measurements (Fig. 55B). For example,

Examination A at 1 P.M.: 4.0 cm of dilatation
Examination B at 2 P.M.: 7.0 cm of dilatation

At face value, the slope here is 3.0 cm/hr, based on the 3.0-cm advance in 1 hour. Ordinarily, this is entirely acceptable. However, we might take into

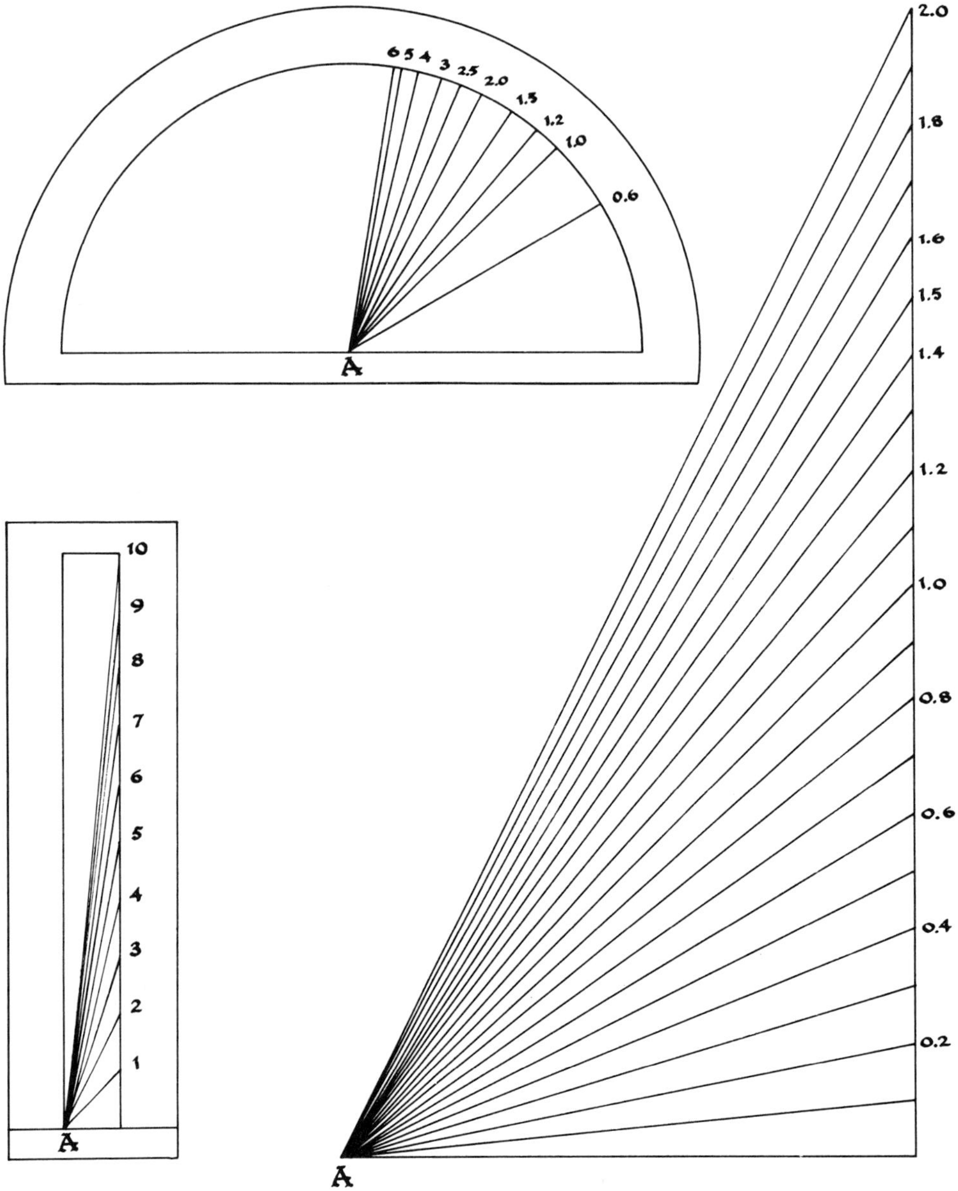


*Fig. 53.* Aids for measuring slopes of cervical dilatation of fetal descent. The basic principle of each allows one to read the rate of change (in centimeters per hour) based on the angle the curve makes with the horizontal. For use in practice they require the graphic form to be devised so that each horizontal hourly time division is equal in size to each vertical centimeter cervical dilatation division. The bottom straightedge is aligned with any horizontal line on the graph to provide a direct reading of the slope when the line being measured passes through point A on the device.

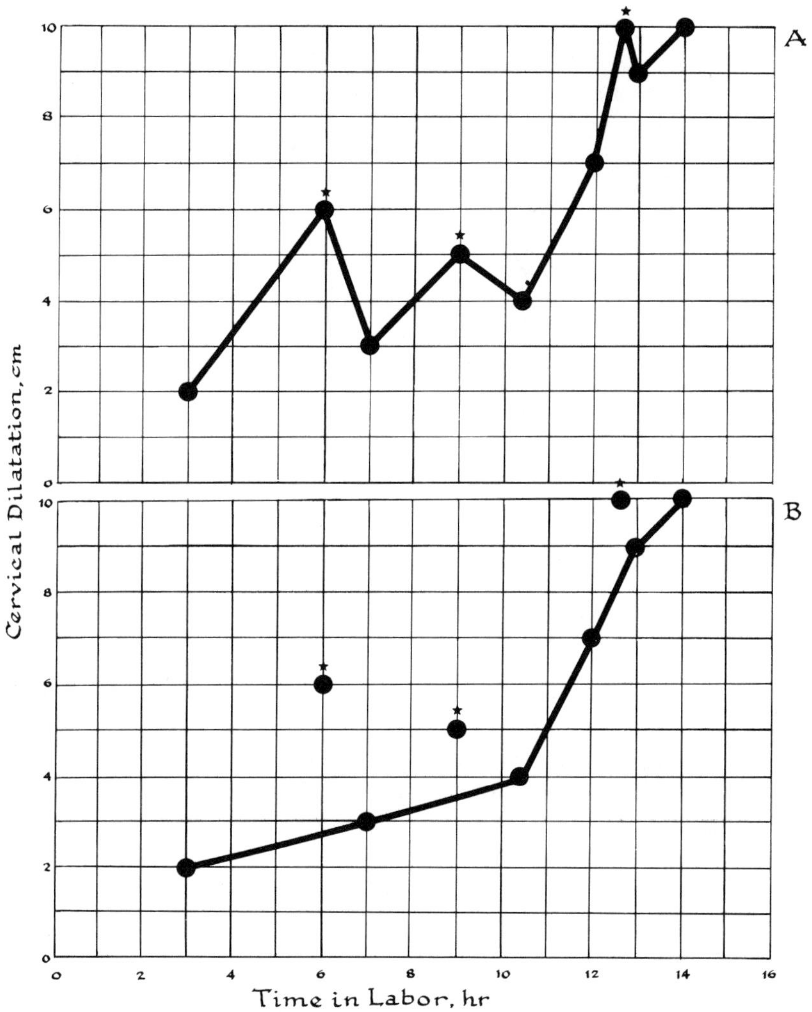


*Fig. 54.* Pattern of cervical dilatation traced when estimates made over a period of time by several different individuals are entered. **A.** Regressive points (*asterisks*) characterized by subsequent observations that suggest they were unduly optimistic or actually in error. **B.** When only nonregressive points are considered, a meaningful curve evolves. Joining the nonregressive points by straight lines yields an acceptable (and in this case, normal) dilatation pattern.

account that these observations were made by different examiners. We cannot rely entirely on the comparability of their estimates. It is possible that observer A regularly reads too high, while observer B reads too low, or vice versa.

Let us, therefore, examine the possible extremes of the slopes based on

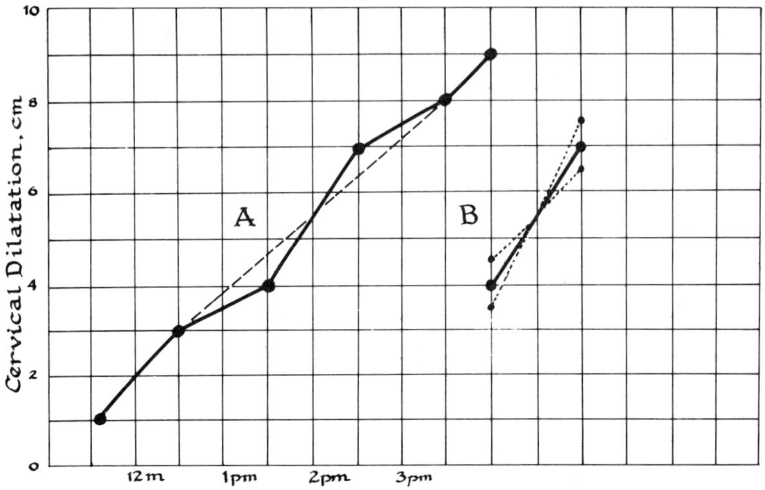


*Fig. 55* Correcting for possible inherent errors of measurements includes (**A**) smoothing or (**B**) taking into account the extent of the error for each observation (see text). The probable minimum and maximum range of the true slope (*dotted lines*) is based on the assumption that either reading may be as much as 0.5 cm in error in either direction.

interobserver errors. The 4.0-cm reading might be as low as 3.5 or as high as 4.5 cm (assuming a maximum likely error of 0.5 cm); likewise, the dilatation at examination B might range from 6.5 to 7.5 cm. At the high end of the slope range (3.5 to 7.5 cm in 1 hour), we obtain a rate of 4.0 cm/hr; at the low end of the spectrum (4.5 to 6.5 cm), the rate is calculated at 2.0 cm/hr.

Since both extremes are within reasonably normal limits, the issue is academic for this patient. However, such is not always the case. Whenever the lower hypothetical limit falls into the abnormal range, it is important that the patient be watched carefully. Subsequent examinations usually clarify the course, showing the true rate of progression on the smoothed curve. The further advanced the labor, the more likely for the pattern to be clearly identifiable.

## *DYNAMIC INTERPRETATION*

Stepwise programmatic analysis of labor progression will almost invariably provide the kind of information necessary for early diagnosis of labor aberrations. It is obvious that serial examinations are necessary. What is not so clear is the frequency and timing of such examinations. On the one hand, we intuitively prefer to minimize the number of vaginal or rectal examinations in deference to the patient's comfort and perhaps morbidity; on the other hand, without timely observations, we cannot follow the course of labor adequately. Spacing of examinations is rarely critical.

The minimum information necessary for evolving a pattern is the time of onset of labor and two observations during the course of the active phase. If the latter are sufficiently separated in time, they can be used to construct the inclination of the phase of maximum slope rather accurately. This in turn can be extrapolated in a retrograde fashion to provide an indication of when the active phase began (and the latent phase ended); or it can be projected forward in time to designate when the deceleration phase and second stage ought to begin. We have discussed such measures extensively before (see Chapter 16) as they relate to the formulation of a trial of labor.

It should be clear that the more rapidly labor is progressing the more frequent the examinations will have to be, in order to provide sufficient information to reconstruct the curve later or to trace it as it evolves. In gravidas whose labor is developing slowly, the interval between examinations should be rather long.

In practical terms, 2-hour intervals usually suffice for the average labor and will be ample for purposes of detecting abnormalities as they arise. Much more frequent examinations will be required to detect the excessively rapid progress of precipitate labors, so that even half-hourly examinations may not be enough. For diagnosed protraction disorders, an examination every 3 to 5 hours may serve our purposes adequately. Needless to say, these are not rigid rules. Examinations may be interspersed whenever the situation appears to demand them or may be delayed if it is clear that the clinical situation warrants it.

Given enough information, a systematic approach to evaluating the dilatation and descent curves can be accomplished. It involves a series of logical considerations at every examination. These can be formulated into a series of questions.

1. What is the cervical dilatation at this time?
2. Has there been any change since the last examination?
3. What is the magnitude of the change?
4. Does the magnitude exceed the error inherent in the examination?
5. If it exceeds the error, what is the rate of change per unit hour?
6. If less than the error, are there preceding examinations for use in evaluating significant change?
7. If no change has occurred, was there foregoing active dilatation?
8. If no prior dilatation, does this represent the latent phase?
9. What is the duration of the latent phase to this point?
10. Is the duration excessive as yet?
11. If prior dilatation has occurred, does this represent secondary arrest of dilatation?

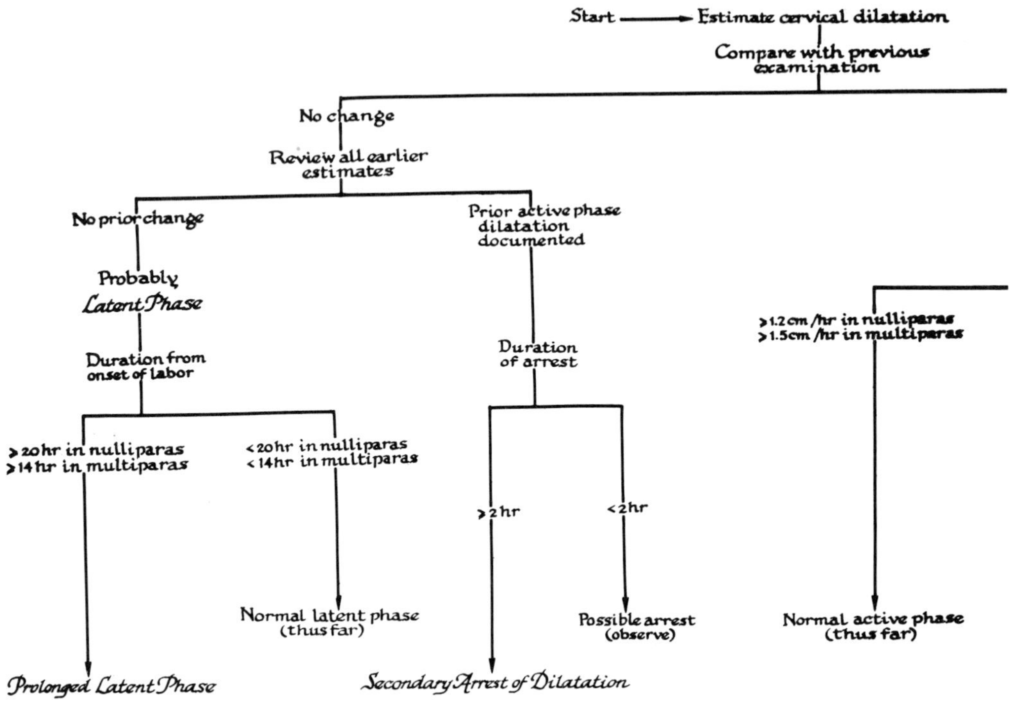


*Fig. 56.* Paradigm of logic sequence diagnosing labor aberrations associated with disordered dilatation patterns. The evaluative observations continue in Figure 57 for purposes of diagnosing descent disorders.

12. If there has been change since the last examination, is it of sufficient magnitude to suggest that the patient is in the latent or the active phase?
13. If in the active phase, is the rate abnormally slow?
14. If abnormal, is this a protracted active-phase dilatation pattern?
15. If there has been prior active dilatation, does this represent the deceleration phase?
16. What is the duration of the deceleration phase to this point?
17. Is the duration excessive as yet?
18. If in the deceleration phase, has active descent begun?

This leads us to a similar series of questions concerning progress in fetal descent. The first six questions listed above apply with equal impact to evaluating fetal station, of course. In addition, we may continue as follows:

1. If there has been no change in the fetal station, has the patient entered the deceleration phase of dilatation?
2. If in the deceleration phase, has there been any foregoing descent in labor?

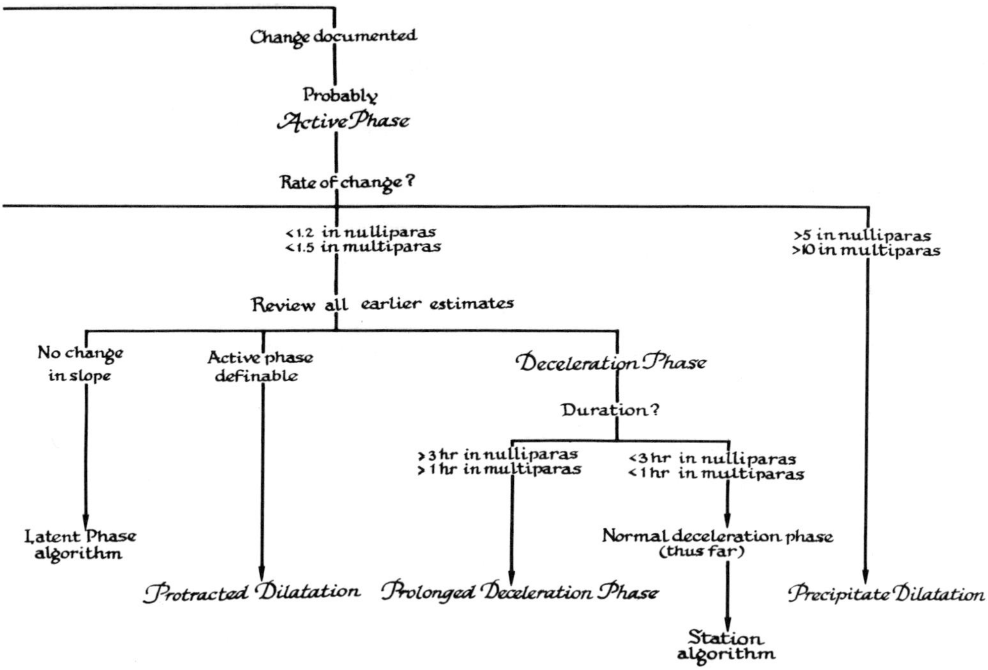


3. If no foregoing descent, is this failure of descent?
4. If there has been foregoing descent, does this represent arrest of descent?
5. If there has been a change in fetal station, is the rate of change abnormal?
6. If the rate is abnormal, does this represent protracted descent?

This series of questions represents the logical decision considerations that every clinician utilizes—either overtly or intuitively—in arriving at the correct diagnoses of normal or abnormal labor processes for the gravidas under his or her care. The framework of this logical sequence has been used to help formulate on-line interactive digital computer programs for purposes of diagnosing both dilatation and descent disorders (Sokol et al, 1973a, 1974b). This followed upon the development of an earlier computer program capable of diagnosing some labor disorders, but on a retrospective basis (Friedman and Kroll, 1971c). Such programs have much to commend them, but cannot do more for the clinician than he or she can do at the bedside. Although comparison of computer technology with the clinical graphic method showed good diagnostic correlation and accuracy, computer logic tended to fail more often. Thus, the simple graphic method appears to offer considerable advantage in terms of cost, applicability, and accuracy.

## *DIAGNOSTIC SEQUENCE*

The flow of diagnostic logic is displayed in Figures 56 and 57. These algorithms are presented to provide a system for developing meaningful diagnoses of all the dilatation and descent disorders we can define objectively. They detail the series of steps one generally takes in arriving at such diagnoses. Those with some experience in this discipline evolve this sort of stepwise approach intuitively. For our purposes here, we shall at this time show the dynamic sequence we utilize more or less routinely.

At each examination (after the first), the estimate of cervical dilatation is compared with the immediately preceding estimate (Fig. 56). If there has been no change, all prior examinations are reviewed to determine whether or not there has been any evidence of foregoing active-phase progression. If none, we may assume the patient is still in the latent phase. Parenthetically, we may have to consider the possibility of secondary arrest of dilatation here if the dilatation is advanced and the labor has not been conducted under our observation (see Chapter 21). The duration of the latent phase from onset of labor is measured in order to assess for the abnormality of prolonged latent phase. If it exceeds 20 hours in a nullipara or 14 hours in a multipara, the diagnosis is confirmed.

If there is documentation of preceding active-phase dilatation, then one must consider that the situation may represent secondary arrest of dilatation. If there has been no change in the cervix for a period of 2 hours or more, the diagnosis is justified. If less than 2 hours, arrest is a possibility, but additional observation will be necessary for verification.

Returning to the original estimate of dilatation, we may find it changed from the prior examination. We generally will assume the active phase to be in progress under these conditions. We can then measure the rate of change (see above) and use that information to tell us whether or not the active phase is normal. If excessively rapid (greater than 5 cm/hr in nulliparas or 10 cm/hr in multiparas), a precipitate dilatation pattern exists. If abnormally slow (less than 1.2 cm/hr in nulliparas or 1.5 cm/hr in multiparas), there is probably a protracted active-phase dilatation pattern.

This last can be verified by reviewing all earlier entries on the curve. A clearly defined foregoing change in slope identifies the beginning of the active phase and supports the diagnosis of protraction. If there has been no evident change in slope, it is more likely that the patient is still in her latent phase of labor after all.

A third possibility is that there is documentation of prior active dilatation presaging the expected slowing of dilatation as the normal deceleration phase is entered. In this case, the duration of deceleration is determined; if it exceeds normal limits (3 hours in nulliparas, 1 hour in multiparas), prolonged deceleration phase is diagnosed. The station algorithm becomes operative once the labor has reached the deceleration phase of dilatation.

The fetal station sequence (Fig. 57) is used during the deceleration phase and second stage as a measure of progression. Each estimate is compared with

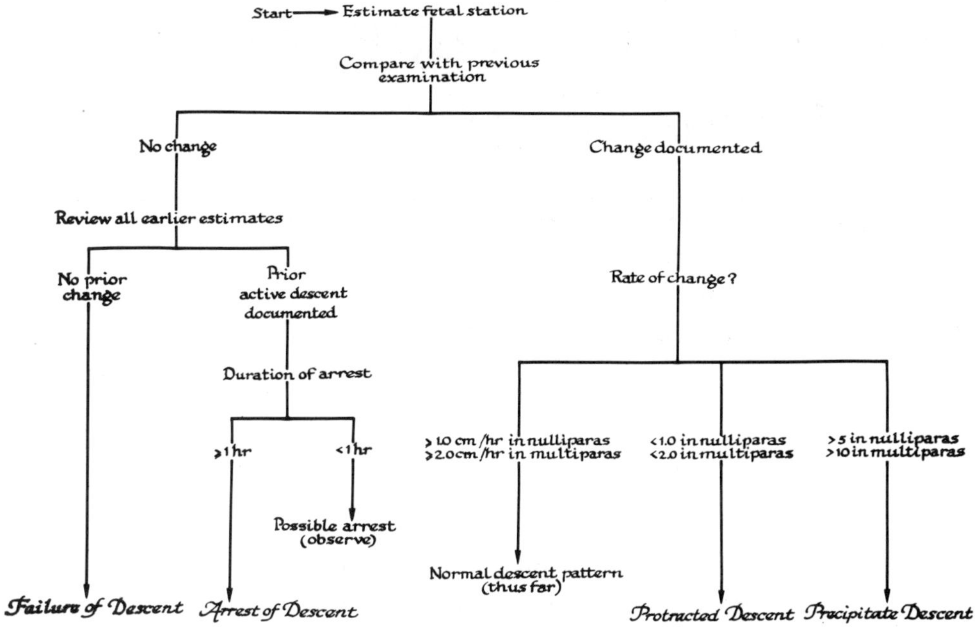


*Fig. 57.* Continuation of the diagnostic algorithm in Figure 56, showing logic for diagnosing descent disorders after the dilatation curve has entered or passed its deceleration phase.

the one obtained before it. If there has been no change, we review all preceding values. Failure of descent is characterized by unremitting lack of descent well into the deceleration phase and second stage. If there has been some documented descent earlier, however, cessation of progression at this time signifies the likelihood that arrest of descent has taken place. It is confirmed as such if there has been no advance for a period of 1 hour or more.

Active descent is evident when there is clear change in fetal station. When found to occur, the rate of change should be ascertained. Again, the rate will define whether the pattern is normal or not. If it exceeds normal limits (5 cm/hr in nulliparas or 10 cm/hr in multiparas), it represents precipitate descent. If it is very slow (less than 1 cm/hr in nulliparas or 2 cm/hr in multiparas), one may diagnose protracted descent.

By going through these steps at each examination, we will be able to uncover abnormalities as they arise. Patients with significant disorders may then be promptly evaluated (see Chapter 22) and have appropriate management regimens instituted (see Chapter 25). In those instances where the diagnosis is not so clear-cut, the patient can be flagged as being at significant risk and observed more carefully for the development of the overt disorder.

# Differential Diagnosis and Evaluation

## CHAPTER 21

Practical means are discussed for differentiating among the several pairs of labor disorders that may manifest similar patterns when observed only over a short interval of time. In addition, issues relating to the poorly defined clinical conditions considered under the terms "soft-tissue dystocia" and "failure to progress in labor" are clarified. The important problem of pelvic dystocia is systematically reviewed to yield the steps recommended for evaluating fetopelvic relationships meaningfully. This utilitarian approach includes antepartum and intrapartum clinical assessment, plus attention to the labor pattern as it unfolds, followed by a dynamic form of cephalopelvimetry in combination with objective radiographic studies for those specifically requiring them. The practical nature of this approach is stressed.

Some of the differential diagnostic quandaries sometimes faced by the obstetric attendant were discussed superficially in Chapter 8. We emphasized that most of the difficulties encountered in making accurate diagnoses could be avoided by intelligent sequential evaluations and careful examination of the dilatation and descent curves as they developed. Such problems will be dealt with in more detail here, concentrating on helpful clues for characterizing specific abnormalities of labor.

While definitive pathognomonic features of labor aberrations may not be readily available—besides the labor curve, of course—it is often possible to construct a logical case for a diagnosis based on such factors as the uterine contractility and its changing pattern, the nature of and change in cervical consistency and effacement, and the fetopelvic relationships. In addition, the patient's subjective and objective responses to sedation, anesthesia, and uterotonic stimulation may be equally valuable in this regard.

Although we have placed no prior emphasis on the significance of the contractile pattern in defining the several labor abnormalities, we will dwell on its potential value for differentiating disordered labors from each other, particularly when documentation of prior patterns of dilatation and descent are unavailable. In those situations in which reconstruction of the labor curves is neither possible nor feasible (because prior recordings are not available or are considered unreliable), it is imperative that all other available data be taken into consideration. While this may strike one as a self-evident truth, it is surprising how seldom it is adhered to in practice.

## *TRUE LABOR VERSUS FALSE LABOR*

Much has been written to help characterize and distinguish between true and false labor. However, there are no fixed and uniformly applicable rules that can be used at the bedside. It is generally expected that the contractions of false labor will recur at irregular and infrequent intervals and that they will be relatively weak and of short duration. Moreover, contractions of false labor are said to be felt by the patient more in the abdomen than in the back. They are reputed not to be affected by activity such as walking. Pain out of proportion to the intensity of the contraction is also thought to be distinctive.

These features may indeed apply in selected instances. In actuality, of course, false labor contractions commonly recur quite frequently, and they may be very intense, very long, and very painful; in a word, they need not comply with any of the common clinical criteria heretofore suggested. Thus, it is seldom really possible to tell them apart from true labor contractions.

In practice, we openly acknowledge the limitations of our diagnostic capabilities. We accept the impossibility of prospective distinction between true and false labor. This being the case, we only need to make the assumption that the condition characterized by uterine contractions that continue uninterruptedly represents labor. If the contractions should continue beyond the prescribed limits of the normal latent phase and not result in cervical dilatation, we are justified in diagnosing the abnormality of prolonged latent phase. Appropriate treatment may then be instituted. Since the management program recommended for this disorder (see Chapter 24) takes into account the possibility that false labor may exist, this arbitrary decision proves to be valid. The wisdom gained by hindsight—when the contractions finally stop altogether—makes the situation clear.

As we have seen (Chapter 9), false labor can be diagnosed retrospectively in about 10 percent of patients with prolonged latent phase. However, we must realize that we cannot distinguish them from those with true dysfunctional labor during the course of the latent phase as long as the uterus continues to contract regularly. The therapeutic measure we utilize for providing much needed rest for these patients—namely, large doses of narcotic-analgesic agents—will usually provide us with the answer in due course. Those in false labor should not resume their contractions when they awaken from this regimen. The therapeutic trial thus aids us in making a meaningful differentiation.

Even under ideal circumstances, the diagnosis of true labor or disordered labor cannot be made clinically until after active cervical dilatation has begun. Because of the characteristically abnormal rate of active-phase dilatation that may occur in association with the protracted active-phase pattern, it will be feasible to ascribe the foregoing state of prolonged latent phase to the dysfunctional state that is now documentable. However, while the patient is still within the latent phase, there are no signposts to help in prognostication.

Clinically, the uterine contractions may be well within normal limits, or they may be desultory, or even hyperactive, without giving the slightest clue as to what the forthcoming events of a particular labor will be. We recognize that many patients with abnormal labor contractility—as defined by weak, infrequent, and/or short uterine contractions—may have perfectly normal dilatation patterns. In contrast, some patients whose contractions seem normal will present a definitely abnormal dilatation and descent pattern after the active phase has been entered. On this basis, any real distinction between the several differential diagnostic possibilities is very difficult to make at best, except perhaps by hindsight.

Whereas the pattern of contractions may not help us, the degree of prelabor soft-tissue preparation may (see below). It does take a nicety of clinical judgment to be able to define and characterize subtle degrees of soft-tissue resistance. Nevertheless, gross evaluation of the cervix can determine readiness for induction of labor with reasonable degrees of accuracy. It should follow, therefore, that an obviously "unripe" cervix—that is, one that is long, closed, tough, and rigid—is not likely to be encountered in a patient who is in early labor. This is particularly so if that labor began spontaneously and was unassociated with such intrinsic labor-initiating complications as systemic or local infection, ruptured membranes, and placental abruption. We should hasten to add, however, that it is certainly possible for true labor to begin even in the presence of poorly prepared pelvic soft tissues, as evidenced by the large numbers of such patients found among those who developed prolonged latent phase (Chapter 9).

For the patient with a long, closed, thick, or rigid cervix that refuses to dilate or change to any significant degree despite apparently active uterine contractions, we must entertain the possibility that the patient is not actually in labor. When the "latent phase" in these patients becomes abnormally prolonged, they present diagnostic dilemmas. Since false labor and true dysfunction cannot be distinguished prospectively under these conditions in any manner that even approaches objectivity, the patient should be given the opportunity to show her ability to respond to sedation and the rest that it offers her. Administering large doses of narcotics effectively rests the uterus. After a suitable interval, during which contractions should cease, the patient almost invariably clarifies her earlier condition. If the contractions do not recur, it is now quite clear that she had an episode of false labor earlier. Under this circumstance, no further treatment is necessary.

In the majority of cases (85 percent), active dilatation begins promptly after the patient recovers from this interval of rest. These patients thus declare themselves as having been in true labor. Usually, no further difficulties occur. For the small residual group whose contractions begin again, but without substantial progress in cervical dilatation, oxytocin stimulation is usually quite effective—provided it is not contraindicated. The therapeutic trial of effective rest has given us a utilitarian means for differentiating true labor from false.

## *SOFT-TISSUE DYSTOCIA*

Perhaps the prevailing confusion about disorders of labor progress caused by soft-tissue factors stems from our innate inability to define normal labor. Indeed, labor aberrations associated with pathologic states of maternal soft tissues have received very little attention in recent years. Cervical dystocia, for example, is treated in a very cursory manner in the latest editions of obstetric textbooks.

The term soft-tissue dystocia refers to abnormal or pathologic labor secondary to anomalies of the soft parts of the pelvis, in contradistinction to difficulties related to the bony pelvis. It has been said (and is undoubtedly still true) that the soft tissues are much more often the cause of dystocia than the bony pelvis (Greenhill and Friedman, 1968). This refers to disturbances of uterine activity, usually manifested by weak and infrequent contractions of short duration.

In any series of patients who ostensibly have dystocia are (1) some experiencing essentially normal labor progress, perhaps misinterpreted as desultory by a misguided or impatient attendant; (2) some in false labor, indistinguishable except in retrospect; (3) some with prolonged periods of prodromal labor, commonly not given the opportunity to demonstrate their potential for normal later progress; (4) some with the major aberrations of protracted active-phase dilatation, or secondary arrest of dilatation, or arrest of descent.

We now recognize that these several variations or abnormalities of labor do not and cannot in any way be considered to represent unique disorders with specific causes. It is clear that they must be distinguished from each other by the clinician so that the most appropriate management regimen can be embarked upon in each instance. Of specific interest here are those manifesting labor aberrations brought about by soft-tissue factors. Let us try to determine if they can be flagged objectively.

How do soft-tissue problems manifest themselves? It is possible that abnormally slow progress after the active labor has commenced may be a direct result of dysfunction of the uterine powers. Negligible myometrial activity might produce this pattern. The cause of uterine dysfunction, however, is a matter of considerable conjecture. Only occasionally can we provide a clear-cut answer.

Consensus holds that debilitating diseases, fatigue, anemia, neurologic disorders, anxiety, anatomic uterine factors such as leiomyomata uteri and scars, fetal malpresentation, and uterine overdistention from multiple pregnancy or hydramnios may be either causative or contributory. We have seen in the series of foregoing analyses presented in this volume that there is little supporting documentation for most of these contentions. Moreover, it is difficult at best to ascribe a specific cause to a given case.

Attempts to quantitate normal uterine contractility have failed to provide any practical means for assessing motive force in such patients. As we have seen, even the most delicate, objective, physiologic measuring apparatus cannot distinguish true from false labor, let alone normal from abnormal labor. Occasionally, weak contractions characterize a "typical" case of uterine dysfunction, which is associated with minimal or absent progression in dilatation and descent. In actuality, this contraction pattern may be identical with the weak contractions of the gravida whose labor progression is normal. We have all seen multiparas, for example, who undergo rapid dilation of the cervix and evacuation of the uterus as a consequence of relatively poor uterine contractions that are quite effective in overcoming the negligible resistance of the birth canal and soft tissues.

True cervical dystocia is exceedingly uncommon. While the diagnosis may be applied in about 1 in 700 patients (Greenhill and Friedman, 1968), most of these cases represent obvious misdiagnoses. Indeed, when labor patterns are objectively scrutinized in these cases, they usually prove to be well within normal limits. Very few exhibit the characteristic cervical rigidity or inability to dilate with effective uterine contractions—hallmarks of true cervical dystocia. In fact, careful perusal of the labor course usually raises serious doubt as to the appropriateness of the diagnosis. Even gravidas with cervical scarification may not have had their potential for dilatation tested sufficiently. Usually, in those cases in which a trial of adequate labor is permitted, vaginal delivery can be effected. With rare exceptions, it is likely that any dystocia due to cervical factors can be overcome by adequate labor.

The "catchbasket" diagnosis of cervical dystocia, used to encompass a spectrum of labor variations, is fortunately falling into disuse. This seems to be the result of the growing appreciation among obstetricians of the physiologic mechanisms of labor and its normal variations. As we become more sophisticated in understanding the pathogenesis of labor abnormalities, we find less and less need for esoteric and cryptic designations such as this. This is further reflected in that we are seeing few cases in which the cervix is designated as the cause for labor difficulties. In the past, attempts to effect delivery through an incompletely dilated cervix were not uncommonly justified by a tenuous designation of cervical dystocia. This was usually applied by the physician whose own impatience deserved to carry the full burden of responsibility instead.

It is conceivable that spasm of the cervix may occur in those rare instances in which the cervix contains enough smooth muscle to effect contraction. However, this is an exceedingly unlikely situation. It is far more probable that myometrial dysfunction—specifically, inadequate contractility to overcome whatever degree of resistance the soft tissues present—is the root cause. Since the cervix is composed largely of fibrous connective tissue with minimal amounts of muscle, any real difficulties encountered by effective uterine contractions in dilating the cervix might be attributable to pathologic resistance. This can occur, of course. It is evidenced by reports of uterine rupture, sacculation, and delivery through the anterior wall of the cervix in badly neglected cases. The extreme rarity of true cervical dystocia, however, should be borne in mind at all times.

Attempts have been made to determine whether specific changes can be recognized in the anatomic, morphologic, and biochemical status of the cervix in such conditions. Investigations have not as yet uncovered any information of value. Usually, the cervix is entirely normal on the basis of clinical and laboratory study. The exception to this generalization involves the rare instances of cicatrization that can result from surgery, cautery, infection, trauma, or neoplasm. In its minor form, this condition may present as cervical conglutination. It is readily and effectively treated in most instances by initiating the dilatation process digitally. Merely inserting the examining finger into the cervical os will disrupt the encircling fibrous band sufficiently to permit the active centrifugal retraction process to begin. Once begun, rapid dilatation can be expected.

The more serious form is manifested by arrest of dilatation, usually between 4 and 8 cm. This alleged form of cervical dystocia is very difficult to distinguish from arrest of dilatation due to other causes (see below). The practice of invoking Dührssen's incisions, once deemed appropriate under such circumstances, deserves to be mentioned only for its historical interest. We must emphasize the very limited usefulness of this procedure. Today, it should be stringently avoided because hazards to both mother and fetus are great.

This technique cannot serve as a substitute for excellent obstetric judgment and evaluation of the individual case. The patient who ought to be given the opportunity to dilate her cervix in response to additional labor should not be subjected to the major risks that are attendant on this operation. Similarly, the infant who cannot negotiate an inadequate birth canal should not be forced to do so by ill-advised vaginal operative manipulations. Since secondary arrest of dilatation and prolonged deceleration phase are so commonly associated with insurmountable fetopelvic disproportion, forceful attempts to effect vaginal delivery by cutting the cervix and applying vigorous instrumental traction to the fetal head are clearly inappropriate.

Even under ideal circumstances, alternative means should be sought. This is particularly relevant in view of the risks of Dührssen's incisions and the dubious nature of the condition for which they are done. In the presence of cephalopelvic disproportion, the resulting secondary arrest of dilatation is more properly handled by expeditious cesarean section. In the absence of disproportion, oxytocin infusion overcomes the arrest pattern in nearly all cases (see Chapter 24).

## LATENT PHASE VERSUS PROTRACTED DILATATION

In Chapter 20, we alluded to the difficulties sometimes encountered by attendants who cannot readily distinguish between the normal cervical changes occurring during the latent phase and the extremely slow rate of dilatation of the abnormally protracted active phase. This pertains most especially to the patient who is first seen after an interval of labor that has not been conducted under observation. The differential diagnostic dilemma involves the patient who is found to have progressive cervical dilatation occurring at a rate that is less than the critical limits for the maximum slope of active-phase dilatation, namely, less than 1.2 cm/hr in nulliparas or 1.5 cm/hr in multiparas.

Without knowing what the pattern of progression was earlier in the course of that labor, we would have difficulty determining whether this represents a protracted active-phase dilatation pattern or a perfectly normal progressive latent phase of labor (Fig. 58). It would have been helpful if the patient had been observed sequentially earlier in the course of this labor so that one could detect the change in rate of dilatation from the latent phase to the phase of maximum slope. However desirable such information may be, it is unfortunately not always available in the world of real patients.

There is a prevalent practice in some areas to insist that the patient remain at home as long as possible after labor begins. While this reduces problems of bed occupancy and diminishes the incidence of gravidas admitted in

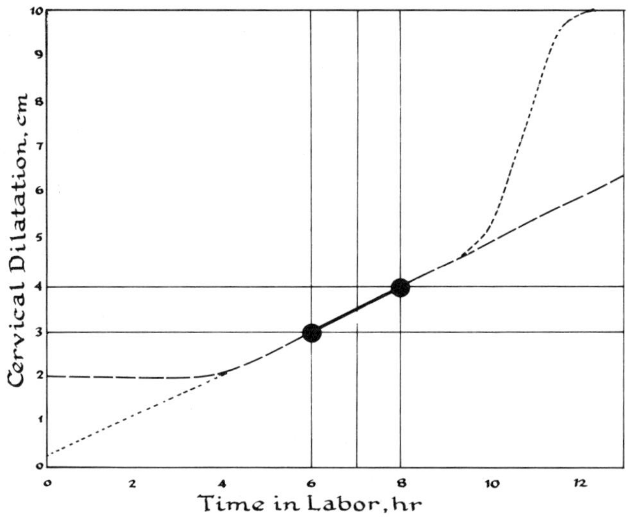


*Fig. 58.* Differential diagnosis between the latent phase of normal labor (*dotted line*) and an abnormally protracted active-phase dilatation pattern (*broken line*) is sometimes difficult when based only on isolated information (*solid line and closed circles*), although the slope of 0.5 cm/hr here would suggest it is probably merely latent phase.

false labor, it is counterbalanced by an increase in precipitate deliveries at home or en route. Moreover, it reduces the possibility for adequate fetal surveillance by monitoring and, in this situation, for tracing the early labor pattern in detail. Without such documentation, the differential diagnosis is sometimes difficult to make.

If the contractile pattern can be determined to have changed, this can be helpful, but it is not necessarily reliable. If the cervix is particularly pliable and the contractions are substantive—that is, strong, frequent, and of long duration—certain inferences can be made. Such conditions suggest an optimal state for rapid progression during the course of the active phase; failing this, it is likely that the slow progression seen thus far represents latent phase only. Contrariwise, if the cervix is unfavorable or contractions are unimpressive, one would not expect much change to take place during the normal latent phase; therefore, any dilatation encountered might be construed to represent active-phase progression, albeit abnormal.

Moreover, we have seen how the rate at which dilatation is occurring may clarify the issue by relating that progression to the contractile forces. Ordinarily, although cervical dilatation may occur during the latent phase, it is negligible or even absent. Sometimes, when the contractions are particularly vigorous and the soft parts are soft and yielding, especially in multiparas, dilatation may be progressive. It rarely advances with a rate as high as 0.6 cm/hr (see above). In nulliparas, a rate of dilatation in the latent phase of this magnitude would be very unusual indeed.

Therefore, unless there is evidence to the contrary, one should assume the condition to be a protraction disorder. The management principles outlined in Chapter 24 then apply. Cephalopelvic disproportion should be ruled out and extreme conservatism used to minimize analgesia and anesthesia. This will tend to avoid inhibiting the expectedly slow progress of labor. At the same time, one should offer appropriate supportive measures for these patients.

If the condition were actually the latent phase, no harm would have been done by this approach. In due course, the expected acceleration would take place and the error in diagnosis would become obvious. By minimizing the inhibitory effects of exogenous agents, one would not have prevented the normal evolution of the labor process.

An error made in the opposite direction—namely, to diagnose prolonged latent phase when a protraction disorder actually exists—might compound the situation somewhat. By administering large doses of narcotic analgesics for the purpose of resting the uterus (as recommended for prolonged latent phase), one will readily produce a secondary arrest of dilatation in a patient with protracted dilatation pattern. This disorder carries a much poorer prognosis (see Chapter 23) and is considerably more difficult to manage. If possible, it is best avoided. Therefore, as a general rule, it is better to assume the worse condition to exist when the differential diagnosis between latent phase and protraction disorder cannot be made with clarity.

Once again, it should be stressed that one can readily make the distinction between these two conditions on the basis of the foregoing pattern of progression. Characteristically, if one can identify a change in the slope of dilatation, one has sufficient evidence to warrant considering the patient to have entered the active phase. With such documention, an abnormal rate of dilatation demands a diagnosis of the more serious disorder of protracted active-phase dilatation pattern.

To repeat, the foregoing course of labor may be helpful here. As a general observation, measurable latent-phase dilatation occurs only with the most efficient varieties of labor, and even then only infrequently. On the other hand, some patients with protracted active-phase dilatation patterns present with a hypotonic or dyskinetic contractility state. If this should be the case, the distinction tends to be fairly easy.

Some physicians search for objective changes in contractility as a means for identifying the beginning of the active phase. Unfortunately, this usually proves to be a vain effort. There are no distinguishing manifestations in contractility pattern, either objective or subjective, to serve as milestones to identify the onset of the active phase. If we were not to trace the dilatation pattern, we would have no means for determining precisely when the active phase begins. We should note that, although there is no characteristic change in the contractions associated with the passage from latent to active phase, the situation is quite different when the dilatation curve reaches the deceleration phase. We have seen (Chapter 6) that this point in time—frequently designated "transition"—is accompanied by rather impressive and easily recognizable manifestations. These include increased intensity and frequency of contractions and markedly increased awareness of the contractions by the patient. Such awareness may take the form of suddenly increased discomfort associated with reflex nausea and vomiting. We have shown that this transition marks the beginning of active fetal descent, as the fetal presenting part distends the upper vagina and stretches the peritoneum of the posterior cul-de-sac (see Chapter 5). No comparable events occur at the time of the earlier transition from the latent phase to the acceleration portion of the active phase.

## *LATENT PHASE VERSUS SECONDARY ARREST*

Difficulties occasionally arise when a patient has experienced some cervical dilatation prior to coming under observation in labor. Without knowledge of when this dilatation occurred and by what mechanism it took place, the attendant faces a dilemma. He or she does not know whether the patient is still in the latent phase (having begun labor with some degree of prelabor cervical dilatation) or is in the active phase as a consequence of more recent active dilatation up to this point. A subsequent observation—say, 2 or 3 hours later—might clarify this situation or confound it. If this second examination shows the cervix to be further dilated, we can assume that the patient is in the active phase. If progression is occurring at a normal rate, routine management is in order. If abnormal, the patient can then be managed according to the principles outlined in Chapter 24.

However, if no further dilatation has occurred by the second examination, the situation is somewhat more critical. One must make the differential diagnosis between a normal latent phase with some prior dilatation and the far more serious disorder of secondary arrest of dilatation (Fig. 59). Only if the earlier labor has been well documented by means of serial observations can one be certain that the active phase has been entered, as shown by the upswing of the dilatation curve. In the absence of such documentation, the differential diagnosis can be made only by inference.

Sometimes, the contractile pattern may be helpful, particularly if it has changed spontaneously or has been influenced by some adverse exogenous factor acting on it. If there has been no discernible change in contractility other than that which is expected in terms of progressive enhancement with time, it is likely that the patient is still in the latent phase.

Nevertheless, in the absence of clear evidence that one is not dealing with secondary arrest of dilatation, it is probably the wiser decision to assume that this disorder is present. On this basis, one should proceed to evaluate for cephalopelvic disproportion and follow the program of management outlined for arrest patterns (see Chapter 24). Again, it is better to err on the side of conservatism in diagnosis because of the major risks inherent in overlooking this disorder if it does exist and in delaying definitive therapy.

The error in the opposite direction—that is, diagnosing secondary arrest of dilatation when the patient is merely in the latent phase—carries essentially no risk to the patient. She will have her pelvis evaluated radiologically (with

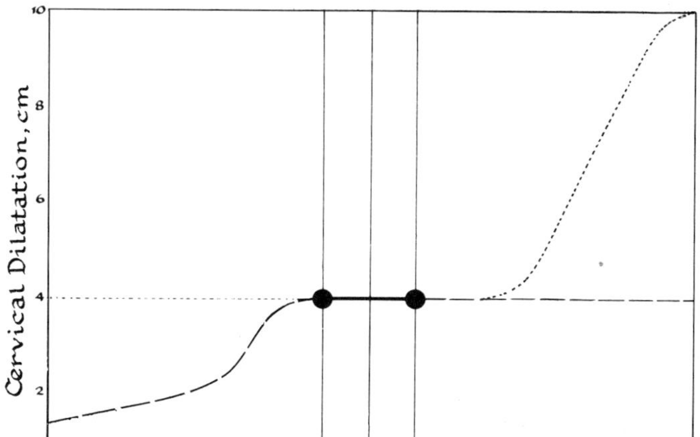


*Fig. 59.* Secondary arrest of dilatation (*broken line*) is occasionally difficult to distinguish from the normal latent phase in a parturient who began labor with some degree of dilatation (*dotted line*), unless there has been some documentation of the course of the earlier labor pattern. It is usually better to assume in these circumstances that an arrest disorder exists.

the minimal hazards this might provide to the fetus) and perhaps be subjected to uterotonic stimulation. The latter is an acceptable form of therapy for this disorder, since cephalopelvic disproportion is unlikely to be present. Generally, this will result in effective progress leading to uncomplicated vaginal delivery.

Sometimes, the problem of differential diagnosis can be resolved profitably by examining all available clinical information. For example, if the patient presents with a history of a brief period of preadmission labor in which the contractions were mild, or demonstrated only the minimal progressive change in intensity characteristic of the normal early latent phase, this might well establish the situation we now face as being most likely the latent phase. On the other hand, a prolonged period of intensive labor preceding hospital admission, perhaps now slowing due to sedation or anesthesia, may indicate that the more ominous secondary arrest pattern actually exists. Whenever foregoing active-phase dilatation has been documented (by the change in the slope of the dilatation curve), secondary arrest of dilatation is readily diagnosed and verified.

## *PROTRACTED DESCENT VERSUS ARREST OF DESCENT*

Earlier (Chapter 20), we reviewed the serious kinds of error resulting from misinterpreting the molding that the impacted fetal head may undergo, as if it were actually descending in the birth canal. Whereas protracted descent is a serious labor disorder, arrest of descent carries a still more ominous prognosis (see Chapter 23). Usually, they can be easily differentiated from each other on the basis of their distinctive descent patterns. Occasionally, however, a fetal head that is fixed in the pelvis may appear to be descending when it is not (Fig. 60). This comes about, of course, as a result of the elongation of the cranial vault with molding.

To add a note of confusion, descent and molding can (and often do) occur concurrently. It is possible, therefore, for the forward leading edge of the fetal skull to appear to be advancing in the pelvis when in fact no true descent is taking place. Periodic verification that descent is occurring should be accomplished by means of suprapubic examinations to ensure that the palpable portions of the base of the fetal skull are actually entering the pelvis (see Chapter 6).

Here, an error in diagnosis can be very serious indeed. Intracranial trauma will almost certainly result if arrested labor is long neglected. Laceration of the tentorium cerebelli or the falx cerebri may be a consequence of extreme degrees of molding. When such tears occur they may disrupt the major veins or venous sinuses of the cranial vault and produce devastating hemorrhage. In addition, progressive thinning of the lower uterine segment can take place in a patient with obstructed labor. This can lead ultimately to uterine rupture. Rarely, ischemic necrosis of the maternal tissues interposed between fetal head and bony pelvis can also occur, resulting in such

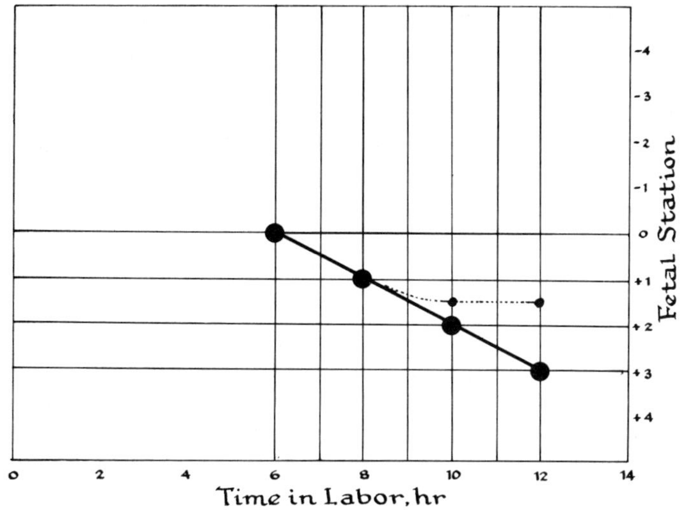


*Fig. 60.* Protracted descent (*solid line*) must be differentiated from arrest of descent (*dotted line*) on the basis of suprapubic assessment of descent to ensure that the advancing station reflects true descent and not merely molding of a fetal cranium that is fixed in the maternal pelvis.

problems as urethro- or vesicovaginal fistula. It is imperative, therefore, that arrest of descent be detected as early as possible so that we can act to prevent the excessive molding and uterine thinning that can be expected if labor is allowed to continue.

Traumatic instrumentation at delivery can further compound this problem. This is especially the case if the forces are misdirected (as in a brow-mastoid application of forceps). The same pertains to traumatic disimpaction of the fetal head at the time of cesarean section. This difficult operative maneuver is frequently delegated to the least experienced member of the obstetric team. If the intravaginal forces are not evenly distributed in the attempts to dislodge the head, trauma will result. It is generally better under these circumstances to apply forceps through the uterine incision and deliver the fetal head by this means rather than persist in uncontrolled and forceful manual manipulations.

In view of the serious nature of this possible error in diagnosis—that is, diagnosing protracted descent when an arrest of descent has actually occurred—every effort must be made to ensure that the documentation of fetal descent is based on objective fact. Careful assessment of fetal station by means of sequential vaginal examinations, coupled with simultaneous suprapubic verification, is mandatory when descent is occurring at an abnormally slow rate. The issue is not relevant if the slope of descent is within normal limits (1.2 cm/hr or more in nulliparas and 1.5 cm/hr in multiparas), because the factitious descent associated with molding appears to be incapable of achieving this rate.

It is only when the forward leading edge of the fetal presenting part advances at such exceedingly slow rates that the differentiation between protraction and arrest becomes problematic. Unless one can clearly document that the head is indeed descending, one must make the assumption that it is not. To assume it is descending means that the diagnosis of protracted descent applies and that watchful expectancy is acceptable under these circumstances.

Not being alerted to the possibility that an arrest pattern may actually be present, the obstetric attendant may fail to pursue definitive evaluation of the cephalopelvic relationships, thereby perhaps delaying the disclosure of an insurmountable bony impediment. The error in this regard is much more serious than that of diagnosing arrest of descent when in fact the labor pattern is one of protracted descent. Here, one would strive to ensure that disproportion is definitively ruled out before allowing the labor to progress much further. The only hazard is inherent in the radiation necessary for radiographic cephalopelvimetry.

This is in sharp contrast to the much more serious perils attendant upon the failure to recognize an arrest pattern (see above). The results of such misdiagnoses to both mother and fetus are clearly unacceptable. Therefore, as with the other differential diagnostic problems, it is better to assume that the disorder with the poorer prognosis is present if their distinction cannot be resolved.

## *PELVIC DYSTOCIA*

Even though pelvic dystocia is one of the more serious obstetric problems faced by the clinician, too little is known about its evaluation and management. It is most important that we learn to understand the nuances of evaluating fetopelvic relationships and to recognize early signs of impending problems before irreversible fetal or maternal damage occurs (Friedman, 1976). We must use all the clinical and laboratory sophistication our discipline has to offer because the stakes are so great in terms of infant trauma, neurologic and developmental damage, as well as mortality.

Radiographic pelvimetry is a very useful adjunct to the evaluation of the fetopelvic relationship, but it must be recognized to be as limited as any other laboratory tool when used alone. When the objective information that it provides is considered along with all the other information available to us, it offers meaningful insights. Such other data are derived from abdominal and digital pelvimetric examinations, assessments of the dynamic thrust of the fetal presenting part within the birth canal, all weighed together with the evolving course of cervical dilatation and fetal descent. Means are at hand for all practitioners to evaluate and manage pelvic dystocia critically. This applies especially to those with a keen grasp of the dynamism of the process of labors that are complicated by cephalopelvic disproportion.

We can detect dystocia if we approach the gravida in an orderly sequence (Fig. 61). This involves four different steps: (1) the screening of all antepartum patients with the aim of identifying all who have pelvic dimensions so small that they warrant flagging with guarded prognosis; (2) intrapartum reevaluation to focus more carefully on those with still greater likelihood of having obstructed labor; (3) the subsequent detection of those specifically developing the disordered labor patterns that are most often associated with cephalopelvic disproportion, namely, protraction and arrest aberrations; (4) the use of dynamic clinical pelvimetry in combination with radiographic cephalopelvimetry, a step designed to provide a means for designating patients for a trial of further labor or, alternatively, for cesarean section. With such a systematic approach, we should be able to optimize the outcome for all cases.

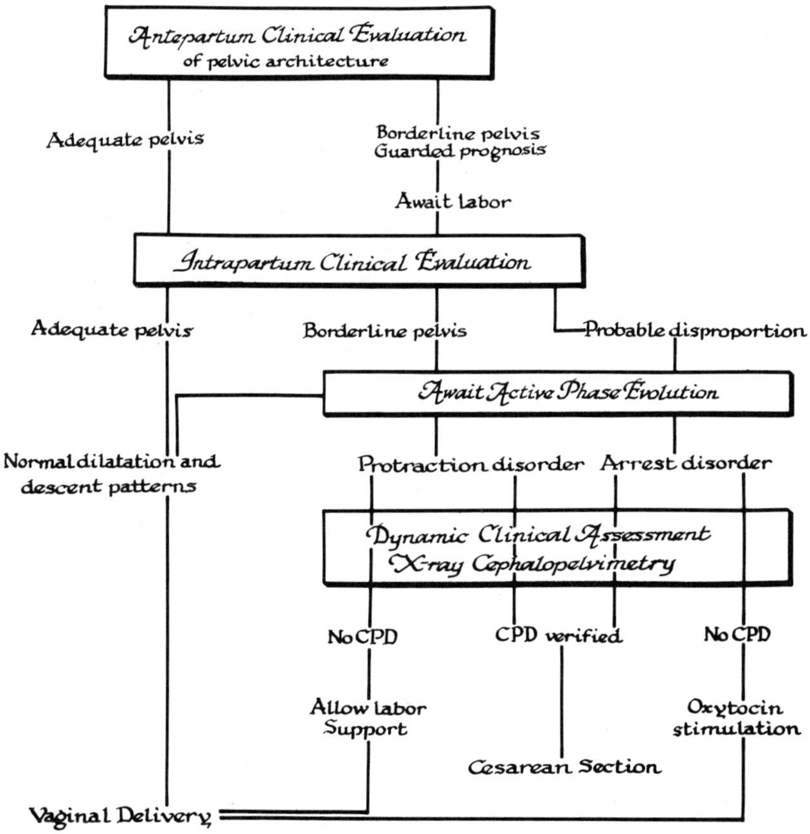


*Fig. 61.* Flow diagram for use in evaluating all gravidas for cephalopelvic relationships beginning in early pregnancy and progressing through labor in an orderly sequence, shown with probable outcome based on findings.

## *Antepartum Screening*

Every patient who presents for antepartum management should be carefully evaluated to determine the adequacy of her pelvis for vaginal delivery. Digital pelvimetry should be an essential part of the complete physical examination at the very first visit. The skills required for performing this examination properly must be developed by every physician early in his or her career. Attention should be directed to the details of physical relationships of the pelvis in regard to both shape and dimensions. External measurements are valueless. If the physician carries out the vaginal examination in a systematic manner, a good assessment of the size and shape of the pelvis will be obtained.

Gravidas can then be classified into three groups. (1) The largest group, approaching 90 percent of the gravid population, are those with an ample pelvis that has good architectural structure and dimensions that are adequate for the delivery of an average-sized baby; (2) a very small group of about 1 to 2 percent includes those with a pelvis that is clearly inadequate to permit passage of any but a small or premature fetus; (3) the remaining patients have a "borderline" pelvis with one or more dimensions foreshortened or with a distorted configuration that makes the prognosis unclear.

It is well beyond our scope to review the details of an adequate assessment of the bony pelvis, but it is imperative that this type of examination be carried out in every instance. The physician should assess specific features and develop a routinized manner for noting the essential landmarks and measuring the critical dimensions. Even with limited experience, one develops a good "mind's-eye view" of the normal pelvis. Deviations from this normal become apparent, particularly when important dimensions are constricted. Using such information, the physician can quite readily designate the patient as having an adequate, borderline, or poor pelvis.

Much useful clinical information can thus be obtained by means of simple but comprehensive examination of the pelvis early in pregnancy. Anatomic details should be thoroughly known to every practicing obstetric attendant. Any physician who feels insecure in this knowledge should correct the deficiency at once by reviewing standard sources and studying pelvic models.

## *Intrapartum Reevaluation*

Pelvic examinations done late in pregnancy, and especially during labor, tend to yield considerably more information than those done earlier. The maternal soft tissues are much more elastic and less resistant. The patient tends to be more cooperative and relaxed, especially between uterine contractions. This is, therefore, an especially good time to evaluate fetopelvic relationships in detail.

Every patient in labor should be studied carefully to ascertain whether disproportion exists between the fetal head and the bony pelvis. Up to this point in pregnancy, pelvic evaluation reflects the examiner's subjective perception of the pelvis with reference to a fetal head envisioned to be of average size. Now, for the first time, an ideal reference structure is available for determining pelvic adequacy—namely, the very fetal head that must traverse the birth canal. For the most part, the same dimensions and characteristics of the pelvic architecture are studied as in the examination done earlier in pregnancy. However, these can now be gauged more meaningfully against the dimensions of the presenting fetal head. Special attention, of course, should be paid to those patients previously considered to have a guarded prognosis because of constricted pelvic capacity.

The history of prior labors may or may not be useful. The patient who has had a previous dysfunctional labor may have a normal pelvis that will present no special difficulties in the current labor. More likely, however, one who has had a long, hard precedent labor, a difficult forceps delivery, or a baby with evidence of birth injury may be at considerably increased risk. This is particularly the case if the fetus is now larger than any delivered before. Such patients are candidates for disproportion and should be watched very closely.

Of equal importance are patients who have had a prior uncomplicated labor and delivery and who, because of such good obstetric performance, tend not to be supervised carefully in subsequent labors. Their management is often delegated to the least experienced member of the obstetric team. This is a common practice, contributing to delays in recognizing labor problems and in effecting appropriate action. Excessive delays are the unfortunate results of erroneously held impressions that once a patient has had a vaginal delivery, she will follow suit in subsequent pregnancies. Although cephalopelvic disproportion is uncommon in multiparas, it occurs with sufficient frequency to warrant constant vigil (Sogolow and Friedman, 1967).

The nullipara who enters labor at term with an unengaged fetal head is suspect. About 5 percent of nulliparas present in this manner at the onset of labor. Cesarean section can be anticipated under these circumstances in 36 to 39 percent as a consequence of associated cephalopelvic disproportion (Burke et al, 1958; Friedman and Sachtleben, 1965d).

All aspects of the evaluation described for antepartum clinical screening should be repeated in detail for the parturient. Much new information can thus be acquired to aid in her assessment. For example, factors relating to presentation and position of the fetus are of obvious importance, along with an evaluation of the degree of ossification and the configuration of the fetal head. One can gain an impression of the firmness of the bones, the sharpness of the parietal contours, the size of the fontanelles, the extent to which the cranial plates overlap during uterine contractions, and the width of the cranial dome. These items tend to be only of limited usefulness, however, unless they are shown to be extreme variations from the norm. When extremes are encountered, they will serve as important signals that a serious dystocic problem probably exists.

## Assessing Labor Progression

We now recognize that most labors associated with cephalopelvic disproportion are characteristically dysfunctional (see Chapter 16). Most often, they take the form of one or more of the arrest patterns, namely, secondary arrest of dilatation, prolonged deceleration phase, arrest of descent, or failure of descent. When these disorders are encountered in the course of a labor, cephalopelvic disproportion must be considered to exist until it can be definitively ruled out. We have shown that the combination of documented disproportion and one of these arrest patterns demands cesarean section without further trial of labor. Obviously, the documentation necessary should be obtained in as objective a manner as possible. We must recognize the limitations of subjective digital evaluations. Appropriate dynamic clinical and radiographic pelvimetry becomes essential, therefore (see below).

As we have shown, detection of the patterns of arrested labor can be fairly routine in those institutions in which cervical dilatation and fetal station are sequentially plotted for all laboring patients. Abnormal patterns are readily recognized by anyone who has any experience in following the tracings. As detailed in Chapter 16, once the patient has entered the active phase of labor, the linear maximum slope of dilatation can be projected upward toward full cervical dilatation. Any deviation to the right is immediately detected.

When 2 or more hours have elapsed without further progression, secondary arrest of dilatation is diagnosed. Similarly, arrest of descent can be identified promptly—during the deceleration phase of the dilatation curve or more usually, in the second stage—if progressive descent ceases for 1 hour or more. A prolonged deceleration phase exceeds the critical limit of duration (3 hours in nulliparas or 1 hour in multiparas) at the end of the active phase, prior to the beginning of the second stage. Descent should be in active progress by the time the dilatation curve has reached the beginning of the deceleration phase. If descent is not occurring by this time, failure of descent can be diagnosed and the possibility of disproportion, strongly considered.

In addition, protracted active-phase dilatation or protracted descent patterns are also frequently associated with disproportion, although only one-half as often as the arrest patterns. The association between protraction disorders and disproportion is not as clear as with the arrest disorders. Nonetheless, those patients presenting with a protraction aberration should also be evaluated for bony obstruction.

## Dynamic Cephalopelvimetry and Radiographic Evaluation

Once it is recognized that the patient in labor is at risk for cephalopelvic disproportion, careful reevaluation should be undertaken. Two essential features of such reevaluation include a dynamic form of assessment—to determine the "thrust" of the fetal head in the birth canal—and radiographic cephalopelvimetry for purposes of comparing pelvic capacity with fetal head volume more objectively. The physician tries to determine by as direct a method as possible if the fetal head is likely to pass through the pelvis. When the patient is in active labor, the fetal head tends to be closely applied to the pelvic inlet (and midpelvis, if more deeply engaged), making evaluation of the cephalopelvic relationships especially meaningful.

Abdominal examination is too often ignored in this regard. It can be important for ascertaining whether the plane of the biparietal diameter of the fetal head has actually passed through the inlet (see Chapter 6). Using the symphysis pubis as a landmark, one can determine the level of the fetal head in reference to the pelvic inlet. This method is not as accurate as vaginal assessment of the station of the forward leading edge of the fetal presenting part with reference to the plane of the ischial spines. Nevertheless, it is recommended as a fine adjunct for ensuring that perceived descent is true descent and not merely a reflection of the molding of the fetal cranium (see above).

Additional relevant information can be obtained by palpating the fetal head with fingers of one hand placed intravaginally and those of the other, suprapubically. With the head forced down into the inlet by a uterine contraction, the anterior parietal boss projects onto the posterior surface of the pubis. Any overriding here suggests inlet disproportion. If the fetus is presenting in an occiput posterior position, the forehead will be prominent anteriorly over the symphysis.

A most important dynamic test of the pelvic capacity to accommodate the specific fetal head is the Müller–Hillis maneuver (Hillis, 1938; Müller, 1896). Müller described the procedure in which an assistant forces the head down into the inlet. With fingers inside the vagina, the physician determines how far into the pelvis the fetal head will advance. Hillis simplified the maneuver by evaluating the fetal descent while applying uterine fundal pressure with one hand placed on top of the uterus and the other intravaginally. Optimal results are obtained by carrying out this maneuver during a uterine contraction. This approach is more reliable after the cervix is well dilated, because the maternal soft parts, if resistant, may prevent the head from engaging under the limited amount of downward pressure that one can exert safely.

Observing the thrust of the fetal head during a uterine contraction while simultaneously applying pressure to the uterine fundus immediately tells the observer whether the head is tightly fixed in the pelvis or is capable of additional caudad movement. It will give the clinician a good appreciation of whether or not additional space is available for descent. If the fetal head appears to flex and rotate in the mechanisms we recognize to be best suited for the pelvis, it is reasonably certain that effective contractions will eventually succeed in furthering descent and, barring other difficulties, ultimately effect vaginal delivery.

Radiographic pelvimetry has clear-cut advantages over digital pelvimetry in terms of the objectivity it provides. However, there is appropriate reluctance to resort to this examination because of the potential radiation hazards to both mother and fetus. The hazards from low-dosage irradiation have been seriously questioned (Oppenheim et al, 1975). Clearly, when radiographic survey is propery indicated, the benefits in terms of the information gained in labor may far outweigh any theoretical risk. We must stress, however, that radiography should be reserved for those cases in which it is obviously essential. Moreover, it should be held in abeyance until the patient is well in labor and the course of labor has indicated a problem known to be associated with cephalopelvic disproportion, as we have just detailed.

Exceptions to this constraint include the nullipara in labor with an unengaged vertex presentation and all gravidas with a breech presentation. Among the latter, the course of labor and its variations may be entirely insufficient to forewarn the physician of impending problems in fetopelvic relationships. Thus, it is important that pelvic adequacy be determined as early in labor as possible. Only if it is entirely clear that the pelvis will be ample for delivery of this fetus should labor be permitted to proceed. Conservatism along these lines has liberalized the indications for cesarean section, and as a consequence the outcome in breech deliveries has much improved in recent years.

Although radiographic cephalopelvimetry is a valuable adjunct to the evaluation of labor progression, it has recognized shortcomings. It is merely a laboratory aid and cannot be expected to provide irrefutable answers. Of the many techniques currently in use, none has been found to provide more reliable or precise measurements than any other (Weinberg and Scadron, 1946). Nonetheless, the Ball technique (Ball, 1936a, b; Friedman and Taylor, 1969; Klapholz, 1975; Friedman, 1976b) does offer a unique advantage in its intrinsic capability for measuring fetal head size. It is especially recommended on this basis as well as for its simplicity and relative freedom from technical drawbacks. By simple triangulation methods, corrections can be made for distortion resulting from dispersion of x-rays from the point source. All important pelvic dimensions can be obtained and corrected, and then converted to volume capacities. At the same time, the head circumference can be measured, corrected, and converted to volume for purposes of comparison with the previously defined pelvic capacities. This approach is equally applicable, with a high degree of accuracy, to the fetal head in breech presentations.

This special attribute of the Ball technique is not shared by any other radiographic pelvimetric method. Certain others can provide accurate measurements of the biparietal diameter but only in limited circumstances, as when the fetal head presents precisely in an occiput anterior, occiput posterior, or occiput transverse position. These instances occur only in about 5 percent of cases. This severe limitation undoubtedly explains why radiographic pelvimetry has not been uniformly accepted everywhere. Without the all-important fetal head dimensions for reference purposes, even the most accurate objective measurements of pelvic capacity provide little meaningful information unless they show extreme diminution in the transit space. Since the Ball technique has overcome this significant shortcoming, it deserves wider application.

If we are to employ radiographic pelvimetry in an optimal manner so that it yields the most information with the least hazard, we are well advised to limit its use to gravidas in whom it is clearly indicated. The argument that most patients who are subjected to radiographic pelvimetry are shown to have normal pelvic measurement is based on indiscriminant use of the technique. When used in the manner we have described (see above), more than one-half of the patients with arrest patterns who are subjected to radiographic studies will have clear evidence of cephalopelvic disproportion (Friedman and Sachtleben, 1976). These patients can be delivered by cesarean section. Those without disproportion are treated conservatively with uterotonic stimulation and can be expected to deliver vaginally unless further problems occur. The objective data provided by radiographic pelvimetry in these cases readily distinguish those that warrant cesarean section from those that do not.

It is important to emphasize that close surveillance must be undertaken by means of combined fetal heart rate and uterine contraction monitoring in all patients allowed to labor under these circumstances. This recommendation is made because these fetuses have been found to be at somewhat increased risk of dying (see Chapter 23). The associated abnormal labors should, therefore, be considered to place the fetus in jeopardy. Continuous monitoring techniques appear to be capable of detecting those fetuses presenting evidence of intrauterine hypoxia. While a discussion of the techniques and the meaningful patterns of fetal response are beyond our scope here, these details should form an integral part of all obstetric management programs involving the care of women with disordered labor patterns.

The sequential systematic approach for evaluating all pregnant women will aid the physician in detecting cephalopelvic disproportion. By periodically searching for objective evidence relating to pelvic capacity and fetal head size and by observing relevant data on labor progression, the obstetric attendant can bring an enlightened understanding to this problem.

## *FAILURE TO PROGRESS IN LABOR*

This last part of our discussion of differential diagnosis concerns the vague condition termed "failure to progress in labor." It clearly comprises several dissimilar and often unrelated disorders that must be differentiated and managed according to guidelines that are appropriate for the specific abnormality (Friedman, 1974b). The patient who does not progress in labor is acknowledged to be a source of great concern to the physician. The objective approaches to evaluating progressive cervical dilatation and fetal descent that we have outlined here have proved useful in helping the clinician understand when labor progression is adequate and to recognize critical abnormalities. The nonspecific designation of failure to progress tends to obscure such recognition, rather than aid it.

It is now possible to make accurate differential diagnoses in patients whose labors are characterized by failure to progress. As stated, they are not a homogeneous group. They may present with any of several distinct labor aberrations, including normal or prolonged latent phase, secondary arrest of dilatation, arrest of descent, prolonged deceleration phase, or failure of descent. These have been adequately defined in the foregoing material and we need not review them here once more. Nonetheless, it is important that the obstetric attendant identify the specific pattern so that he or she may be apprised of possible etiologic factors, response to therapy, and prognosis. This will permit selection of the specific management program for each patient according to the type of labor aberration she has.

Perhaps most important in this regard is the misdiagnosis of failure to progress in a patient who is in the latent phase of an otherwise normal labor. We have not heretofore addressed ourselves to this issue in our discussions of differential diagnosis. Before it became widely appreciated that progressive cervical dilatation does not have to occur in the normal latent phase, this erroneous diagnosis was more commonly made than it is now. Based on the error (labeled failure to progress, or primary inertia, or some other nondescript term), these patients were often subjected either to superfluous uterotonic stimulation or ill-advised and inappropriate cesarean section. If the labor is allowed to evolve, an interval of observation will generally reveal the true nature of the condition. The expected acceleration in cervical dilatation will occur as the active phase is entered, provided progress is not being delayed by the inhibitory effects of analgesic or anesthetic agents.

The graphic portrayal of the labor progression is especially useful in these patients. It permits us to recognize the several distinctive disorders that comprise failure to progress in labor as they arise. This gives us the opportunity to delineate which abnormal pattern, if any, is specifically present in a given labor. The definitive diagnosis having been made in this way, we can proceed to seek and critically evaluate etiologic factors so that an appropriate program of management can be initiated, which will most likely yield good results for both mother and infant.

## *EVALUATION FOR CAUSATION*

Once the diagnosis of the specific labor abnormality has been made, it is imperative to evaluate the patient thoroughly for causative or contributory factors. This will permit one to choose an appropriately effective program of management. To begin with, extensive examination is needed in order to determine the patient's general physical condition and the obstetric situation prevailing. Attention should be directed toward fluid needs and electrolyte balance. The patient's psychological state must be appraised, especially noting anxiety and fears. The role of the psyche in labor progression has not been defined, but there can be little doubt that it is important in clinical management. The status of uterine contractility, cephalopelvic relationships, fetal lie, presentation, and position, attitude, and synclitism must all be critically evaluated also.

The search for probable etiologic factors will be directed according to the type of aberration encountered. One's index of suspicion should be oriented to the direction indicated by the kinds of situations and conditions that have heretofore been recognized as commonly associated with the particular abnormality. These are detailed at length in the various chapters dealing with the specific aberrations (see Chapters 9 through 12). They will be touched on here only briefly.

Excessive sedation is perhaps the most common factor associated with prolonged latent phase. There can be little doubt that well-intentioned and sympathetic, but ill-advised sedation and anesthesia given too early in labor—that is, before the latent phase is terminated—will prolong labor unnecessarily. The latent phase is particularly sensitive to these agents, as we have seen. We are referring, of course, particularly to the effect that sedation has on the patient's sensorium and uterine functional integrity, rather than to the type and dosage of medication used. If recognized as contributing to the delay, one can allow the inhibitory effect to abate.

Similarly, patients who begin labor with the cervix unprepared—that is, thick, uneffaced, rigid, and undilated—will perforce have a long latent phase during which the cervix is undergoing the necessary preparation for subsequent active dilatation. When this phenomenon is encountered, one can expect the latent phase to be prolonged. Appreciating this relationship gives the physician enough insight to permit him or her to forewarn the patient and her family of the likelihood that labor will be prolonged, reassuring them that this will not be a threatening problem.

The protraction disorders are often associated with minor malpositions, which are probably inconsequential. More importantly, excessive sedation and cephalopelvic disproportion are frequent factors. In all such cases, combined digital and radiographic cephalopelvimetry (see above) should be performed. The shortcomings of these diagnostic procedures notwithstanding, the information they provide is often critically important and can be of inestimable aid in evaluating the problem at hand.

An additional causative or contributory factor in protraction disorders is conduction peridural anesthesia, especially when it is improperly administered. By this we mean that it has been given too early (during the latent phase), to too high a level (above the tenth thoracic dermatome), or in conjunction with excessive preanesthetic analgesia, a preexisting labor abnormality, or cephalopelvic disproportion. Although this form of anesthesia is an excellent means for relieving the pain of labor and delivery, its use is best restricted by these conditions.

The most serious cause of arrest patterns is cephalopelvic disproportion. It is found in about one-half of the cases. Therefore, it is absolutely mandatory to rule out bony dystocia in these cases before proceeding with any form of treatment. Once again, the limitations of available pelvimetric techniques must be kept in mind. In those patients who do not have disproportion, arrest patterns may be associated with malpositions, excessive sedation, improperly administered conduction anesthesia, or most commonly, with combinations of these. Arrest patterns often follow a protraction disorder if anesthesia or excessive sedation has been administered.

It is clear, therefore, that the clinician's approach to the management of the several kinds of disorders must take into account the findings that are uncovered in an extensive pretreatment evaluation. Therapy (Chapter 22) is prescribed and will be modified according to the factors uncovered during such thorough investigation.

# Therapeutic Issues

## CHAPTER 22

The range of therapeutic options for managing the patient with abnormal labor is assessed, together with discussions of preinduction priming and the principles and practices of induction of labor. Wherever appropriate, specific applications of each treatment method are stipulated.

The practice of obstetrics provides a paucity of possible therapeutic options. They are limited in number and types. In order of aggressiveness, our treatment armamentarium for labor problems is confined to watchful expectancy, therapeutic rest, stimulation of the uterus by specific uterotonic agents, and measures aimed at terminating the pregnancy expeditiously, either by the vaginal or by the abdominal route. As we shall see (Chapter 24), each of these is singularly applicable to a given set of labor disorders. In this chapter we will review each modality in turn for purposes of providing some insights into the kinds of problems likely to be benefited. We will concentrate on the clinical criteria for making an appropriate choice, based on previous clinical observations of efficacy.

For completeness, we will also deal with considerations of priming in anticipation of the induction of labor, as well as matters relating to induction of labor itself. On the subject of uterotonic stimulation, elective and therapeutic stimulation will be discussed as it relates to use of oxytocin and other available agents. The controversial issue of amniotomy as an ostensible stimulatory practice will also be reviewed.

### *PREINDUCTION PRIMING*

It has been demonstrated both in vitro (Brummer, 1971) and in vivo (Gillespie, 1972) that the human gravid uterus responds with enhanced effect to oxytocin stimulation after it has been exposed to prostaglandin $E_2$ ($PGE_2$). In addition, $PGE_2$ has been shown to be unexpectedly efficacious in inducing labor when conditions for induction are unfavorable (Anderson et al, 1971; Calder and Embrey, 1973; Friedman and Sachtleben, 1974a). These observations have suggested the possibility that changing the unfavorable cervix with $PGE_2$ may be feasible and advantageous prior to the use of oxytocin for indicated inductions of labor (Beazley, 1972a; Embrey, 1971).

Priming the cervix implies the creation of favorable changes such that subsequent labor induction will be readily accomplished. The need for an agent that will safely and effectively prime the cervix has long been recognized. Unfortunately, this need is as yet unsatisfied by any available means. If $PGE_2$ could have been shown to be useful in this regard, it might have served to considerable advantage in certain high-risk situations where preterm pregnancy termination is advisable in the interest of either the mother or the fetus.

Studies have been carried out on a double-blind basis to assess the potential effect of $PGE_2$ in changing the condition of the cervix prior to oxytocin induction of labor. Conflicting results have been reported from investigations conducted under essentially identical circumstances. Gravidas were preselected by the criterion that the cervix was considered to be unfavorable on the basis of prelabor pelvic evaluation showing a Bishop Score (see below) of less than 6. On a random basis, patients were assigned to receive either $PGE_2$ or placebo. The active medication consisted of 0.5 mg of $PGE_2$ administered orally in two-tablet doses (1.0 mg) at 3-hourly intervals for three doses. The Bishop Score was reevaluated prior to each priming dose and subsequently, prior to initiating the active induction with oxytocin. Intravenous oxytocin infusion was begun between 8 and 12 hours following the last priming dose of medication or placebo. The oxytocin was delivered at a rate of 2 mU per minute at first, and the rate of infusion was increased at approximately 30-minute intervals until adequate uterine contractions were produced to simulate strong clinical labor. If active labor was not in progress after 10 hours of infusion, the induction was deemed to be a failure.

When the coding was broken at the conclusion of one such study (Friedman and Sachtleben, 1975a), it was found that the control and study groups were remarkably alike. This comparability applied not only to their composition (with regard to parity and initial Bishop Scores, for example), but also to the favorable change that had occurred in the Bishop Score over the course of the priming and subsequently, prior to the oxytocin induction (averaging 1.5 points in both groups). The frequency of perceived uterine contractions was the same, as was the incidence of spontaneous onset of labor during the priming period, and the rate of successful inductions. Moreover, there were no differences in the dosage of oxytocin stimulation needed to induce active labor or to effect delivery. The duration of oxytocin stimulation and the interval from onset of priming to delivery were also quite comparable.

Contrary evidence was presented in a similar study (Weiss et al, 1976). Here, the control group showed no significant change in the cervical condition as measured by the Bishop Score, whereas those receiving active drug generally did change their Bishop Score by an average of more than 3 points. Similar differences were seen in the frequency of spontaneous onset of labor during the priming phase, as well as the rate of failure of oxytocin inductions subsequently. However, in successfully induced patients, the response to oxytocin—as expressed by the duration of labor from onset of induction to delivery and the mean dose of oxytocin required for the induction—was almost the same. It should be emphasized, however, that the effect reported in this study may have been invalidated because the treated patients were not entirely comparable to the controls in terms of their Bishop Score distributions. The priming effect of $PGE_2$, therefore, remains to be verified.

Despite the attractive hypothesis that $PGE_2$ might be effective as a means for enhancing subsequent myometrial responsiveness to oxytocin stimulation as a consequence of its ability to prime the previously unresponsive uterus, objective documentation of the effect in clinical usage is not as yet available. It is conceivable that our failure to verify this action may have been due to factors relating to inadequate dosage, insufficient duration of the priming stimulus, or unduly short priming-to-induction delay. Nevertheless, if oral $PGE_2$ is capable of producing some form of priming, ripening, or enhancement, the effect is at best subtle and is, therefore, of little real clinical value for gravidas at term with unfavorable conditions for induction (these constituting the constraints of the studies cited above).

## *INDUCTION OF LABOR*

The practice of elective initiation or augmentation of labor without clearly defined indication has become increasingly popular in recent years. The proponents of such discretionary measures emphasize that elective induction has many potential advantages. For example, the patient is well rested; she is psychologically prepared for labor. This implies that she has not been coerced to accept the procedure, but is positively motivated toward it. Elective induction, moreover, ensures that the patient's stomach is empty, provided of course that oral intake has been restricted for at least 8 hours before the induction is undertaken. This is an important consideration in reducing the risks of anesthesia. The patient can also avoid last-minute transportation difficulties and those difficulties attendant upon the disposition of older children. Allowing the patient time to organize family and work responsibilities is especially advantageous for today's career-oriented woman. For the mother with a history of excessively rapid labors, induction averts the possibility of delivery at home or en route to the hospital. It is alleged that patients whose labors are induced have the benefit of somewhat better equipped and staffed daytime hospital services. Similarly, they can be assured physician attendance and availability. All tend to ensure the patient's peace of mind.

## Risk versus Benefit

Induction of labor, however, is not completely devoid of hazard. While serious complications are uncommon in well-conducted inductions under optimal circumstances, the hazards of induced labor must nevertheless be kept in mind at all times. Toward this end, the practitioner should continuously weigh the benefits against the potential risks, especially when undertaking elective induction of labor.

No one would question attempting to induce labor, even under suboptimal circumstances, in a patient whose clinical picture suggests that continuing the pregnancy will subject her or her fetus to considerable harm. Here the relative risks of induction are far outweighed by the perils of allowing the pregnancy to continue. When such strong indications do not exist, however, the burden of responsibility rests on the physician who induces labor and who thereby exposes the patient to a possible risk that may or may not be justified by the potential advantages of the procedure.

In current clinical practice, elective induction is acceptable and can be rationalized, provided the risks are minimized. Care in selection of patients, with particular attention to avoiding a premature delivery, will ensure success. Additionally, it is imperative that the physician have a detailed knowledge of the procedures for inducing labor and their possible hazards. He or she must be knowledgeable about the appropriate means available for detecting and correcting adverse effects when they arise. The constant presence of experienced personnel is likewise essential.

Means for avoiding overstimulation and its serious effects on both mother and fetus will be discussed in detail below. The hazard of prematurity in induction of labor is a real risk, based on our inability to estimate fetal weight and size correctly by physical examination alone. Objective measures for assessing fetal maturity are now available and should be used whenever doubt exists.

## Prerequisites

The conditions influencing the success of induced labor are twofold. One encompasses the extrinsic factors dealing with the milieu in which the induction is to be done, and the other involves intrinsic factors within the patient. Both are critical insofar as safety and efficacy are concerned (Bishop, 1958; Niswander and Patterson, 1963). Needless to say, suitable facilities must be at hand to deal with any complications that might arise. There must be adequate numbers of well-trained personnel. It is absolutely essential that the attending physician be present at all times. It is equally imperative that the patient be emotionally and physically prepared. Efforts should be made to ensure that she is near term, both by dates and by estimated fetal size.

Reliable means for assessing the maturity of the fetus address developmental parameters as well as physiologic functions. Cytologic examination of the amniotic fluid will show a sharp increase in the percentage of cells containing lipid substances (staining orange with 0.1 percent Nile blue sulfate) after 38 weeks of pregnancy. This appears to be related to the functional maturity of the sebaceous glands from which these cells may arise. Creatinine concentration levels in amniotic fluid also rise abruptly, most often with levels in excess of 2 mg per 100 ml after the thirty-seventh week. Minute amounts of bilirubin are detectable in amniotic fluid by spectrophotometric analysis. The level falls progressively with gestational age, usually disappearing by the thirty-sixth week. Radiographic techniques search for the appearance of specific epiphyseal centers of ossification and can measure fetal skull and long bones for purposes of verifying fetal maturity. Most often used is the distal femoral epiphysis, which ordinarily appears toward the end of the thirty-sixth week. Radiation hazards to the fetus, however, must be considered.

A preferable approach for obtaining reasonably good fetal biparietal diameter measurements is ultrasound examination. This method is more reliable when obtained serially. Still more useful are the amniotic fluid lecithin–sphingomyelin ratio determinations. Rapid increase in lecithin content—apparently derived from the maturing fetal lung—is noted after the thirty-fifth week of pregnancy. This valuable measure of functional lung maturation has been shown to be a very sensitive indicator (Gluck et al, 1971). When the ratio is greater than 2, the fetal lung is likely to be sufficiently mature to ensure that the infant will not develop respiratory distress after birth.

There are certain conditions that tend to preclude induction within acceptable standards of clinical practice. These include fetopelvic disproportion, unfavorable fetal position or presentation, placenta previa, fetal distress, and a previous uterine incision from cesarean section, hysterotomy, myomectomy, or metroplasty. Moreover, induction should not be undertaken in a patient with breech presentation whose pelvis cannot be definitively demonstrated to be adequate for that fetus. Where it is obvious that no fetopelvic disproportion exists, however, breech presentation per se does not constitute a contraindication to induction. Less binding contraindications include grand multiparity and uterine overdistention from multiple pregnancies or hydramnios. Even though problems only rarely arise with induction under these latter circumstances, appropriate conservative obstetric practice suggests that they be observed as contraindications unless overriding and extenuating circumstances exist.

## *Bishop Score*

Selection of patients by objective criteria to indicate whether they are ready for a successful induction of labor is important. Ideally selected patients run minimal risks from the induction procedure. Their induction rarely fails to yield an essentially normal labor and delivery. Generally speaking, labor should be expected to be inducible if the cervix is soft and yielding, particularly at the internal os, with a moderate amount of effacement and dilatation. A most useful scoring system has been devised by Bishop (1964) as a means for predicting the success of induction. The system evaluates five relevant factors: cervical dilatation, effacement, and consistency, as well as station of the fetal head and the position of the cervix in relation to the vaginal axis. A value of 0 to 3 is assigned to each factor according to its degree of "ripeness" (Table 62). The value assigned to each factor is added to yield the total score, ranging from 0 to 13. The higher the score, the more inducible the labor. In a large series of oxytocin-induced multiparas (Friedman et al, 1966), no failures were encountered with scores of 9 or greater; 5 percent failures occurred in women with scores of 5 to 8; and 20 percent failures, in those with scores of 0 to 4.

*Table 62. PRELABOR STATUS SCORING SYSTEM FOR EVALUATION OF INDUCIBILITY**

| Factor | Score 0 | Score 1 | Score 2 | Score 3 |
|---|---|---|---|---|
| Cervical dilatation (cm) | Closed | 1–2 | 3–4 | 5+ |
| Cervical effacement (%) | 0–30 | 40–50 | 60–70 | 80+ |
| Fetal station | –3 | –2 | –1, 0 | +1, +2 |
| Cervical consistency | Firm | Medium | Soft | |
| Cervical position | Posterior | Midposition | Anterior | |

* Modified from Bishop EH: Obstet Gynecol 24:266, 1964.

While useful as an index of inducibility, the Bishop Score is incapable of predicting fetal weight (Niswander et al, 1967). The Bishop Score, therefore, cannot serves as a means to avoid the induction of labor and the inadvertent delivery of a premature infant. The other more objective means described above should be used for this purpose to rule out prematurity. These means may be applied either routinely where readily available or at least in every instance where fetal maturity is in doubt (Cowett and Oh, 1976).

## Methods

A great many methods for inducing labor have been used over the years. Most have been discarded largely because of their ineffectiveness, unacceptable hazard, or lack of control. The test of time and wide clinical usage have proved the value of those techniques remaining in popular clinical use today. These include amniotomy and oxytocin, alone or in combination. More recently, use of prostaglandins has been shown to be effective in this regard as well.

*Amniotomy.* The success of amniotomy in initiating labor depends primarily on the preparedness of the cervix. When patients are properly selected, amniotomy usually initiates labor, although most series report about 10 percent failure rates. The principal drawback to amniotomy is the possibility of infection with ascending amnionitis. This is particularly the case if labor does not begin in a reasonable period of time. Prolapse of the umbilical cord can also occur and is seen especially in the patient with an unengaged fetal presenting part. The risk of failure of amniotomy and its associated complications, notably infection, limit its application to inductions that are clearly indicated for medical reasons. Such problems tend to be too large a price to pay in patients induced electively.

In elective induction it is preferable to attempt to initiate labor by pharmacologic means rather than to subject a patient to amniotomy, thereby committing her to delivery within a relatively short time. If labor cannot be initiated successfully by amniotomy, cesarean section will likely prove to be necessary. If pregnancy had been allowed to continue without interference in these patients, spontaneous labor might have occurred in some future time and may have resulted in an otherwise uncomplicated vaginal delivery. Of course, this constraint does not apply when medical indications warrant the timely termination of the pregnancy. Here both oxytocin and amniotomy in combination are clearly justified to expedite labor and delivery.

*Oxytocin.* Pharmacologic uterotonic stimulation with oxytocin (Pitocin or Syntocinon) is valuable for inducing or augmenting labor. However, because there is no way to predict precisely how sensitive the individual gravid uterus will be to a given dosage, the drug must be administered with extreme caution. When first given, even infinitesimal amounts may cause sustained tetanic contractions without forewarning. Thus, stringent precautions must be taken whenever oxytocin is being administered to the pregnant woman. We have earlier outlined the prerequisites and contraindications for its use. Only if all attendant personnel retain a healthy respect for this agent and continually bear in mind its serious effects when mishandled can its safety be reasonably assured.

Ideally, oxytocin should be administered intravenously in dilute solutions by critically controlled means. It is recommended that it be given by an infusion pump mechanism, either in the form of the syringe injection variety or the peristaltic type, if available. These devices will help avoid the problems frequently encountered with standard intravenous infusions in which the flow rate varies considerably and may be difficult to control. This is particularly so when the patient changes position and intermittently occludes venous return in the infusion arm.

The rate of infusion controlled by pump is not directly affected by the size of the needle, the caliber or flow in the vein, or the drop size. Moreover, continuous counting and rechecking the drip rate is superfluous by this method. The rate of infusion can be increased or decreased rapidly, as needed. If such equipment is unavailable, intravenous infusion by drip method is acceptable, although clearly less preferable. Continuous attention to drip rate is necessary to ensure that dosage level is maintained and that neither underdosage nor overdosage (especially the latter) occurs.

In usual clinical usage, 10 units of oxytocin are added to 1,000 ml of 5 percent aqueous dextrose. This solution, when properly mixed, delivers 1 milliunit (mU) of oxytocin with each 0.1 ml given intravenously. Acknowledging that drop size may vary between infusion sets, we can calculate that an infusion rate of eight drops per minute will administer approximately 0.5 ml, or 5 mU per minute; at 16 drops per minute, 1 ml, or 10 mU per minute. The recommended physiologic dosage of oxytocin needed for the initiation of labor at term is usually around 2 mU per minute (Theobald, 1955). It very rarely exceeds 16 mU per minute (Caldeyro-Barcia et al, 1957). Pregnancies induced prior to term may well be less sensitive and require large doses to effectively stimulate uterine contractions. One can readily recognize how difficult it would be to try to maintain a standard infusion of about three drops or 2 mU per minute in the usual clinical situation without an accurate control of flow rate.

The intravenous infusion of oxytocin must begin at a very slow rate. If given by standard infusion technique, this initial rate should not exceed six to eight drops per minute, initially. Under no circumstances is the needle to be flushed with a bolus of the oxytocin solution. A two-bottle technique is preferable here. The first infusion is a solution of 5 percent dextrose in water containing no oxytocin; the second bottle contains the aforementioned oxytocin concentration and is attached in a secondary fashion, perhaps by a Y connection, to the tubing of the first bottle. In this manner, the needle can be inserted and checked with impunity, and the oxytocin can be clamped off and discontinued at any time without disturbing the intravenous infusion.

After the infusion has begun, the patient is observed continuously for uterine response in terms of intensity, frequency, and duration of contractions. She must be watched for alterations in fetal heart rate and for changes in her own vital signs. The optimal clinical features to look for include moderate to strong contractions recurring every 2 to 3 minutes and lasting 45 to 60 seconds. It is essential that the uterus relax completely between contractions. At no time should the patient be unattended during the course of the oxytocin infusion. At every 15-minute interval during oxytocin administration, the rate of oxytocin flow, the frequency and character of contractions, and the fetal heart rate should be recorded on the patient's chart. Subsequently, if adequate uterine contractility has not been achieved, the rate of infusion may be increased by four drops per minute. Again, the patient's response is observed until stabilized for 15 to 30 minutes and the relevant information recorded. If the contractions are still inadequate, the drip can be increased again by four drops per minute and the process repeated as often as needed until strong clinical labor is achieved.

Once the patient has been titrated and her optimal oxytocin dosage determined, it is essential that she be observed continuously and without interruption. It may be necessary to reduce the dosage in the event that excessive contractility develops. Not infrequently, as labor evolves, the uterus appears to become increasingly sensitive to exogenously administered oxytocin. It is necessary under these circumstances to reduce the infusion rate or even to stop it entirely. Because of the short half-life of circulating oxytocin (around 3 to 4 minutes), its biologic effects are rapidly dissipated. Therefore, if uterine contractions become excessive, the infusion can be stopped immediately and the uterotonic effect of oxytocin will usually diminish rapidly.

Maximum rates of administration have been set arbitrarily. Because almost all gravidas at term can be induced with infusion rates of 16 mU per minute or less (the equivalent of 24 drops per minute of the above solution), this dosage is usually considered by many to be the upper limit for use without consultation. Whereas higher dosages may be effective in resistant cases, that the cases are resistant suggests one of two situations: either they are not truly ready for induction—that is, conditions are unfavorable for successful induction under optimal circumstances—or the labor to follow will be complicated and difficult. Furthermore, high dosages are more commonly associated with hypercontractility. Although the uterus in such cases has demonstrated its relative insensitivity to low dosages of oxytocin, the uterus is still capable of overreacting vigorously to high dosages. Thus, the limits placed on permissible rates of infusion are not really critical. Instead, the limits are based on the experience that inductions requiring greater speeds of infusion often fail or are complicated.

In actuality, the amount of oxytocin needed to produce good uterine contractions may occasionally be large. This is particularly so when induction begins before the cervix is ready (see Bishop Score, above). For example, this applies when there is a strong medical indication for induction prior to term. The limit of dosage should, therefore, be considered merely as the rate of infusion that produces good contractions, bearing in mind, however, that the more oxytocin required, the less it is likely to succeed.

As to duration of infusion, most patients become rather exhausted after 8 hours of oxytocin infusion. Generally, the patient's trial should not be extended beyond this unless urgency dictates. If necessary, the procedure may be repeated at daily intervals until labor supervenes, although this is not considered good practice without overriding indications to justify this aggressive pursuit. What constitutes failure will depend on the vigor or enthusiasm with which one attacks the problem, within broad limits. For purely elective inductions an air of reasonableness must prevail, logically curtailing the duration of one's attempts to induce labor according to the patient's physical and emotional tolerance. As stated, this should rarely exceed 8 hours of strong, simulated clinical labor. Avoidance of failure can be accomplished by a process of patient selection. We have already alluded to the use of the Bishop scoring system. By weighting the several observable factors that define inducibility, one can determine in advance what the likelihood of failure will be.

If contractions become excessive, particularly if they exceed 90 seconds in duration or if they are associated with any evidence of fetal hypoxia, the infusion must be discontinued at once. The diminished uterine blood flow from the excessive contractions produced by oxytocin infusion can cause fetal hypoxia. When the infusion is appropriately monitored on a continuous basis, this effect can be noted by the characteristic late deceleration patterns of the fetal heart rate, in rapid response to the transient hypoxia. It has been shown that about 27 percent of fetuses subjected to oxytocin infusion in labor develop these deceleration patterns characteristic of the hypoxia of uteroplacental insufficiency (Schifrin, 1972). This occurs even without apparent uterine hypertonus, although the incidence of late decelerations almost doubles in the presence of overt hypertonus. When oxytocin infusion is superimposed on peridural anesthesia, the incidence of such hypoxic patterns increases to 40 percent.

Additionally, simultaneous monitoring of uterine activity is equally important. External tocodynamometry will provide a more objective check on the frequency and duration of uterine contractions than can be achieved by intermittent abdominal palpation. External monitoring of contractions, while useful in this regard, cannot offer the additional advantages that internal intrauterine pressure monitoring affords in terms of its ability to measure both uterine resting tonus and the intensity of uterine contractions. These two factors are of considerable importance during the course of uterotonic stimulation with oxytocin. Should the uterine resting tonus increase beyond 15 to 20 mm Hg, the uteroplacental circulatory exchange will be impeded because the average intervillous space pressure is 15 to 20 mm Hg. Actual measurement of contractile intensity, moreover, gives the physician important information relating to the uterine sensitivity to oxytocin, because it permits him or her to anticipate impending hypercontractility that could lead to fetal hypoxia.

There is strong support for the recommendation that fetal heart rate and uterine contractility be monitored whenever uterotonic stimulation is undertaken for induction or for stimulation of labor. The introduction of this important technologic advance for instantaneous and continuous beat-to-beat fetal heart rate surveillance has vastly improved the level of fetal "intensive care," and is apparently capable of ensuring optimal outcome in such high-risk circumstances as stimulation and induction of labor.

The quintessence of prevention of complications in inducing labor is diligent attention to details during observation and administration of oxytocin. It is mandatory that patient monitoring be carried out at all times by knowledgeable professionals so that uterotonic response can be determined on a continuous basis. The drip or pump rate of oxytocin infusion must be watched critically and adjusted according to the observed response. The optimal clinical features of strong, simulated labor, in which the uterus relaxes completely between contractions, should be sought.

Overstimulation should be assiduously avoided by careful titration of the oxytocin dosage and uterine response. Management of hypercontractility deserves to be stressed again. Such hypercontractility must be managed expediently to avoid its adverse effects on the fetus. Thus, if contractions exceed 90 seconds in duration, or if there is evidence of fetal hypoxia in the form of late deceleration of the fetal heart rate, the infusion must be discontinued at once. Perhaps the only other method consistently effective in alleviating uterine tetany is surgical anesthesia with open-drop ether, chloroform, or halothane. Unfortunately, these measures are not always immediately available. By the time they are instituted, the offending contraction pattern has usually subsided spontaneously in response to withdrawal of the oxytocin.

Continuous monitoring of uterine contractility and fetal cardiotachometry are appropriate, if available. Clearly, they should be used whenever possible, especially during such high-risk situations as induction and stimulation of labor. Besides these fine advances in technology, perhaps the best approach to preventing complications is avoiding induction except under ideal circumstances, where the criteria of inducibility are most favorable, where no contraindications exist, and where all prerequisites are met.

*Prostaglandins.* Clinical use of prostaglandins for induction of labor has been extensively discussed in Chapter 19. These agents will undoubtedly prove to be useful for this purpose when they are released for clinical practice. The precautions we have outlined for use of oxytocin in labor must apply equally for the use of prostaglandins. It will perhaps be even more important to consider the constraints about observing contraindications, monitoring the labor and the fetus, and ensuring appropriate environment and techniques with prostaglandins. This is so because, while they are effective, their therapeutic index (the ratio between toxic dose and effective dose, a measurement of their margin of safety) is small.

More important than the gastrointestinal side effects, including nausea, vomiting, and diarrhea, is the occasional unexpected hypercontractility that has been encountered. Oral $PGE_2$, for example, has been shown to be effective at relatively low levels of drug administration in terms of both its capability to induce labor and its potential to effect a labor that progresses normally or is enhanced to an acceptable degree (Friedman and Sachtleben, 1974a; Friedman et al, 1975b). Undesirable side effects, on the other hand, are encountered with increasing frequency and intensity as the dosage schedule increases.

Hypercontractility must be considered to be an adverse reaction of major significance. Whereas it is more likely to occur in association with excessively large doses, it has been observed even with the administration of small amounts. The latter appears to be the result of an unusual degree of uterine sensitivity, comparable to that sometimes seen with oxytocin stimulation. Indeed, reports of prolonged hypercontractility have appeared from time to time in association with all effective uterotonic agents, most especially when given by routes of administration other than carefully regulated intravenous infusion.

Contrary to such experiences, however, the episodes of hypercontractility seen with $PGE_2$ were short-lived and generally unassociated with evidences of fetal distress. With rare exceptions, they appear not to require any form of active intervention. We should justifiably be concerned about hypercontractility, nevertheless. This effect cannot be ignored and must be guarded against. Thus, the same precautions, caveats, and attention to detail are necessary during the administration of $PGE_2$ as we have described above for intravenous infusion of oxytocin.

*Sparteine.* Essentially the same principles apply to the use of sparteine sulfate. Once rather popular, this agent is no longer widely employed for labor induction because of isolated reports of tetanic contraction and uterine rupture coincident with or following its administration. The incidence of such complications, however, is apparently very small. Nonetheless, since uterine response to this drug can be variable and unpredictable, sparteine sulfate must be used with caution.

It is administered intramuscularly in 75-mg doses hourly until labor is established, for an average of three doses. Care must be taken to ensure that hypercontractility is averted or recognized promptly when it arises. It is likely that the adverse effects attributed to this agent in the past were the result of failure on the part of attendant personnel to respond promptly to developing hypercontractility by reducing or eliminating subsequent dosages of the drug. Because sparteine is still available and approved for clinical use, it is mentioned here for completeness.

## *AUGMENTATION OF LABOR*

The introduction of carefully titrated oxytocin infusion for purposes of stimulating the desultory labor has been shown to be an important advance in obstetrics over the past several decades. There can be little doubt that its use has contributed major benefits to this discipline, especially when applied under appropriate conditions. However, oxytocin is not without hazard. It is well recognized that serious complications can result if it is used inappropriately. We have already reviewed some of the prerequisites for its use (see above) and the precautions to be taken to minimize risk.

It must be emphasized here that, while it is possible to reduce the peril to mother and fetus considerably, it cannot be eliminated altogether. This being the case, it becomes imperative to weigh the benefits against the risks in each instance. Thus, there appears to be little justification for electively augmenting a labor that is progressing normally. This practice is unfortunately common, but it cannot be condoned.

Indeed, there have been proposals urging that active management be undertaken in essentially all labors to provide assurance that no labor will exceed 12 hours, even among nulliparas (O'Driscoll et al, 1970, 1973). It would appear intemperate to commit oneself inflexibly to early delivery. Whereas the results reported with this practice have thus far been good, the potential for much harm exists if it were adopted universally.

There can be no objection to the replacement of a passive concept of labor management with intensive care and personalized supervision of the laboring patient. However, to go beyond this approach for purposes of aggressive augmentation of all labors that are not progressing adequately (with cervical dilatation of at least 1 cm/hr) suggests that many patients in whom such stimulation is inappropriate or even contraindicated will be at risk. These include those in the latent phase, those with protraction disorders recognized to be generally unresponsive to such stimulation, and those with arrest disorders who are likely to have serious concomitant problems relating to cephalopelvic disproportion.

The hypothesis upon which this practice is intuitively based—namely, that a labor of normal duration produces a better maternal and fetal prognosis (Barber et al, 1972)—is entirely unverified. One must continually ask what the cost of such augmentation is, particularly in terms of maternal and fetal damage. This applies, of course, especially to situations in which excessive or abnormal uterine activity is produced, which may lead in turn to precipitate labor and delivery, fetal hypoxia, birth asphyxia, abruptio placentae, cervical laceration, or uterine rupture. Although these are uncommon occurrences, they constitute real complications.

Despite this general denigration of the practice of routine uterotonic stimulation of normal labor, there are some clearly defined indications for this practice. These will be reviewed in detail in Chapter 24. Oxytocin is appropriate specifically for those dysfunctional labor disorders that are known to respond favorably to such stimulation. They fall into two recognized groups: (1) patients with abnormally prolonged latent phase—without progressive dilatation after the onset of labor for 20 hours in nulliparas or 14 hours in multiparas—who persist in the latent phase after an adequate trial of therapeutic rest; (2) gravidas with arrest patterns—including secondary arrest of dilatation, prolonged deceleration phase, arrest of descent, and failure of descent—who clearly have no evidence of cephalopelvic disproportion. Exceptionally, patients with prolonged latent phase with concomitant conditions militating against the delay that would result from a program of rest will also tend to benefit from augmentation of labor.

Those parturients with protraction disorders are best served by withholding oxytocin. On the one hand, it will not enhance the rate of dilatation or descent; on the other, it may subject the patient or her fetus to substantial hazard with no compensating benefits. As to the patient with an arrest disorder occurring in association with disproportion, uterotonic stimulation is clearly contraindicated because of the extremely poor prognosis for vaginal delivery. To stimulate the labor under these circumstances puts both mother and fetus in jeopardy. The prognostic outlook for such cases will be discussed in depth in Chapter 23. Thus, uterotonic stimulation should not be used electively in normal labors or on a routine basis in labors that are deemed to be desultory or inert, unless it can be shown that specific disorders amenable to such stimulation are present.

Perhaps a word is in order about the use of amniotomy as a stimulatory device in labor. Amniotomy is documented to be effective in initiating labor when conditions are suitable for labor to begin (see above and Chapter 17). However, it cannot be shown to be effective in augmenting a labor that is already in progress. This statement stands in sharp contradistinction to the generally held clinical impression that amniotomy serves to stimulate labor progression. We have reviewed the illogical basis for our misconception in this regard in Chapter 17. We can recognize that the expected acceleration of cervical dilatation that normally takes place as labor enters the active phase of the first stage is often too readily attributable to the amniotomy done in the latent phase. Indeed, the criteria that are generally used for selecting patients for elective rupture of the membranes in labor are the same criteria as those characterizing the patient who is about to enter the active phase.

With the advent of more or less routine internal fetal heart rate monitoring—a technique requiring amniotomy—this issue is becoming moot. While there are acceptable indications for amniotomy during the course of normal labor (such as internal fetal monitoring, scalp blood sampling, management of abruptio placentae or the second twin, and in preparation for forceps application), amniotomy for purposes of uterotonic stimulation is rather dubious. As discussed (Chapters 9 through 12), moreover, amniotomy cannot be demonstrated to be effective as a therapeutic measure for any of the specific labor dysfunctions we have heretofore defined.

## *THERAPEUTIC REST*

It was once common practice to subject laboring patients to large doses of narcotic-analgesic medication for purposes of providing "twilight sleep," a method now roundly denounced with full justification because of its adverse effect on the neonate. The recommendation here (see Chapter 24) to invoke therapeutic rest by using such agents must not be misinterpreted to mean that we are advocating a return to this unacceptable practice for routine labor management. There is ample evidence to support a policy aimed at minimizing the administration of such agents in labor. What is offered instead is a means for providing much-needed rest to the patient with a prolonged latent phase (and only under this condition). Secondary gains are derived from the insight this approach provides toward making accurate diagnostic differentiation between false labor and the latent phase of true, but abnormal labor.

As we have seen (Chapter 9), placing the uterus at rest for an interval of 6 to 10 hours by administering large doses of narcotics will give the patient an opportunity to recover from the exhausting experience of her nonprogressive labor pattern, while simultaneously giving the physician the opportunity to correct any electrolyte imbalances or fluid deficiencies. Moreover, when the patient awakens, she is very likely to have already entered the active phase and be well on her way toward evolving active dilatation and progressive descent.

Concerns over the potentially adverse effect of the narcotic-analgesics on the infant can be allayed by the realization that circulating and tissue drug levels will have had ample time to be cleared by the time the delivery takes place. Recall that the medication is given only in those cases with prolonged latent phase, 20 hours having elapsed without progress in the nullipara, or 14 hours in the multipara. Unexpectedly rapid progress is unlikely to take place at once. Furthermore, any subsequent progression is inhibited rather effectively by the use of these agents. Finally, when the patient awakens after 6 to 10 hours, she still has many hours to go before she will be ready to deliver. Thus, by the time the baby is born, the effect of the medication has long since abated.

In our experience, such infants do exceedingly well in the neonatal period. The only exceptions we have encountered thus far were offspring of gravidas to whom it was found necessary to administer more than two doses of analgesia in order to try to stop uterine contractions. Unfortunately, it was determined too late that these women were already entering the active phase at that time. Because the patient had not been examined prior to each dosage, the physician did not recognize the error. The labor was not inhibited and delivery took place during the time that the medication was still in effect. The result was a depressed infant requiring the use of narcotic antagonist to correct the adverse effect of the morphine. Although the babies did well, it is important to recognize the need to assess the patient carefully to ensure that the active phase has not been entered and that delivery will not occur imminently. While such an occurrence is very unusual, it is best guarded against. Our stipulation of the dosage schedule, limiting administration to two doses spaced 20 minutes apart, stems from this experience.

One further note is relevant in this regard. We have spoken here of resting the uterus, implying that this was the mechanism of action of this approach. In actuality, tocodynamometric observations clearly demonstrate that the contractions generally continue, although usually very much attenuated and not perceived by the patient (or the attendant observer). Whereas we do not know how sedation brings about its beneficial effect when used as treatment for the prolonged latent phase, we have clear objective evidence that it does work empirically. To engage in polemics about our conjectures regarding the mechanism would be an unrewarding exercise at this time because of the very limited state of our knowledge concerning myometrial function.

## *EXPECTANCY*

Watchful expectancy is very unpopular among action-oriented obstetricians. There is perhaps ample historical justification for decrying an attitude that can be interpreted as neglect. Many of the obstetric catastrophes of the distant past were undoubtedly based on inappropriate inaction for uncommonly long periods of time when intervention was clearly in order. It is fervently hoped that we will never return to a time when patients with gross malpresentations or overt cephalopelvic disproportion will be subjected to such unacceptable practices. We have come a long way from that era when both mother and fetus were compromised by the trauma associated with uterine rupture, aseptic tissue necrosis, and intracranial tentorial or falx laceration with hemorrhage, among others.

While we decry such extremes of neglect, we must be equally on guard against extremes of active intervention (see above). Indeed, there appear to be well-defined circumstances under which expectancy is entirely appropriate. Specifically, certain dysfunctional labors with characteristic protraction disorders—that is, protracted active-phase dilatation pattern or protracted descent—are best managed in this way (see Chapters 11 and 24). Among patients with protraction disorders, those who do not have associated cephalopelvic disproportion can be expected to continue their dilatory course of dilatation and descent without interruption, provided no inhibitory conditions are superimposed. We recognize that such labors are especially sensitive to the deleterious effects of narcotic-analgesics, for example; thus, such agents should be avoided or, at least, minimized.

As long as the courses of dilatation and descent follow the extrapolated projection of their early labor curves, these patients can be allowed to continue in labor. Should arrest develop, intensive evaluation (more appropriately, reevaluation) must be undertaken to ensure that an underlying insurmountable bony dystocia has not been overlooked. Thus, these patients are not being neglected, but rather they are being intensively observed to ensure that they are following their expected pattern of progression. The observers should be alert to such deviations in order to mobilize all necessary resources at once for purposes of determining the cause and correcting it, if possible (for example, by allowing inhibitory sedation or anesthesia to abate).

Unless one can be assured that disproportion does not exist, it is far better under these circumstances to consider terminating the labor here by cesarean section. The pitfalls centering around the difficult distinction between protracted descent and arrest of decent with cranial molding have been discussed extensively (see Chapter 21). It is most important for every obstetric attendant who may be called upon to assess progressive fetal descent to be familiar with the nuances for making this distinction creditably. Failure to recognize that progressive descent has actually stopped—even though it may appear to be continuing due to molding—may subject the fetus and the mother to serious risk. Here the distinction between acceptable expectancy and unconscionable neglect becomes clear.

## *ABATEMENT*

A special subcategory of watchful expectancy is that in which we may specifically direct our attention to allowing the effects of exogenously administered inhibitory agents to abate. We are referring here to analgesic and anesthetic agents particularly. Their ability to deter the course of some labors has been detailed earlier (see Chapter 19). We now recognize that the latent phase of dilatation is perhaps the most sensitive period during the course of labor insofar as inhibitory effect is concerned. The active phase is far less responsive to equianalgesic levels of drug, provided the course is normally progressive. If the pattern of dilatation in the active phase is protracted—that is, less than the critical limits established here (see Chapter 10) —one can generally anticipate that the labor pattern will respond adversely to either peridural anesthesia or narcotic-analgesic medication. The normal second stage is usually almost totally unaffected by such measures, although the terminal part of the normal descent process can be delayed somewhat by peridural anesthesia unless the patient is able to augment expulsive forces voluntarily. More importantly, the problem of protracted descent is readily compounded by an arrest pattern if conduction anesthesia or a large amount of analgesic agent is given.

If it can be ascertained that labor progress has been inhibited by such measures aimed at relieving discomfort, allowing their effects to abate may redirect the dilatation and descent patterns toward normal (or back to the condition prevailing before the inhibitory influence was invoked). This applies, for example, to those gravidas with prolonged latent phase disorders in whom it is clear that the latent phase is iatrogenically inhibited through the intermedium of well-meaning, but ill-advised sedation. We generally recommend that such patients be subjected to therapeutic rest by means of the very same agents, but in much larger doses for the purpose of resting the uterus as well. In certain selected and exceptional instances, of course, it may be equally justifiable merely to allow the sedation previously given to abate. We should emphasize, however, that such women tend to be rather exhausted and, therefore, they usually deserve (and profit from) the benefits of rest.

A more frequent occurrence in which this approach tends to be useful is that of the gravida with protraction disorder—either protracted active-phase dilatation or protracted descent—who becomes secondarily arrested following the administration of analgesics or anesthesia. It is perhaps too easy here to ascribe the arrest to the agent that was given, and this may prove to be a trap for the unwary. Whereas the post hoc relationship may seem likely, it becomes essential in this sequence of events to ensure that one is not overlooking cephalopelvic disproportion as the underlying true proximal cause of the arrest.

The correlation between disproportion and the development of both protraction and arrest patterns has been exhaustively detailed (see Chapters 10, 11, and 16). Even though one has what appears to be an obvious reason for the arrest pattern to develop (in the analgesia or anesthesia), one must always be on the alert for the possibility that bony dystocia is also present. Thus, when arrest occurs, evaluation of the fetopelvic relationships must be undertaken at once, while simultaneously allowing the more obvious inhibitory agents to abate.

Among patients with arrest of descent (Friedman and Sachtleben, 1976), more than one-half were determined to have well-documented fetopelvic disproportion. Among those others with adequate pelvic dimensions, the best delivery prognosis was seen in those cases in which the apparent cause of the arrest was either peridural anesthesia or excessive sedation, and in which these agents were allowed to abate expectantly. Those who demonstrated further progression in the descent pattern were assured of an atraumatic vaginal delivery (spontaneously or by low forceps). However, not all of them advanced further in labor; their delivery prognosis was not so optimistic, less than one-half delivering vaginally. Nevertheless, the overall delivery prognosis for the abatement program was better by far than for comparable patients with arrest of descent who were managed by uterotonic stimulation, by expectancy (but no abatement), or by immediate delivery procedures.

Insofar as the fetal outcome was concerned in these cases, the incidence of birth trauma was considerably lower among those managed by abatement than those handled by any other treatment regimen. It is clear from these observations that allowing inhibitory anesthesia or sedation to wear off has a definite place in the obstetric armamentarium. It should be considered a positive measure in these clearly defined circumstances; its passive aspects need not debase its therapeutic importance.

There is a natural reluctance on the part of obstetric attendants to withdraw medication or anesthesia from the laboring patient once these have been instituted. Indeed, our *raison d'être* centers around helping such patients by relieving their discomfort. They are certainly deserving of whatever pain alleviation we can offer, provided it does not simultaneously incur hazard. Where it is likely that a disordered labor pattern has resulted from the use of such agents, the patient is better served by allowing her pain to return (with her full understanding of the rationale) than by permitting her and her fetus to suffer the consequences of the abnormality. The dire prognostic outlook for the offspring of gravidas with major labor aberrations, particularly those delivered by operative vaginal procedures, will be discussed in detail in Chapter 23. Most women faced with this dilemma will opt for safety rather than comfort. We the obstetric attendants should do likewise.

## *EXPEDITIOUS DELIVERY*

Provided neither mother nor fetus is placed in any jeopardy, normal spontaneous delivery is an appropriate goal for all parturients. In current obstetric practice, true low forceps procedures are also acceptable—when strictly defined as an application "to the fetal skull when the scalp is or has been visible at the introitus without separating the labia, the skull has reached the pelvic floor, and the sagittal suture is in the anteroposterior diameter of the outlet of the pelvis" (Hughes, 1972).

For those cases in which neither spontaneous nor low forceps delivery is likely to be accomplished without the risk of fetal death or serious damage, no other option appears to be available to us today except cesarean section. Even in the hands of technically very skilled obstetricians, midforceps operations can sometimes be traumatic. Midforceps operations as a means for terminating an abnormal labor carry an especially poor prognosis for the fetus and the surviving infant (see Chapter 23). Therefore, we are hard pressed to justify their continued use.

Most obstetric units today have ample facilities and supporting personnel for performing cesarean section expediently and safely. There is no doubt that cesarean section, although relatively safe among major surgical procedures, subjects the patient to greater hazards than does spontaneous or low forceps delivery, principally including those of anesthesia complications, infection, and blood loss. The length and degree of discomfort and physical impairment during recovery are also quite different.

Thus, we are under obligation not to undertake cesarean section without clear-cut justification in the form of substantial benefits either to the mother herself or, more relevant in regard to management of major labor disorders, to the fetus. By contrast, midforceps operations appear to provide neither the low maternal risk of spontaneous or low forceps delivery nor the low fetal risk of cesarean section. As a consequence, midforceps must be considered to constitute an unacceptable alternative.

It is imperative to realize that we are not advocating that physicians resort directly to cesarean section in every instance of abnormal labor. Moreover, cesarean section is not the only recourse for the physician who contemplates undertaking a midforceps procedure. Circumstances will dictate what else might (and should) be done. For example, the patient with arrest of descent resulting from peridural anesthesia (but with no evidence of cephalopelvic disproportion) could well be permitted to labor further if the anesthesia is allowed to abate or, alternatively (but less preferably), if uterine contractility is augmented with oxytocin. If the fetus can be shown to be in good condition, as documented by internal fetal heart rate monitoring (and scalp blood sampling, if necessary), there should be no concern about allowing the descent process to continue almost without regard for the duration of the second stage. As long as progress is being made and the fetal condition is uncompromised, there is no reason for operative intervention.

Similar scenarios can be constructed for other situations in which the physician might be confronted with a decision concerning delivery. As a general rule, unless there are strong maternal or fetal indications to effect delivery at that given time, further labor can be permitted to evolve, provided of course that vaginal delivery remains a viable option. If the conditions prevailing are such that vaginal delivery cannot be expected to take place, further delay is inappropriate. The programs of management relating to specific labor disorders, leading either to uncomplicated vaginal delivery or operative cesarean section, are described in Chapter 24.

# Prognostic Outlook

## CHAPTER 23

The expected results are detailed for both mother and baby, based on the outcome obtained for each group of dysfunctional labor patterns. The innocuous nature of prolonged latent phase stands in sharp contrast to the more ominous impact of protraction, and especially arrest abnormalities. Postarrest progression proves to be an especially useful index of prognosis during a trial of oxytocin stimulation for an arrest disorder. The intrinsic fetal risk of the labor pattern is clearly enhanced by operative vaginal delivery procedures. Midforceps operations, which appear to carry an adverse fetal prognosis even after normal labors, are especially hazardous to the fetus if they are undertaken following protraction or arrest disorders. Long-term results show persistent effects among surviving infants.

We have made some rather important observations concerning delivery and fetal outcome. Abnormal dilatation and descent patterns under the influence of prescribed treatment plans have frequently been found to serve in the capacity of prognostic indicators. Their practical value in this role cannot be overestimated. This holds particularly in situations where extremes of action appear to be completely warranted or just as clearly interdicted. An example of a case in which cesarean section is unquestionably called for is one with coexistent arrest pattern and cephalopelvic disproportion. At the other extreme, an instance in which the choice of treatment should be conservative is that of the patient with prolonged latent phase. Here, abdominal delivery for purposes of primary treatment of the labor aberration is patently improper. It is the relative difference in prognostic outlook that determines how these decisions are to be made. Let us examine the factors that affect delivery and fetal prognosis for the several types of abnormal labor patterns separately. These will help us to evolve meaningful management programs (see Chapter 24) aimed at optimizing results.

## *DELIVERY PROGNOSIS*

In our discussions dealing with each of the defined labor disorders, we alluded to differences in outcome data. Having stratified our material according to treatment modalities, we were in a position to assess which therapy was most appropriate, based on the best results achieved. These results in turn now serve to provide us with information on prognosis. They give us insight into what types of delivery specific patients will likely be subjected to as their labors evolve. The principles upon which these assessments are based form the essence of similar forecasting systems in other medical disciplines. Delivery prognosis here is based on evaluations of the results obtained under clearly defined circumstances among gravidas presenting with specific dysfunctional labor patterns.

### *Prolonged Latent Phase*

Among patients with prolonged latent phase, we can anticipate an overall cesarean section rate of well under 10 percent. This immediately implies that cesarean section invoked to terminate a labor in the latent phase would be unwarranted nine times out of ten, provided the only problem recognized to exist is this abnormal labor pattern. Furthermore, we can recall that about one-tenth of these patients are actually in false labor, although we cannot identify them prospectively. To subject such patients to major abdominal surgery under this circumstance would constitute an exceedingly aggressive act and one without clear justification.

If the active phase is permitted to evolve in patients with prolonged latent phase, those few who actually deserve operative intervention will become known in due course. We have seen (Chapter 9) that most patients with this disorder, if allowed to labor, will go on to have perfectly normal active-phase patterns. Most of these represent gravidas who were excessively sedated during the course of the latent phase or whose latent phase was prolonged because they began labor with unprepared pelvic tissues, especially the cervix.

The several possibilities of progression that can occur after the latent phase has ended are illustrated in Figure 62, together with their frequencies of occurrence. As just stated, most of them enter a normal active phase and proceed uneventfully into a normal descent pattern to deliver vaginally. A very small number of those patients who enter the active phase with normal maximum slopes of dilatation later become secondarily arrested. In terms of prognostic outlook, therefore, the chances of continued normal

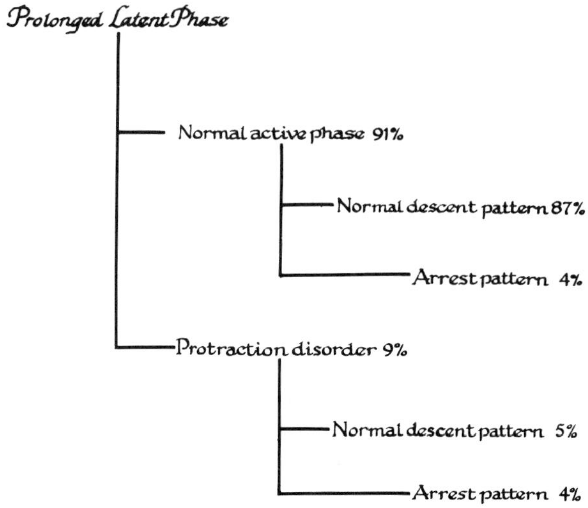


*Fig. 62.* Prognostic outlook for labor course following successful termination of prolonged latent phase, indicating the optimism that should generally prevail.

progress in labor outweigh the possibility of arrested labor by a factor of nearly ten to one if a normal active-phase pattern follows the termination of the prolonged latent phase.

Among those gravidas with prolonged latent phase who subsequently develop an abnormally protracted active-phase dilatation pattern, somewhat less than one-half become secondarily arrested later in the first stage. Here one can forecast that arrest is more likely to result if the active phase is already abnormal. These results are not unexpected. In fact, they appear to be the same (or even somewhat better) than seen in association with protraction disorders that are not preceded by prolonged latent phase (see below).

As to the labor patterns that might be expected after prolonged latent phase, the overall frequencies included more than one-half who continued uninterruptedly with normal progressive dilatation and descent, about one-fifth who developed protraction disorders and continued in these dilatory patterns to delivery, and the remaining one-fifth who became secondarily arrested. These are the results if the type of treatment program is not considered.

We recognize (see Chapter 9) that either oxytocin infusion or therapeutic rest is equally effective in terminating the prolonged latent phase in about 85 percent of cases. It is clear that selection has a great deal to do with this, since large numbers of patients in false labor will dilute the material considerably and provide a relatively lower cure rate. Similarly, the outlook in a series containing many patients with prolonged latent phase due to excessive sedation will be much brighter. We may, therefore, expect variations in results among population groups. Nevertheless, a general feeling of optimism should prevail insofar as the labor prognosis for prolonged latent phase is concerned.

As to delivery outcome, we have already noted the low overall cesarean section rate. There is little doubt that, in the final analysis, the outcome will depend largely upon the patterns of active-phase dilatation and second-stage descent that follow the termination of the abnormal latent phase. Indeed, delivery frequencies (Table 63) relate directly to the subsequent labor course. Among patients with prolonged latent phase who proceeded into a normal active phase, for example, essentially all can be expected to deliver vaginally. None should require cesarean section unless, of course, other critical problems arise. It is clear that few delivery complications need be anticipated if dilatation and descent take place normally after a latent phase disorder. On the other hand, if a protraction disorder should develop, operative vaginal or abdominal delivery is much more likely. Furthermore, the prognosis for operative delivery becomes still worse should an arrest pattern develop.

*Table 63. DELIVERY OUTCOME BY LABOR PATTERN FOLLOWING PROLONGED LATENT PHASE*

| *Pattern* | *Spontaneous and Low Forceps* (%) | *Midforceps* (%) | *Cesarean Section* (%) |
|---|---|---|---|
| Normal dilatation and descent | 92 | 8 | 0 |
| Protraction disorder | 74 | 21 | 5 |
| Arrest disorder | 38 | 23 | 39 |
| Combined protraction and arrest | 35 | 23 | 42 |

We must strongly reemphasize that the majority follow a perfectly normal pattern. One cannot predict with any degree of certainty which patients with prolonged latent phase will or will not progress normally. In view of these considerations, we cannot condone the practice of resorting to cesarean section as a primary method of treating the patient with prolonged latent phase. Needless to say, cesarean section might be warranted on the basis of some other problem that exists concurrently, but this labor pattern must never be construed to represent a legitimate indication for cesarean section by itself.

In our experience, most of the patients with prolonged latent phase who subsequently came to cesarean section were those who developed later arrest disorders. Since we lack the clairvoyance to identify these patients in advance, we cannot predetermine which few will require cesarean section and which of the many others will be able to deliver normally. On this basis, it seems reasonable to allow these patients with prolonged latent phase to proceed into the active phase and do demonstrate their capabilities to evolve a normal pattern and deliver vaginally. This approach is particularly pertinent, since we have shown that there is no increase in fetal or maternal morbidity or mortality if such a program is undertaken. The prognosis for the fetus will be discussed in more detail below.

### *Protraction Disorders*

Prognosis for delivery in protracted active-phase dilatation and protracted descent disorders depends on two considerations: (1) whether or not an arrest pattern supervenes and (2) how aggressively the delivery process is managed. We have seen (Chapter 10) that nearly two-thirds of patients with protraction disorders that are uncomplicated by subsequent arrest patterns will progress to uneventful delivery. In contrast (Table 64), if an arrest pattern should occur subsequently, there is a fourfold increase in the expected cesarean section rate. Except in those cases with cephalopelvic disproportion—a factor that will usually and predictably compound the protraction pattern by superimposing an arrest disorder—there seems to be no reliable signpost to help us foretell which patients will continue uninterruptedly in their abnormal protraction pattern and which ones will later arrest. It seems reasonable to presume, despite this lack of forecasting ability, that the prognosis remains rather good as long as continued progress is maintained along the extrapolated projection in a protraction pattern.

*Table 64. DELIVERY OUTCOME IN PROTRACTION DISORDERS BY EVOLVED PATTERN*

| *Pattern* | *Spontaneous and Low Forceps* (%) | *Midforceps* (%) | *Cesarean Section* (%) |
|---|---|---|---|
| Unremitting protraction | 65 | 25 | 10 |
| Subsequent arrest pattern | 39 | 18 | 43 |

More will be said concerning the risks to the infant in association with protraction disorders (see below). We have already alluded to the real hazards that appear to accrue to these babies when the protraction pattern is terminated by potentially traumatic operative vaginal delivery procedures (see Chapter 10). Besides this peril, there appears to be no substantially increased risk to either mother or infant from the labor condition itself, provided of course that no ill-advised measures for stimulation or traumatic delivery are undertaken. Expectancy, therefore, is recommended (see Chapter 24). This approach has generally been found to be associated with good outcome.

### *Arrest Disorders*

The arrest patterns reviewed in Chapter 11 represent particularly serious abnormalities. Collectively, they yield an especially poor prognosis for vaginal delivery. We now appreciate that about one-half the patients with these disorders ultimately require cesarean section because of the high frequency of associated cephalopelvic disproportion of insurmountable degree. Despite this association, it is also quite clear that the prognostic outlook is very favorable for the patient with an arrest disorder whose pelvic relationships are adequate. More than four of every five such gravidas deliver vaginally.

These considerations notwithstanding, the course of labor following an arrest pattern is very useful in providing a prognostic forecast. The several types of progression that can occur following arrest are illustrated in Figure 63. We can see that less than one-quarter of those permitted to labor after the arrest showed no additional progress. The overall cesarean section rate in this nonresponsive group exceeded 80 percent. Among the remaining three-quarters of patients who progressed further in labor, a small number arrested again. These comprised 5 percent of this subgroup or 3 percent of the total. All the others continued to advance without interruption.

Thus, from the prognostic viewpoint, about one-half the labors with arrest patterns may be expected to return to normal in due course. When one eliminates those patients with bony dystocia in whom further trials of labor are clearly unwarranted, one improves the prognosis to an expectation exceeding 70 percent of gravidas who will progress in subsequent labor without further problem. In other words, in the absence of high degrees of disproportion, three-quarters of the patients with arrest patterns may be expected to exhibit subsequent normal progress in labor.

We have seen (Chapters 11 and 16) that delivery outcome may be predicted with some accuracy on the basis of the subsequent course of labor following an arrest. Indeed, if there is any additional progress in dilatation

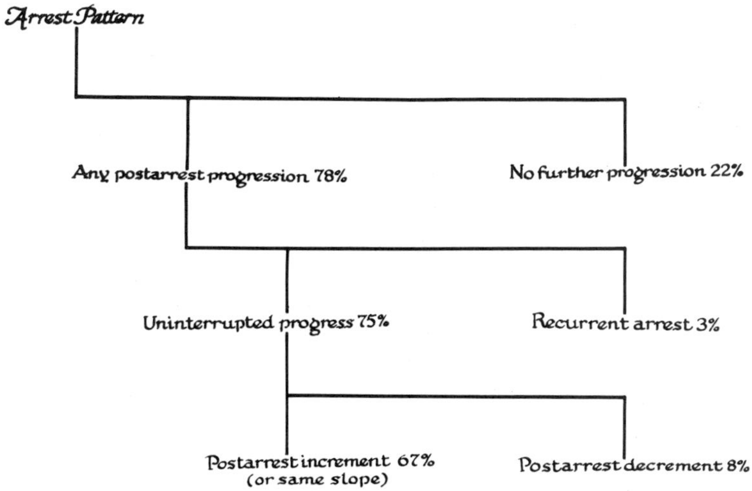


*Fig. 63.* Labor progression expected following arrest patterns in the absence of documentable cephalopelvic disproportion, showing the good results usually seen, especially if adequate postarrest progression occurs.

or descent at all after a documented period of arrest, the likelihood that cesarean section will be necessary is less than 7 percent. Thus, if any additional progress in dilatation occurs in response to a trial of labor, prospects for vaginal delivery improve considerably. Under these circumstances, one may expect normal delivery in about 65 percent of cases. In addition, early experience shows a potentially correctable high rate of midforceps, at about 25 percent. This may be attributed to understandable, but not necessarily excusable, impatience on the part of the physician near the end of these long, tedious labors.

A valuable adjunct here is comparison of the rate of progression before arrest with the rate after arrest. We find that the outcome improves progressively with the increment in slope. The more rapid the postarrest slope, the fewer cesarean sections are required. If the two slopes are the same—that is, if there is no increment—or the postarrest slope is less steeply inclined than the prearrest slope, the end results at delivery are considerably worse than those following a positive increment. In the group without any increment, one in six required cesarean section, whereas those with a positive increment were subjected to cesarean section only 4 percent of the time. Similarly, a positive increment of less than 2 cm/hr was associated with a section rate of 6 percent, while there were no sections done in cases with increments greater than this critical point.

The midforceps rate fell correspondingly and inversely with the rising rate of normal uncomplicated deliveries. Indeed, no midforceps procedures were necessary in labors with increments of 3 cm/hr or greater. The optimism that positive increments generate in prognostic outlook appears to be warranted in the 80 percent of cases in which they are encountered, excluding those with documentable cephalopelvic disproportion.

## *Trial of Oxytocin*

We encounter paramount difficulties in trying to specify the limits of a trial period of stimulation in arrested labor. The obstetric literature contains numerous reports attesting to the efficacy of oxytocin stimulation in abnormal labors. The weight of much collective clinical experience suffices to justify our continued use of this beneficial agent for these purposes (see Chapter 19). From the practical viewpoint, however, there is a paucity of specific data to indicate (1) the minimum period of stimulation that we should persist in (in the absence of further progress) before the therapeutic trial should be declared a failure, (2) the degree of response to be expected in the form of additional dilatation or descent after stimulation in order for us to justify continuing the trial, and (3) the outcome we can expect according to the degree of response that is elicited. These issues are obviously interrelated and therefore will be dealt with here as relevant to prognosis. Our studies (Friedman and Sachtleben, 1963a, 1976) have provided clinically useful information in this regard.

Patients treated with oxytocin for arrest patterns are obviously preselected in that those with severe degrees of cephalopelvic disproportion (and many with lesser degrees as well) are justifiably delivered by cesarean section with no attempt to stimulate labor. We must understand, therefore, that a trial of oxytocin applies almost exclusively to situations in which arrest of dilatation or descent takes place in the absence of significant recognized bony dystocia. The findings of comparable studies undertaken in the face of overt disproportion have already been detailed (see Chapter 16).

To aid us in prognostic forecasting, we learn that responsive patients demonstrate the effect of therapy unfailingly within 7 hours. The response we are seeking here, of course, refers to postarrest dilatation or descent, not delivery. Overall, in the absence of documented disproportion, a success rate of 91 percent is readily achievable. We conjecture that success rates as high as 97 percent could be accomplished with astute attention to preselection and maintenance of adequate stimulation, in terms of both duration and degree. Among those who respond with postarrest progress, response is seen in less than 2 hours in 76 percent and within 4 hours in 93 percent.

In our experience, many of the cases in which 4 or more hours of stimulation have elapsed before expected progressive dilatation occurred are deemed likely to have responded earlier if sufficient exposure had been given. For example, for much of the period prior to the response, the uterine contractions that are produced in many of these cases are clearly suboptimal. It is important to note that the duration of the trial of oxytocin stimulation should, therefore, be timed not by the interval of the infusion, but rather according to the period during which good active labor is being simulated; that is, we have produced regular, strong uterine contractions, lasting 50 seconds or more and recurring at least at 3-minute intervals. If these criteria are observed, all responses are likely to be seen well within a period of 4 hours.

As to ultimate outcome, it is clear that any progressive dilatation or descent in response to stimulation promptly improves the outlook. Among oxytocin failures, 90 percent require cesarean section. This contrasts sharply with 71 percent normal vaginal deliveries among those responding with additional dilatation or descent following the interval of arrest.

We can find no differences in delivery outcome according to the duration of stimulation required to produce its effect. Our findings show that the relative delivery rates remain essentially constant, regardless of how long it takes for the oxytocin infusion to become effective. There are some interesting differences, however, according to the degree of cervical dilatation and level of station at which the arrest occurs. The incidence of successfully treated labors does not vary greatly in this regard. However, the subsequent course of labor in patients who respond to therapy is substantially better in those whose dilatation arrests early in the active phase. This holds true for both the postarrest rate of dilatation and the outcome at delivery. The average increase in maximum slope is greater for those arresting, say, at 4 cm, than for those arresting at 7 or 8 cm. Although the section rate remains fairly constant in the various subgroups, the frequency of midforceps procedures increases markedly and, simultaneously, the incidence of uncomplicated vaginal deliveries decreases with advancing degrees of dilatation at arrest.

A rough index of the ultimate outcome is found in the absolute value of the postarrest slope after successful response to therapy (Table 65). The broad spread of the data negates the practical value of this observation. Nevertheless, there is little doubt that the relative prognosis for normal vaginal delivery is directly related to the absolute rate of postarrest progression. For example, all patients with labor patterns in which the second slope is more than 4.0 cm/hr deliver normally. In contrast, only one-third of those with postarrest rates of 1.0 cm/hr or less deliver spontaneously or by low forceps. A relationship is thus established between the progression brought about by treatment and the end result at delivery. Although this correlation is clear, it lacks the precision required for a definitive and utilitarian prognostic tool.

*Table 65. DELIVERY OUTCOME IN ARREST DISORDERS BY RESPONSE TO OXYTOCIN*

| *Postarrest Slope (cm/hr)* | *Spontaneous or Low Forceps (%)* | *Midforceps (%)* | *Cesarean Section (%)* |
|---|---|---|---|
| No response (zero slope) | 0 | 10 | 90 |
| ≤1.0 | 33 | 56 | 11 |
| 1.1–2.0 | 71 | 23 | 6 |
| 2.1–3.0 | 75 | 20 | 5 |
| 3.1–4.0 | 67 | 33 | 0 |
| 4.1+ | 100 | 0 | 0 |

Further refined, this material proves very useful when the postarrest slope is compared with the prearrest slope. The relative increase in the maximum slope after successful therapy shows good correlation with outcome. Quantitatively, the greater the increment, the greater the likelihood of normal vaginal delivery (Table 66 and Fig. 64). Where the change is 0.5 cm/hr or less, only one-third deliver normally; this figure improves somewhat (to almost one-half of normal deliveries) if the postarrest slope is 1.0 cm/hr greater than the prearrest slope. More pertinently, cesarean section is rarely indicated among those with increments of greater than 1.0 cm/hr. In fact, all appear to be done for factors not related to the labor or the therapy. Moreover, no sections at all are found to be necessary in those whose increments are more than 2.0 cm/hr. It is also noteworthy that midforceps rates decrease sharply with increasing postarrest increments, reaching acceptably low levels in those with increments of greater than 1.5 cm/hr. With increments of more than 2.5 cm/hr, all patients can be expected to deliver normally, without exception.

*Table 66. DELIVERY OUTCOME IN ARREST DISORDERS BY CHANGE IN SLOPE*

| *Slope Increment** *(cm/hr)* | *Spontaneous or Low Forceps* *(%)* | *Midforceps* *(%)* | *Cesarean Section* *(%)* |
|---|---|---|---|
| ⩽+0.5 | 33 | 60 | 7 |
| ⩽+1.0 | 47 | 43 | 10 |
| >+1.0 | 84 | 14 | 2 |
| >+1.5 | 94 | 6 | 0 |

* Increment refers to the difference between prearrest and postarrest slopes in response to oxytocin infusion administered for treatment of arrested labor.

On the basis of these data, we can recognize a critical transition point above the increment of 1.0 cm/hr in postarrest slope. It is clear that labors with large increments carry better prognoses than those with small ones. Of even more importance is the observation that nearly all patients can be predicted to deliver normally if they respond after an arrest pattern with a slope that is more than 2.0 cm/hr greater than the corresponding prearrest slope.

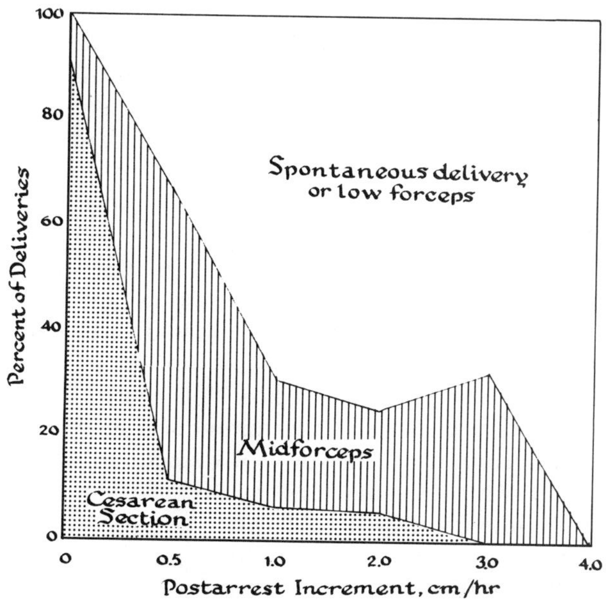


*Fig. 64.* Delivery outcome as related to postarrest slope increment in nulliparas who have arrest disorders unassociated with cephalopelvic disproportion and are treated with uterotonic stimulation. The greater the response relative to the slope before arrest, the better the outlook for vaginal delivery. This applies particularly for increments greater than 1.0 cm/hr.

The decisive features of a therapeutic trial of oxytocin in the specific arrest disorders become clear as a result of these observations. Our evaluation here does not concern itself primarily with the special instance of arrest occurring so commonly in association with cephalopelvic disproportion. Indeed, we hold that insurmountable bony dystocia manifesting itself by such labor aberrations is more properly handled by expeditious abdominal delivery. A trial of oxytocin is unwarranted under these circumstances.

The crucial factors in the administration of oxytocin for arrest are those of time and amount. Each patient requires and deserves individual handling. Diligent attention must be paid to uterine responsiveness to oxytocin. The intravenous technique, by infusion or pump, is best suited to the frequent adjustments in instantaneous dosage that are required to produce an optimal labor. The rate of infusion is regulated according to demonstrated uterine response, starting very slowly and increasing gradually until the level required to maintain strong clinical labor is reached. Continuous supervision by qualified personnel is necessary because of the frequent revision of the rate that may be required. Such personnel must be knowledgeable in recognizing and managing any complications that may arise as well. There is as yet no known way to predict with accuracy the sensitivity of any given individual to oxytocin. The contractions that result, however, may be used as a gauge to determine whether the proper level of infusion has been reached.

Simulation of clinically good spontaneous labor is the prime immediate aim of this form of treatment. Many so-called failed trials of oxytocin appear to have resulted from apparent disregard of this principle. In some, error was compounded by the additional shortcoming of insufficient exposure. In others, only the time factor was at fault—that is, not enough time had been allowed for the oxytocin to have taken full effect. There is a prevailing misconception that dilatation and descent must begin and proceed immediately after the oxytocin has been initiated; we now recognize that finite intervals may pass (and usually do) before such progression is actually realized. An optimal period of stimulation to effect strong, active labor and to produce further dilatation in secondary arrest of dilatation appears to be about 4 hours in duration; for arrest of descent, 2 hours. In the absence of cephalopelvic disproportion, essentially all patients should be expected to respond to such treatment if these basic standards are observed.

The only criteria we use for assessing immediate success is the occurrence of progressive advancement in dilatation or descent following the arrest for which the treatment was prescribed. It may be pertinent, therefore, to point out that the 4-hour time limit for an adequate trial of oxytocin is applicable merely to the interval between the initiation of active labor and the beginning of further dilatation or descent. It is appropriate to ignore the time it takes from initiating the infusion until a good contractile pattern is established. Moreover, we must understand that delivery cannot be expected to occur within these very narrow limits.

Nevertheless, the outcome at delivery does appear to be related to certain easily recognizable and potentially useful prognostic factors. The most obvious is that of the successful response to uterotonic stimulation itself. The absence of any response portends an operative delivery, most commonly cesarean section. If any further progress occurs, the outlook becomes considerably brighter. In our series, this represented 94 percent vaginal deliveries, all but 23 percent of which were normal.

The duration of uterotonic stimulation that is required to bring about a positive effect does not seem to influence the outcome. Similarly, the degree of cervical dilatation achieved at the time of secondary arrest of dilatation does not appear to affect relative chances of beneficial effect from stimulation. The dilatation, however, is related to both the immediate and the ultimate results. The earlier the arrest, the greater the dilatation that can be expected to occur after the arrest; moreover, there should be greater expectations for an increase in the postarrest dilatation rate and, as a consequence, a better forecast for uncomplicated vaginal delivery. In later arrests subsequent progression tends to be slower, with smaller increments of slope and greater numbers of midforceps procedures. The frequencies of operative delivery may likely reflect a general feeling of impatience on the part of the obstetric attendants, yielding to the temptation for relatively earlier intervention for purposes of terminating the labor. This is also mirrored in the greater incidence of major and minor trauma, both fetal and maternal, encountered here. Comparable principles apply for the station of arrest in cases of arrest of descent (Friedman and Sachtleben, 1976).

The actual rates of postarrest dilatation or descent are coarse measures of the outcome. The inverse correlation between increasing postarrest slope and decreasing frequency of operative delivery is well demonstrated. The intrinsic practical value of this variable, however, is exceeded by that of the relative change (increment) in slope, comparing postarrest slope with prearrest slope. A sharp, apparently reliable transition has been demonstrated—consisting of a positive increment exceeding 1.0 cm/hr—to indicate the strong likelihood that an uncomplicated delivery will result, barring unforeseen and unrelated obstetric problems.

From the standpoint of delivery prognosis, this factor of postarrest increment is useful and commendably functional. Strict limitations of its use must be kept in mind, nevertheless. It requires accurate information regarding both the courses of dilatation and descent before the labor arrested, and comparable information on the progressive sequential change thereafter. For cervical dilatation, the increment rule is applicable when secondary arrest occurs before the cervix is too far dilated (8 cm maximum) to allow accurate quantitative evaluations of the postarrest slope. Finally, it should not be inferred that this approach in any way condones or recommends a therapeutic trial of uterotonic stimulation merely to test the adequacy of the pelvis, in lieu of pelvimetric studies. Clear distinction must be made as far as management is concerned between arrest due to obstructive fetopelvic disproportion and arrest resulting from other, perhaps less serious causes.

## Overview

The data dealing with delivery prognosis that we have discussed thus far were derived from preselected subpopulations of gravidas presenting with the specific labor aberrations. It is essential that we ascertain whether or not our findings are applicable to the obstetric population at large. Several successful attempts have yielded meaningful relevant information (Friedman et al, 1970; Friedman and Sachtleben, 1971; Friedman, 1973c). In general, the information is confirmatory.

Specifically for nulliparas at term with fetuses in vertex presentation weighing at least 2,500 g, high frequencies of operative delivery are encountered in association with protraction and arrest patterns, but not in association with prolonged latent phase (Table 67). As expected, the types of delivery are not uniformly distributed among the several labor-pattern groups. Spontaneous and low forceps deliveries occur quite frequently in association with normal graphic patterns (68 percent), as well as with prolonged latent phase (83 percent).

*Table 67. DELIVERY OUTCOME BY LABOR ABERRATION IN NULLIPARAS**

| *Labor Pattern* | *Spontaneous* (%) | *Low Forceps* (%) | *Midforceps* (%) | *Cesarean Section†* (%) |
|---|---|---|---|---|
| Normal | 33 | 35 | 31 | 1 |
| Prolonged latent phase | 45 | 38 | 17 | 0 |
| Protraction disorder | 21 | 31 | 42 | 6 |
| Arrest disorder | 12 | 25 | 56 | 7 |
| Combined protraction and arrest | 10 | 23 | 59 | 8 |

* Specifically, those at term with fetus in vertex presentation and birth weight of 2,500 g or greater.

† Excluding all cases subjected to cesarean section for cephalopelvic disproportion prior to the full evolution of their active phase pattern.

By contrast, normal delivery types are much less frequently seen in association with protraction and arrest disorders. Midforceps delivery occurs in a reversed sequence. Labors with arrest patterns are delivered by midforceps more than one-half of the time. Essentially no cesarean sections are required to effect delivery of a labor with a normal graphic pattern or one with prolonged latent phase. For all other patterns there is a section rate of 7 percent, an unexpectedly low incidence. Much higher frequencies of abdominal delivery are generally encountered in patients with arrest patterns.

This discrepancy is probably based on a policy of early evaluation for suspicion of cephalopelvic disproportion and a prevalent aggressive attitude toward termination of labor when major degrees of disproportion are uncovered. In this way, the opportunity is lost in these patients for developing the characteristic arrest pattern. Thus, one finds a low incidence of disproportion and hence a diminished requirement for abdominal delivery in patients whose labor progression traces a pattern of arrest of dilatation or of descent. If those patients who had been subjected to cesarean section for cephalopelvic disproportion early in the course of labor were reinserted into the data matrix in Table 67 and distributed among the several graphic patterns according to their expected concentration in the protraction and arrest categories, the new results for cesarean section rates would resemble those in Table 63 almost precisely.

This material confirms the prognostic significance of the labor pattern after appropriate selection techniques are applied to eliminate various possible confounding influences. Thus, from the prognostic point of view, a labor diagnosis derived by observing the evolution of the dilatation and descent patterns proves to be useful for determining what the delivery outcome is likely to be.

## *FETAL PROGNOSIS*

Perinatal mortality statistics have not changed appreciably during the past decade. Brain injury resulting from either hypoxia in utero or trauma during delivery is second only to prematurity as a cause of fetal wastage, infant morbidity, and neurologic deficiency. It is obvious that if we are to make any further inroads toward improving fetal salvage and optimizing long-term outcome potential, we must try to uncover conditions that will serve as indicators that a high-risk situation exists or is likely to develop. The general concept that prolonged labor contributes to perinatal loss is undoubtedly correct. However, it is not sufficiently definitive to provide the guidelines necessary for identifying those specific patients whose labors deviate from the normal and may, as a consequence, be deleterious to the fetus.

As routine fetal heart rate monitoring becomes more widespread, this matter will perhaps become more or less academic in the future. We are encouraged to believe that early signs of fetal hypoxia, regardless of cause, will then be regularly detectable during labor. This may or may not provide the kind of information that will be necessary to assess how much cranial molding and other mechanical stresses a given fetus will be able to accept without undergoing irreversible damage during the birth process. Until such time as we can be assured that information of this kind is available, we must pursue an objective that allows us to specify those labors in progress that will present the greatest likelihood of causing fetal difficulties.

Important relationships have been uncovered between specific labor disorders, subsequent delivery procedures, and perinatal outcome (Friedman et al, 1969b; Friedman and Sachtleben, 1971; Friedman, 1973c). Observations included assessment of mortality results as well as 1-minute and 5-minute Apgar Scores. Subsequent reports dealt with neurologic and developmental effects of labors on the surviving infants at ages 8 months and 1 year (Friedman et al, 1969c), as well as at 4 years (Friedman et al, 1977).

The findings of these investigations form the basis for assigning relative risk potential to specific labor disorders and delivery procedures.

On the basis of labor patterns examined without consideration for the type of delivery, for example, we find that relatively few infants are lost in association with normal graphic patterns or those characterized by prolonged latent phase (4.9 and 4.0 per 1,000, respectively). With protraction disorders, however, the rate rises to 15.2 per 1,000, and with arrest patterns, to 30.2 per 1,000. Where both protraction and arrest disorders are concurrent in a labor, the perinatal mortality is 29.4 per 1,000.

When examined according to the type of delivery, this time ignoring the labor pattern, we find impressively low rates of perinatal loss for babies born spontaneously (2.2 per 1,000) and those delivered by low forceps (6.2 per 1,000). In contrast, midforceps deliveries are associated with perinatal losses of 18.9 per 1,000.

The overall perinatal mortality associated with cesarean section in comparable patients is somewhat higher than that of low forceps. It is difficult to interpret this rate, however, because we recognize that cesarean section is sometimes done under the kinds of critical emergency conditions or for medical or obstetric complications that would be expected to yield high fetal wastage. Eliminating those sections undertaken electively (repeat cesarean sections), or for indications unrelated to the labor, we obtain perinatal mortality rates falling between those of spontaneous delivery and low forceps. For our purposes here, these will not be included for further consideration.

The relationship between labor pattern and delivery type becomes quite clear when we examine the distribution of fetal and infant deaths as a function of both simultaneously (Table 68). For spontaneous deliveries, we see clearly that there are essentially no losses except in association with arrest patterns. Similarly, low forceps delivery following normal progression or after prolonged latent phase seems entirely innocuous; after a protraction disorder, on the other hand, the mortality rises to 12.0 per 1,000; after an arrest pattern, moreover, it doubles to 24.4 per 1,000, at which level it remains in association with combined protraction and arrest disorders.

*Table 68. PERINATAL MORTALITY BY LABOR PATTERN AND DELIVERY METHOD**

| *Labor Pattern* | *Spontaneous* | *Low Forceps* | *Midforceps* | *Total* |
|---|---|---|---|---|
| Normal | 2 | 3 | 11 | 5 |
| Prolonged latent phase | 0 | 0 | 11 | 4 |
| Protraction disorder | 0 | 12 | 29 | 15 |
| Arrest disorder | 16 | 24 | 38 | 31 |
| Combined protraction and arrest | (0) | 25 | 37 | 29 |
| Total | 2 | 6 | 19 | 10 |

* Rates expressed per 1,000 births, based on data from 3,000 gravidas at term with vertex presentation and birth weight of 2,500 g or more. Parentheses signify rate based on small sample size.

Midforceps operations, in contrast, are associated with 10.8 per 1,000 perinatal mortality, even after normal labors or patterns of prolonged latent phase. Losses nearly triple with midforceps procedures following protraction disorders (28.5 per 1,000) and almost quadruple after arrest patterns (38.3 per 1,000 alone, and 36.6 per 1,000 if arrest follows a protraction abnormality). These data are illustrated graphically in Figure 65, which displays a multidirectional effect of both the labor disorder and the delivery procedure, acting alone and synergistically in combination.

Several clear trends are uncovered by these observations. First, there appears to be little doubt that midforceps delivery subjects the fetus to substantial risk regardless of the labor pattern that precedes it. This applies even across the range of midforceps delivery as liberally defined, including many considered to be relatively "easy" and essentially atraumatic operations by many obstetricians. One might offer the rebuttal that such procedures may have been undertaken to terminate a labor in which the fetus demonstrated evidences of intrauterine hypoxia. However, in actuality,

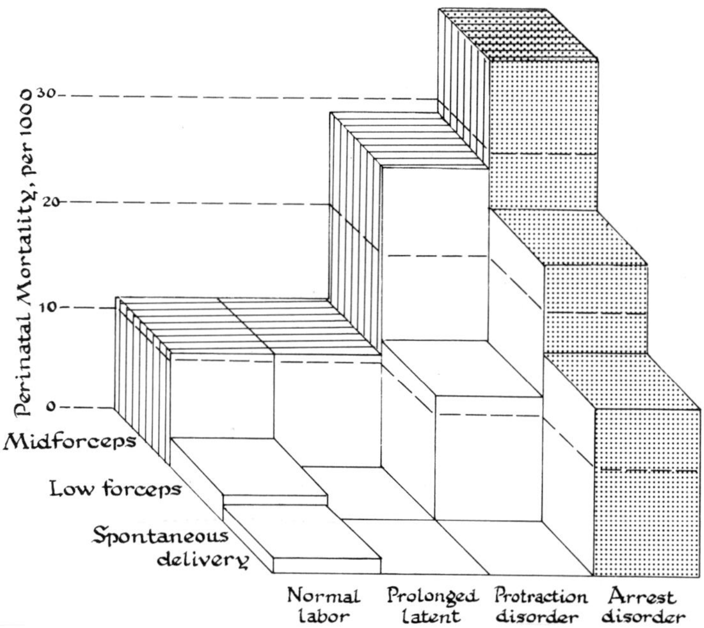


*Fig. 65.* Three-dimensional perspective showing perinatal mortality (*vertical bars*) as it relates to labor disorder (front projection) and type of delivery (side projection). The inherent hazard of midforceps delivery (*cross-hatched*) is independent of the innate risk of arrest disorders (*stippled*), although both act synergistically when applied concurrently. The peril to infants delivered instrumentally after protraction disorders is also seen. Neither normal labor nor prolonged latent phase patterns carry any special risk.

(From Friedman EA: Clin Obstet Gynecol 16:172, 1973)

most of these were done without even marginal justification. Furthermore, infants delivered by midforceps operations are subject to additional increases in mortality when the foregoing labors were characterized by protraction or arrest patterns, or both.

At the same time, certain labor patterns are recognized as not totally innocuous. We see an increment of inherent risk specifically in arrest disorders, even when followed by spontaneous delivery. This is enhanced among infants delivered by low forceps, and especially by midforceps. Babies delivered spontaneously after a protraction disorder do not appear to be in peril, although they demonstrate increased losses in association with any forceps procedure, aggravated in the extreme with midforceps.

The data for distribution of depressed infants based on Apgar Scores at 1 and 5 minutes are essentially the same, as far as they demonstrate increased hazard to the surviving infant from midforceps procedures regardless of the labor pattern. They also show the special inherent risk of protraction disorders when followed by any form of operative delivery. Arrest patterns yielded high frequencies of neonatal depression regardless of the form of delivery, but especially after forceps procedures of all kinds. Thus, the distribution of depressed Apgar Scores parallels the perinatal mortality rates.

It is important to stress that the graphic abnormality of prolonged latent phase did not contribute in any detectable way to perinatal mortality or to the incidence of neonatal depression. Realizing that most labors designated clinically as abnormal—including those diagnosed as uterine inertia, prolonged labor, dysfunctional labor, dystocic labor, and so forth—actually fall into the category of prolonged latent phase, we are at once able to separate out a large proportion of clinically aberrant labors that appear to present no increased risk to the fetus.

Protracted active-phase dilatation and protracted descent patterns, while offering no apparent threat when followed by spontaneous delivery, on the other hand, are hazardous to a degree when accompanied by any form of operative vaginal procedure for the delivery. Thus, the protraction pattern probably does not contribute to the poor results sometimes seen among these infants, but rather such results are obtained as a consequence of the potentially traumatic operative procedures used for the delivery.

Arrest patterns, including secondary arrest of dilatation, arrest of descent, prolonged deceleration phase, and failure of descent, must be considered labor patterns that carry inherent peril for the fetus regardless of foregoing or concomitant labor disorders and regardless of the method of delivery. However, it is clearly shown that the deleterious fetal effect of arrest patterns is augmented by superimposing a potentially hazardous operative delivery procedure, such as midforceps.

When this information became available, it was imperative to pursue investigations of the possible effects of labor and delivery on the surviving infant. Although there is intuitive agreement that abnormal labor may adversely affect growth and development of the resulting infant, little substantiation exists. Bishop and Vollman (1963) were able to show a correlation between the duration of labor and the incidence of neurologic abnormalities of the baby at 1 year of age. Unfortunately, the sensitivity of available techniques for evaluating neurologic and developmental status of infants during the first year of life is open to question. For example, well documented anoxigenic obstetric conditions cannot be clearly demonstrated to increase the risk of neurologic damage for the mature infant. Such conditions include abruptio placentae, placenta previa, and the prolapse of the umbilical cord (Niswander et al, 1966a–d). It has been determined that deficiencies in conceptual ability may result from such insults (Graham et al, 1962), rather than gross motor disabilities. Therefore, we must be particularly conservative in drawing possibly unwarranted conclusions from examinations aimed primarily at uncovering gross motor disorders.

Studies of surviving infants were undertaken at age 8 months, utilizing Bayley mental and motor assessment scores (Bayley, 1933), and at age 1 year, incorporating neurologic examinations (Friedman et al, 1969c). Remarkable uniformity is encountered in the mean Bayley Scores when these data are stratified according to graphic labor pattern. The absence of correlation might be interpreted in one of two ways. First, it is possible that surviving infants are not subjected to increased risks from disordered labors. Second and more likely, one may question the ability of such tests to uncover subtle abnormalities at this age.

When we examine the same data according to the frequency of abnormality, as defined by the incidence of Bayley mental scores of 64 or less and motor scores of 23 or less, we begin to recognize previously undetected trends. For example, there were consistently high motor abnormality rates in association with disordered labors. Similar trends were not encountered in the mental scoring data, raising the issue of whether or not this evaluation system is sufficiently sensitive at this stage of development. If we accept the likely premise that the 8-month and 1-year evaluation techniques are not capable of detecting all varieties of subclinical neurologic and developmental deficiencies, we are forced to concede that the data are inappropriate to provide the answer to the question initially posed, concerning the effect that abnormal labor may have on the infant. While we are unable to demonstrate the deleterious influence that many believe exists, we are certainly unable to show an absence of such an effect. Those trends that are uncovered, although admittedly unconfirmed by statistical analysis, are felt to require substantiation by additional study of these infants over long periods of time to reveal any latent abnormalities in perception and abstract thinking.

Recently (Friedman et al, 1977), such long-term follow-up studies have yielded the data we sought. It has been determined that there are significant adverse effects among offspring delivered by midforceps procedures, as well as those born following labors characterized by one or more of the arrest patterns. Surviving offspring were evaluated intensively at ages 3 and 4 years by means of a battery of speech, language, and hearing tests (scored separately in terms of summary, global, and articulation aspects), as well as a series of psychologic examinations. Specifically, the latter consisted of the Stanford–Binet Intelligence Scale (to provide intelligence quotient raw score and summary code) and summary tests such as the Graham–Ernhart block sort, motor test, and behavioral profile. The objective was to yield clinical impressions of intelligence, fine and gross motor development, concept formation, behavioral rating, and overall summary.

At the outset, it was recognized that other important influences that correlated strongly with such development parameters as intelligence quotient scores had to be taken into account; these included race, parity, and prematurity. The intelligence quotient scores for children whose birth weight was at least 2,500 g were examined separately, thereby nullifying the recognized influence that low birth weight has on this score, simultaneously stratifying by race and parity. When this was accomplished, clear-cut trends were encountered with reference to the several labor patterns that the mothers of these infants had experienced prior to their birth (Table 69).

*Table 69. MEAN INTELLIGENT QUOTIENT SCORES BY LABOR PATTERN AND DELIVERY TYPE**

| *Labor Pattern* | *Spontaneous* | *Low Forceps* | *Midforceps* | *Total* |
|---|---|---|---|---|
| Normal | 108 | 106 | 101 | 105 |
| Prolonged latent phase | (104) | (108) | (101) | 105 |
| Protraction disorder | (106) | (101) | 101 | 102 |
| Arrest disorder | (98) | 101 | 99 | 99 |
| Total | 106 | 104 | 100 | 103 |

* Data limited to children with birth weight of 2,500 g or more, delivered of white nulliparas. Parentheses designate means based on small sample size. Distribution of scores is statistically significant, $p < 0.01$.

Ignoring the delivery procedure, we obtain statistically significant correlation between intelligence quotient and the pattern of labor. Equivalent scores are seen with normal labors and prolonged latent phase patterns; somewhat lower scores occur with protraction disorders, and the lowest scores overall, with arrest disorders. Similarly, the mean intelligence quotient score appears to be correlated with the type of procedure by which the children were delivered. The lowest determinations occurred among those delivered vaginally by midforceps instrumentation. The best scores were found among those delivered spontaneously or by low forceps. The frequency of cesarean sections in this series was quite small, making evaluation of the resulting infants meaningless. However, they generally fared well.

These data suggest that both the labor pattern and the type of delivery may influence long-term outcome adversely. Again, we may pose the question as to whether or not the effects of these factors are independent. We have already shown that the type of delivery chosen for patients with dysfunctional labor patterns is strongly influenced by the pattern itself (see above). Thus, some disordered labors, particularly protraction and arrest disorders, are more likely to result in operative vaginal delivery than others. Therefore, it is mandatory to stratify the data for labor patterns according to the type of delivery.

This accomplished (Table 69), it becomes apparent that the intelligence quotient trends are essentially independent, in that both aberrant labor and operative vaginal delivery influence outcome. This applies particularly to arrest disorders and (to a lesser extent) protraction patterns on the one hand, and midforceps operations on the other. The midforceps effect appears to be exerted uniformly without regard for the labor pattern, although there is a negligible trend suggesting enhancement when associated with arrest disorder. Analogously, there is uniform lowering of scores in conjunction with arrest disorders, regardless of the type of delivery. Protraction disorders were associated with reduced scores only if there was an instrumental delivery.

These findings verify the trends outlined earlier (see above) for mortality and neonatal depression. The results are most impressive among nulliparas, white and black patients considered separately. While the direction and magnitude of trends are similar among multiparas, they cannot be verified statistically because of the relatively small numbers of multiparas who have abnormal labor or are subjected to operative vaginal delivery.

In general, data dealing with other aspects of the 4-year developmental evaluations follow the same pattern. This applies especially to those dealing with gross clinical impressions of intelligence and overall summary of psychologic performance. The 3-year results dealing with the incidence of suspect or abnormal speech, language, and hearing tests are also similar with regard to labor and delivery trends (Table 70), verifying the adverse influence of both midforceps and arrest disorders, apparently acting independently.

*Table 70. SPEECH–LANGUAGE–HEARING RESULTS BY LABOR PATTERN AND DELIVERY TYPE**

| *Labor Pattern* | *Spontaneous* | *Low Forceps* | *Midforceps* |
|---|---|---|---|
| Normal | 6 | 6 | 12 |
| Prolonged latent phase | 6 | 7 | 17 |
| Protraction disorder | 9 | 15 | 23 |
| Arrest disorder | 25 | 30 | 36 |

* Based on data from white children with birth weight of 2,500 g or more, all maternal parity groups combined; in percent frequency of those rated suspect or abnormal.

These long-term prognostic results are not unexpected in view of the findings that relate major disordered labor patterns and associated operative vaginal delivery to increased perinatal mortality. It is clear on this basis that the survivors remain at some continued risk.

# Management Programs

## CHAPTER 24

Systematized approaches are provided for the obstetric attendant faced with a specific disorder in a laboring patient. These programs are synthesized from relationships based on previously developed, objective empirical observations. These programs serve as utilitarian guidelines for clinical practice.

The formulation of meaningful and practical programs of management for the disorders of labor that we have identified rightfully serves as the culmination of our efforts. Whether it was overtly stated or merely implied, our ultimate objective was and should remain the application of clearly stated principles to clinical practice. We began encumbered by conflicting concepts and interpretations of uncontrolled observations characterized by authoritarian and pragmatic dogma. Our analytic process began with the collection of much experiential material; only a fraction of the total has been presented in this volume. We have tried to digest, synthesize, and systematize the massive information available to us. By doing so, we are encouraged to believe that suitable principles of obstetric care for the laboring patient may be evolved.

The programs set forth in this chapter are the end result of such activities. They represent recommendations based on total perspective overviews. Whereas originally devised on the basis of retrospective analysis, each of them has since been shown to be effective in the hands of obstetric attendants, ranging from physician specialists to trained midwives. They appear to be readily grasped, understood, and incorporated into daily practice. They can be applied in almost any clinical milieu. The proof of their suitability for clinical use is in the feedback they yield in good results for both mother and baby.

For the patient with a labor disorder that is correctly diagnosed, the logical choice of the most effective program of management can be based on adequately evaluated etiologic and contributory factors. We have assiduously avoided making recommendations for clinical decisions without supportive evidence in objective form. Considerations dealing with diagnosis, differential diagnosis, and evaluation have been discussed at length in Chapters 20 and 21. Details of the possible therapeutic measures and factors relating to decisions about assigning appropriate choices have been presented in Chapter 22; relevant prognostic factors helpful in this regard appeared in Chapter 23. These discussions should be reviewed in detail by those who wish to understand the subtle nuances comprising the foundations for the material summarized here.

## *PROLONGED LATENT PHASE*

Among therapeutic measures used to combat the problem of prolonged latent phase, we recognize that only two seem to offer any real benefit. Both oxytocin infusion and energetically pursued therapeutic rest are equally effective in terminating the abnormally prolonged latent phase. Amniotomy as a specific method of treatment is generally ineffectual. On the basis of such observations, an outline can be formulated (Fig. 66) for managing these difficult cases.

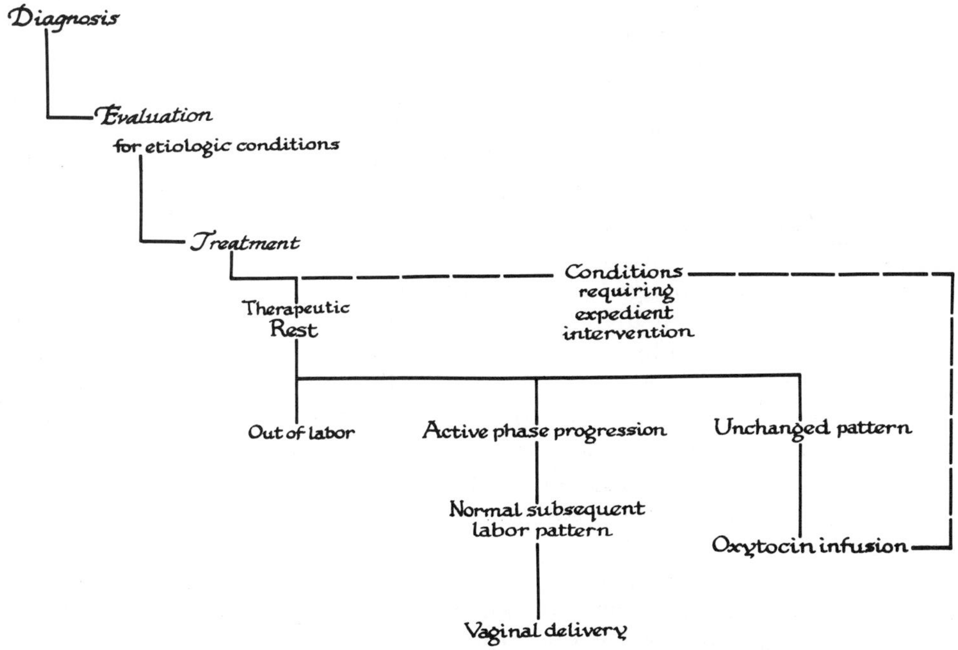


*Fig. 66.* Program of management for patients with prolonged latent phase. The principal recommended approach is support and therapeutic rest by use of large doses of narcotic-analgesics, applicable to all but about 2 percent of gravidas with this disorder. Exceptionally, oxytocin infusion may be undertaken directly if the additional 6 to 10 hours of delay by rest would be clinically unacceptable.

It should be emphasized that suitable search for etiologic factors will reveal those in which unripe cervix, excessive sedation, or anesthesia might account for this abnormality. Evaluations of the maternal pelvis, fetal lie, and position are also obviously important, but it is unlikely that abnormalities relating to these factors will prove to be contributory to the problem. This is not to imply that such abnormalities will not be encountered; rather, they do not occur any more frequently among patients with prolonged latent phase than in the normal population. Thus, they play no role in the development of this disorder.

Selection of treatment is next in order. In general, these patients are physically exhausted and often emotionally depressed or anxious. They tend to be discouraged by their lack of progress despite the long, grueling labor. Since by definition at least 20 hours have elapsed from the onset of labor (14 hours in multiparas), it is reasonable to expect that most of them will be approaching a state of exhaustion. Rest and supportive measures, therefore, are of utmost importance. Attention should be given to replenishing fluid and correcting electrolyte imbalances. The problem should be thoroughly discussed with the patient and her family. Continuing optimistic reassurance is certainly to be recommended, particularly in view of the expectedly good outcome.

Because of the generally poor physical and emotional status of these patients, therapeutic rest should be the treatment of choice. The recommended program under these circumstances involves a determined effort to provide an interval of rest by use of a narcotic agent. We generally prescribe morphine sulfate. The usual initial dose is 15 mg given subcutaneously. If the patient is particularly obese or large-framed, the dose may be increased to 20 mg. The gravida should be carefully reevaluated about 20 minutes after this medication has been given. The important information that should be obtained includes assessment of respiratory rate and depth, cervical dilatation, and uterine contractility.

If the cervix has changed at all from the previous examination (which should have been done just prior to administering the first dose of morphine), one must not administer any additional medication. To do so might constitute a serious error in view of the possibility that the active phase has already been entered. A second dose of morphine given at this time might result in a severely depressed infant at birth. This unusual event has been discussed in Chapter 22. Most often, of course, uterine contractility has been almost completely inhibited and no further progress in dilatation can be detected.

If contractions are continuing and respiration has not been depressed, an additional dose of morphine should be given; for the average patient, 10 mg will usually suffice; for the large individual, 15 mg. By this means, we have attempted to provide a minimum of 6 hours of deep sleep. The narcotic should be given in sufficiently large amounts to benefit the patient by actually stopping labor contractions temporarily, if possible.

As previously stated, our concern about the potentially depressing action of these drugs on the infant's respiratory center can be allayed, since these patients should not be expected to deliver during the time the drug is active. The depressant effects will have worn off long before the infant is born, provided delivery is not effected (say, by cesarean section) for any reason during the 4-hour period following administration of the drug.

Most patients treated in this way go on to have perfectly normal labor patterns. After 6 to 10 hours, the patient usually awakens. At that time, she should be reevaluated. She will demonstrate one of three possible conditions. First, she may be out of labor. This will establish on a retrospective basis that the preceding state was false labor. The difficult differential diagnosis will have been made. No further therapy will be required. Normal labor may be expected to begin at some later time. Second, the patient may be well into the active phase of dilatation—or even in the second stage, although this is rare. Here, the desired result has been accomplished and the abnormally prolonged latent phase has been terminated effectively. Whether this effect has been brought about directly as a result of the treatment administered, or indirectly by the increment of time allowed, cannot be answered. Nevertheless, all but a few patients should be expected to respond in this way.

The third possibility, seen in the remaining patients treated with narcotics for rest, is that the gravida will awaken in the same condition as before beginning therapy. This can be expected to occur in less than 5 percent of the cases thus treated. The original problem, characterized by persistent contractions effecting no active cervical dilatation, will recur and continue unrelentingly. These patients have certainly benefited from the period of rest that was provided. The time lost by the treatment has served this useful function well. In these cases, the latent phase continues without essential change.

It is only among this group that any further aggressive action will be desirable. In order to take advantage of any benefit that has been derived from this period of rest, these patients deserve a course of uterotonic stimulation with oxytocin infusion, unless there is clear-cut contraindication to this form of therapy (see Chapter 19). Most patients respond quite favorably.

Amniotomy, again, does not appear to be of any value in this disorder, contrary to commonly held opinion. Indeed, it may only complicate the situation. Similarly, cesarean section in the latent phase has no place as a primary method for treating the disorder of prolonged latent phase.

A point of contention may arise with regard to the choice of rest for these patients, as opposed to primary use of oxytocin stimulation. We may argue that both therapeutic modalities carry approximately the same potential for success: about 85 percent. We should recall that patients with prolonged latent phase include roughly 10 percent in false labor. They will be recognized as such only after a significant additional period of time has elapsed. With this in mind, if we were to proceed to stimulate this group routinely, we would perforce be attempting to induce labor in this unidentified subgroup. We have discussed the benefits and risks of labor induction (see

Chapter 22) and need not review this matter again here. Nevertheless, it is generally agreed that maternal and fetal risks increase the further one is removed from the ideal situation—namely, one in which all conditions for the induction are optimal. The conditions in patients with prolonged latent phase are generally suboptimal, suggesting that routine uterotonic stimulation subjects many of these patients to unnecessary risk. Moreover, the basic choice between oxytocin stimulation and therapeutic rest appears to be quite optional, neither having distinct advantages with regard to success rate in dealing with this abnormality. Since neither is especially advantageous over the other, we must address the matter of the relative risks they pose. Therefore, we lean very strongly toward a more conservative approach and recommend rest rather than stimulation as the primary mode of attack.

Needless to say, extenuating circumstances might exist, requiring more aggressive intervention. In our experience, this applies in less than 2 percent of cases with prolonged latent phase. As a general rule, any situation in which it would be inappropriate to permit an additional 6 to 10 hours of delay in the labor—for example, documented amnionitis (but not merely ruptured membranes)—would warrant the choice of uterotonic stimulation over the usually more preferable rest program. Thus, exigent circumstances will dictate that the usual course of action be altered and that stimulation be used first instead.

## *PROTRACTION DISORDERS*

We recognize that therapy for the abnormally protracted active phase of dilatation or protracted descent has been uniformly ineffectual in speeding progress. These abnormal labor patterns apparently cannot be improved by any of the stimulatory measures currently available to us. Once the dilatory active phase of dilatation or descent has begun, the slowly advancing process cannot be enhanced. Whereas it is possible to augment uterine contractility in such cases, we are unable to document any real change in the slope of the labor tracing. This is another example of the dissociation between contractility and the work that the uterus is attempting (teleologically) to accomplish, namely, cervical dilatation and fetal descent.

Contrariwise, it is very easy to inhibit progress or even produce an arrest pattern in these cases. Such potentially deleterious inhibitory measures as excessive sedation or peridural anesthesia, for example, readily compound protraction disorders in this way. Thus, it is imperative to recognize when a protraction disorder is present so that these agents can be minimized or avoided. Cephalopelvic disproportion, while doubtfully causative here, is encountered in more than one-fourth of patients with protraction disorders. When documented, cesarean section is the obvious procedure of choice. This will avert the necessity of the patient being exposed to an extremely prolonged additional trial of labor, with its associated risks of ascending infection.

The most characteristic feature of these disorders is their unrelentingly slow progress. Nothing seems to influence its persistence. For those patients in whom disproportion can be ruled out, the basic requisites for management (Fig. 67) include recognition of the disorder, correction of potentially contributory factors, and support. It is essential to recognize the problem and accept the apparent fact that this slowly progressive pattern cannot be prodded. If one appreciates its special characteristics, particularly its refractory nature, one will be less inclined to undertake vain aggressive management.

These patients must be provided all the support they require, with particular attention to fluid and electrolyte needs. In addition, they and their families will benefit from an explanation of the problem and a review of what can be anticipated by way of the subsequent labor course. Patients are much more likely to cooperate, particularly in minimizing demands for

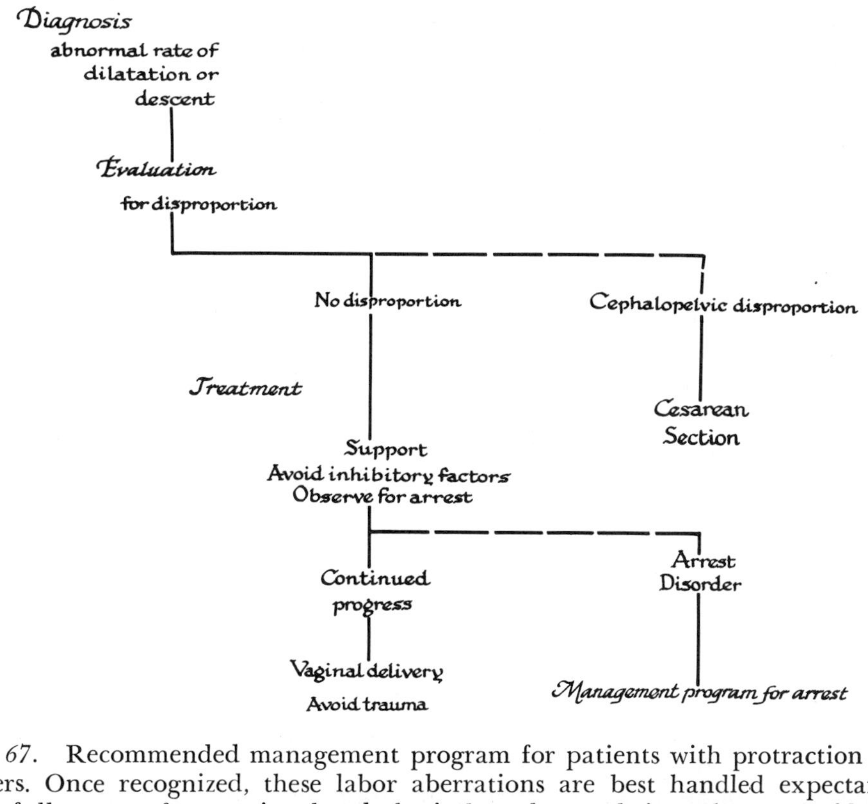


*Fig. 67.* Recommended management program for patients with protraction disorders. Once recognized, these labor aberrations are best handled expectantly with full support for emotional and physical needs, care being taken to avoid anything that may even remotely inhibit progression in these long, slow labors. The documentation of fetopelvic disproportion justifies terminating the labor by cesarean section and averting the difficulties of management here. For those allowed to labor, it is essential to avoid the trauma of instrumentation at delivery.

analgesia, if they understand why it is beneficial to do so. Given such full explanations, anxieties may be allayed.

As to active management, little can be done. One must avoid compounding the problem by impeding progress and unnecessarily complicating the situation with factors that may increase maternal and fetal morbidity in labor and at delivery. Of particular pertinence is the issue of operative vaginal delivery. We must reemphasize that fetal mortality and long-term neurologic and developmental morbidity have been documented as associated with protraction disorders, especially as the result of heroic efforts at instrumental intervention to effect vaginal delivery.

There is great temptation to terminate such lengthy and tedious labors when, at long last, the cervix is fully dilated and the fetal head has begun its slow descent. Generally, one can anticipate continued slow descent and even spontaneous delivery, given enough time for this process to evolve completely. Unless one is willing to invest that time and effort into effecting this good result, one will be tempted to undertake potentially traumatic forceps operation in the interest of foreshortening the labor process. Without some overriding, clearly documented reason for intervention, one cannot justify subjecting mother and fetus to the real risks of operative intervention. By allowing the labor process to continue (under the closest possible scrutiny, of course), one can often realize a much more innocuous spontaneous delivery.

## *ARREST DISORDERS*

There can be no disagreement that arrest disorders are the most serious labor problems we encounter. There is no other dysfunctional labor pattern in which the stakes are as high. Here, the relationship between etiology and treatment is vital. One-half of the patients with arrest patterns show evidence of major degrees of fetopelvic disproportion. The presence or absence of bony impediment separates them into two distinctive groups. Two different avenues of attack apply (Fig. 68); it is critical that the distinction be recognized.

Potential difficulties can be averted if this serious situation is handled expeditiously and aggressively, but with studied care. As stated, most important among factors found to exist in these cases is cephalopelvic disproportion. The significance of this relationship has been previously investigated and discussed (Chapters 11 and 16). Its importance cannot be overstated. In many patients with unsuspected disproportion, the presence of bony obstruction may manifest itself for the first time in labor with the development of an arrest disorder. Therefore, once encountered, arrest patterns require intensive search for possible causative factors, and the factor that carries the most ominous portent is, of course, cephalopelvic disproportion.

In every instance of prolonged deceleration phase, secondary arrest of

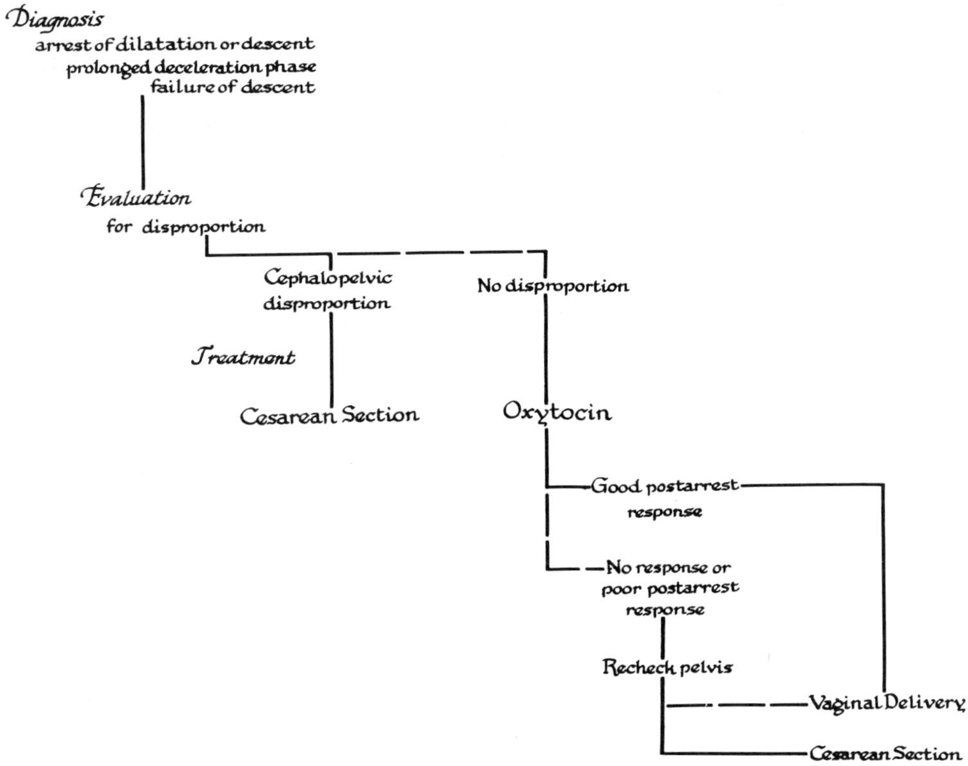


*Fig. 68.* Management schema for gravidas with arrest disorders. The most critical aspect of evaluation in these patients is assessment for cephalopelvic disproportion, because this factor is so commonly associated. When encountered in a patient with an arrested labor, disproportion demands cesarean section. For the remainder, oxytocin is in order and can be expected to yield good results if the postarrest slope is at least as good as the prearrest slope was.

dilatation, arrest of descent, or failure of descent, it is strongly urged that the patient be studied thoroughly by a combination of accurate digital assessment and radiographic cephalopelvimetry (see Chapter 21). It must be established as an absolute rule that no form of therapy should ever be instituted for arrest patterns before the pelvic relationships are adequately investigated. It is equally clear that, in the absence of disproportion, other reversible factors should be identified so that they can be corrected. These most often include excessive sedation or improperly administered peridural anesthesia. Thus, the program of management chosen for these cases will be determined on the basis of objective and thorough evaluation.

Effective treatment for gravidas with arrest disorders primarily includes immediate operative termination for those with disproportion, or uterotonic stimulation for those with a pelvis adequate to accommodate delivery of the fetus. Alternative and generally less preferable approaches, mentioned here for completeness, also include expectancy and rest by narcosis. The choice will depend entirely on the underlying etiology of the condition and on the status of the patient when the diagnosis is verified. We hold that high degrees of cephalopelvic disproportion associated with arrest patterns do not warrant any further trial of labor, in view of the extreme unlikelihood that subsequent vaginal delivery can occur. Moreover, if vaginal delivery should take place, one can expect unacceptably high morbidity and mortality rates, especially if forceps have to be used. The conservative outlook in these cases, therefore, appears to demand abdominal delivery without further labor.

Rarely, expectancy alone may suffice for those few patients in whom arrest follows or appears to result from sedation or anesthesia. Usually, these are patients with preceding protraction disorders in whom the analgesia or anesthesia has inhibited progress acutely. If arrest has resulted from a reversible factor, such as excessive sedation or conduction anesthesia, expectancy to allow abatement of the effect may suffice to accomplish the immediate aim of allowing progressive labor to reinstitute itself. As the inhibitory effects of the deleterious agent subside, one can expect the dilatation or descent pattern to return to its prearrest status; that is, progressive change will be reinstituted at a rate comparable to that seen prior to the arrest. The special intrinsic significance of abatement programs was reviewed in Chapter 22.

Similarly, rest may be in order for those patients who are thoroughly exhausted. Such rest will provide an opportunity to correct fluid and electrolyte imbalances. While therapeutic rest may be necessary on rare occasions for these patients, most will benefit more by uterotonic stimulation instead. This option, therefore, is seldom exercised. Amniotomy as a therapeutic device has not been found to offer any particular advantage in patients with arrest problems. While it is appropriate to rupture the membranes in anticipation of applying a fetal scalp electrode for purposes of internal monitoring of fetal heart rate, which should be done in these circumstances, one cannot expect the amniotomy to enhance progression.

Careful uterotonic stimulation with oxytocin infusion should be undertaken in those arrested labors in which the cephalopelvic relationship is adequate. Once again, it must be stressed that cephalopelvic disproportion should always be ruled out first before undertaking such stimulation. The required optimal duration of stimulation, with the infusion titrated to produce uterine contractions simulating strong clinical labor, is minimally 4 hours for arrest of dilatation (2 hours for arrest of descent), beginning from the time when an adequate contractile pattern has been established. One can expect most patients to respond to this regimen. This provides an optimistic forecast for patients with arrest disorders occurring in the absence of disproportion. Therefore, cesarean section is inappropriate as a primary means of therapy in these cases.

Postarrest progression will provide a useful tool, particularly if it is compared with the slope of dilatation or descent prior to the arrest. Prognosis is worst if no progression occurs. Here, it is likely that cephalopelvic disproportion exists, but was unrecognized. Reevaluation of the patient, with attention to her pelvis and its relationship to the fetus (see Chapter 21), together with review of the radiographic studies, is mandatory. Unless one can rule out disproportion with certainty, it must be assumed to exist under these special circumstances. Moreover, unless one can achieve further progression with attainment of full cervical dilatation and adequate descent of the fetal presenting part to the perineum, vaginal delivery is interdicted.

At the other extreme of response, if the postarrest slope is as good as or better than the prearrest slope, prognosis is excellent. One should expect uncomplicated vaginal delivery here unless some other, unrelated problem should arise. Those patients with arrest disorders who respond to uterotonic stimulation with smaller postarrest slopes (smaller than the prearrest slope) signal a possible problem in fetopelvic relationships. As with those who do not respond at all, they should be thoroughly and carefully evaluated to ensure that the pelvis is adequate. Poor postarrest response can serve as a valuable index of prognosis (see Chapter 23).

## *COMPREHENSIVE PROGRAMMED APPROACH*

A systematized plan for managing patients with abnormal labor is in order. For the patient with prolonged latent phase, once diagnosis is made, one should search for the common etiologic factors of unripe cervix, excessive sedation, or anesthesia. One must recognize that these patients tend to be tired, depressed, and discouraged. They deserve support, both with regard to their growing anxiety and to their rather frequent fluid and electrolyte imbalances. They deserve to be informed and reassured.

We recommend that these patients be rested. Morphine is very effective in stopping the labor temporarily for the purpose of providing a suitable period of beneficial rest. When the patient awakens, she will either be out of labor (indicating by hindsight that we were dealing with false labor), well into the active phase of dilatation (the abnormality having thus been cured), or unchanged. Only if the condition persists will additional therapy be necessary. Provided there is no contraindication, oxytocin infusion should be useful in such cases for terminating the latent phase and producing normal active phase progression.

This program has been shown to be very effective in managing cases of prolonged latent phase. The choice of rest over oxytocin infusion or other forms of stimulation, as previously discussed, is based on the need to provide for the possibility that false labor might exist. In false labor, uterotonic stimulation will unnecessarily increase fetal and maternal risk in the patient who is not prepared physiologically or functionally to enter labor. Amniotomy has not been found to be consistently effective as a stimulatory device when the latent phase is prolonged. It is advisable, therefore, not to perform amniotomy in these cases if the membranes are still intact, because the labor may be false. Moreover, since delivery may not take place for many hours, the ensuing labor may be associated with ascending infection.

Management of the patient with protraction disorder is generally frustrating to the obstetric attendants. We must be cognizant of our inability to improve the dilatory pattern by any of the modes of treatment available to us today. Moreover, we must be wary of compounding the problem by introducing factors that will make the situation noticeably worse. These labors are particularly sensitive to various potentially deleterious factors, including excessive sedation and peridural anesthesia. When these inhibitory agents are used, such patients frequently develop arrest patterns.

It is important to search for contributory factors. When cephalopelvic disproportion is encountered, one may legitimately avoid the travail of the long labor by performing cesarean section. For the remaining patients with protraction disorders who do not have disproportion, support is again vital, with regard to both emotional and physiologic needs.

Basically, it is imperative to recognize the abnormality, to provide essential supportive measures, and to avoid introducing any factor that might even remotely impede progress or jeopardize the outcome for mother and baby in these difficult cases. Most importantly, it is essential to avoid subjecting these "sensitized" fetuses to instrumental delivery. Whereas the outcome for babies born after protraction disorders is good if delivered spontaneously, they tend to do badly if forceps have to be used.

The need for supportive care of these patients during their long, slow labors must not be overlooked. An ideal program includes detailed attention to maintaining nutrition, meeting fluid requirements, correcting electrolyte imbalances, and providing much needed rest and emotional encouragement. As long as progress continues without interruption along the extrapolated dilatation–time and station–time tracing, conservative expectancy and support should be continued. It is most important that the obstetrician not be tempted to interrupt the progressive labor process by operative means. The poor fetal and infant results that accrue from instrumental intervention speak strongly against any such aggressive measures.

There are two primary approaches to the management of patients with arrest disorders. For those with cephalopelvic disproportion, cesarean section is mandatory. For those without bony impediment, uterotonic stimulation is generally in order. Amniotomy has not been shown to be a useful stimulatory influence in these conditions. Similarly, therapeutic rest by narcosis is only rarely effective and then only in association with maternal exhaustion. Occasionally, allowing peridural anesthesia or sedation to abate may be undertaken, where they are clearly etiologic, particularly for arrest of descent. Postarrest progress under these circumstances yields the best results, provided the procedure chosen for the delivery is atraumatic, of course.

Whether to select cesarean section or uterotonic stimulation as the management course must rest on the presence or absence of cephalopelvic disproportion. The choice is primarily determined by the presumptive cause for the arrest. The very serious portent of the combination of arrest pattern and bony disproportion clearly establishes this as a guiding principle. While immediate cesarean section cannot be considered a wholly innocuous procedure either to the mother or to the fetus, it is far less hazardous than attempted or successful instrumental vaginal delivery in the same circumstances.

Thus, it is appropriate first to evaluate the pelvis and the relationship of its dimensions to the fetal head before embarking on any definitive course of action. If careful digital examination and radiographic cephalopelvimetry demonstrate disproportion—as they will in at least one-half of the cases—cesarean section is indicated at once, without further trial of labor. In the absence of fetopelvic disproportion, labor may be allowed to continue with uterotonic stimulation to effect postarrest progress. This should be carried out under continuous monitoring of fetal heart rate, of course.

Postarrest progression, especially if at a rate that is the same as or greater than the prearrest slope, should be viewed as an encouraging prognostic sign. Such progression is almost always seen, where successful, within 4 hours of the beginning of strong contractions in arrest of dilatation, or within 2 hours in arrest of descent. The absence of any further descent, or a postarrest slope that is less than the prearrest rate, signifies the likelihood that there will be a poor end result. This is especially so if one is tempted to try to effect vaginal delivery operatively in these cases. Delivery should be undertaken only if the fetal head crowns. Instrumental vaginal delivery techniques are decried.

One should seek to achieve delivery by spontaneous means, if possible. As long as progress continues and the fetus shows no signs of distress, further labor should be allowed and the patient should be supported until it is possible to effect vaginal delivery atraumatically. The assertion that labor must be terminated if second-stage duration exceeds 2 hours cannot be supported by objective study of the good results achieved (Cohen, 1977). It is not justifiable to terminate labor merely because this arbitrary interval has elapsed. If no advancement takes place, it is probable that unrecognized disproportion is actually present. Unless one can definitively rule out disproportion, cesarean section is indicated here because it is far less hazardous to both mother and fetus than an operative midforceps procedure undertaken in these same circumstances.

In the clear absence of disproportion, uterotonic stimulation is almost always effective in producing further progression in dilatation and descent. We must observe the provision that the rate of infusion will be adjusted to simulate strong, active labor and will be continued for an appropriate period of time. Where oxytocin stimulation fails to correct the labor aberration, one may suspect that it has not been given adequately; that is, the patient has not had the benefit of sufficient stimulation, either because clinically good uterine contractions have not been produced or an insufficient duration of stimulation has been allowed, or both. This suggests that true failures of oxytocin stimulation are rare with arrest patterns except in association with cephalopelvic disproportion. Indeed, if one is sure that the stimulation has been adequate, it is likely that disproportion underlies the failure to achieve progression.

Recapitulating, we recognize that prolonged latent phase may be treated primarily by providing a suitable period of rest through the use of narcotic agents. For those few refractory cases, uterotonic stimulation in the form of oxytocin infusion may be required. As an acceptable alternative in special circumstances interdicting any undue delay, oxytocin stimulation may sometimes have to be used as a primary mode of therapy.

Protraction disorders are best treated by expectancy and support, unless insurmountable bony dystocia provides one with the option to terminate labor by cesarean section. Arrest patterns are managed according to the presence or absence of documented cephalopelvic disproportion. Those with bony impediment should be delivered expediently by cesarean section; those with adequate pelvic dimensions to accommodate the fetus will benefit from oxytocin infusion.

The epitome of this material is shown simplistically in Figure 69, divested of all explanatory trappings. Seven labor disorders are diagnosable (excluding precipitate dilatation and descent, at the opposite end of the scale of abnormal progression). They fall naturally into three distinct divisions based on common etiology, response to therapy, and prognostic outlook: (1) the single disorder of prolonged latent phase; (2) the two protraction dis-

| | | Preferred Treatment | Exceptionally |
|---|---|---|---|
| Prolonged Latent Phase | | Therapeutic Rest | Oxytocin for exigencies |
| Protraction Disorders | | Expectancy and Support | Cesarean Section for CPD |
| Arrest Disorders | With CPD | Cesarean Section | No exceptions |
| | Without CPD | Oxytocin | Rest for exhaustion |

*Fig. 69.* Summary of management recommendations. Labor disorders are divisible into four therapeutic groups, as shown, each with its own distinctive treatment regimen. Those secondary options listed should be held in abeyance and considered to be useful only in truly exceptional circumstances.

orders of protracted active-phase dilatation and protracted descent; (3) the four arrest disorders, namely, secondary arrest of dilatation, prolonged deceleration phase, arrest of descent, and failure of descent. The arrest disorders as a group can be subdivided according to the presence or absence of cephalopelvic disproportion. This yields four separate identifiable sets of labor entities, each managed most appropriately by a different primary approach. Therapeutic rest applies best for prolonged latent phase; expectancy and support for protraction disorders; cesarean section for arrest disorders occurring with disproportion; and uterotonic stimulation, for arrested labors without disproportion.

In an era when decreasing birth rates emphasize the role of obstetrics in optimizing the outcome for every fetus brought to viability, we are under the strongest possible obligation to ensure that we will not undertake any delivery procedure that may cause harm, even if only remotely. Needless to say, we have to weigh the alternatives in order to choose the least hazardous course of action for managing a given disorder. Our recommendations, therefore, are based on objective examination of the results that have heretofore been obtained from management programs embarked upon under a variety of conditions. These were undertaken in an attempt to effect delivery among patients with clearly defined labor disorders.

We have tried to approach the problems of labor and its management objectively. We find that labor can be studied on the basis of the patterns of cervical dilatation and fetal descent, as these patterns evolve with elapsed time in labor. The tracings thus produced serve as useful guides to all obstetric attendants in helping them define the several varieties of abnormal labor. These can be examined individually and collectively. They have offered a means for studying and clarifying etiologic factors, methods of diagnosis, the relative efficacy of available modalities of therapy, and prognosis for the several major aberrations that we now recognize to constitute the range of dysfunctional labors.

Based on this information, it is now possible to formulate a detailed programmatic approach for each group of related abnormalities. The foundation for our recommendations embodies the derived principles of diagnosis, evaluation, and management, as well as prognostic aids resulting from observations of the expected outcome of specific modes of therapy. We have systematized our management programs by dividing the material conceptually for convenience and practicality into diagnosis, evaluation for causes, treatment, immediate results, and outcome. Thus, a programmatic overview approach to the patient with disordered labor, based on the patterns of cervical dilatation and station as set against time, has been formulated for purposes of application to the clinical situation. The practical applications of the organized approach are well documented. It is perhaps a fitting tribute to their usefulness that they have been adopted almost universally.

# Case Reviews

# CHAPTER 25

Illustrative case material follows. We have summarized the relevant details of the course of labor in a series of real patients for purposes of providing examples of specific issues to help clarify evaluation and management principles. While the material has been carefully selected to illustrate specific points, these cases have not all been optimally managed. Detailed critiques spell out where alternative approaches might have been used to advantage. This supplemental discussion should help to put these matters into perspective.

## Case #1

BL is a 25-year-old nullipara at term who had an uneventful antepartum course. Her membranes ruptured spontaneously at 9:30 A.M., and regular uterine contractions began at 10:00 A.M. When she arrived in the hospital at noon, her cervix was 4 cm dilated and completely effaced. The fetus presented by the vertex, position left occiput transverse at station +2. Contractions were occurring at 3-minute intervals, lasting 45 to 50 seconds. She was somewhat uncomfortable, but did not desire to take analgesia. An hour later, the cervix was 5 cm dilated and the fetal station was essentially unchanged. An internal fetal heart rate monitor was applied. It subsequently showed variable deceleration (cord compression) patterns, but with good recovery. Because of increasing discomfort, the patient was reexamined at 1:30 P.M.; the cervix was 6 cm dilated, station again unchanged. Over the course of the next hour, the clinical situation remained the same, and no further cervical dilatation took place (Fig. 70).

The cephalopelvic relationships were checked digitally. An attempt was made to determine whether or not the fetal head could be compressed more deeply into the pelvis at the height of a contraction with Kristeller pressure (the Müller–Hillis maneuver), and it was found that it could be done easily. The patient was observed carefully and was found to resume rapid progressive cervical dilatation, attaining full dilatation by 4:10 P.M. At that time, the fetus was found to have rotated spontaneously to the right occiput anterior position. Moreover, progressive but slow descent had begun. After

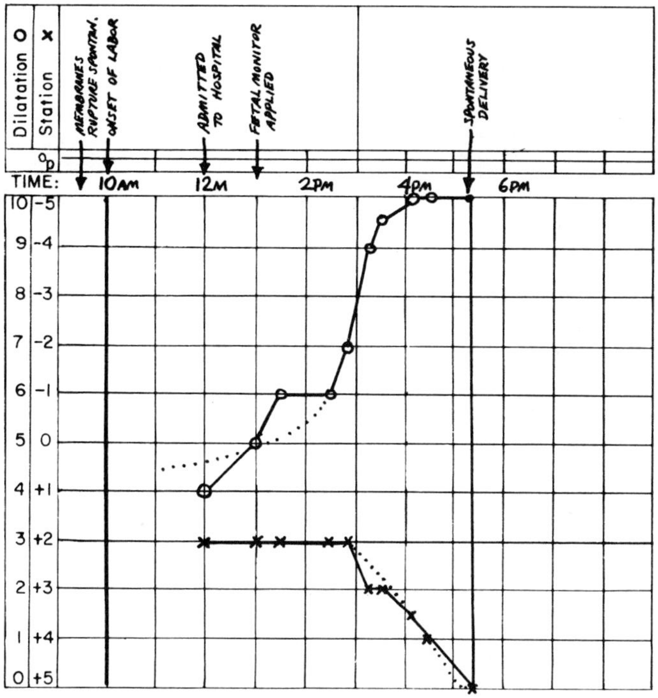


*Fig. 70.* Labor pattern of Patient BL, Case #1.

1 hour of second stage, the fetal head had reached the perineum. A normal, spontaneous, well-controlled and uncomplicated vaginal delivery occurred, with episiotomy and local anesthesia. The baby weighed 3,100 g and did well.

This patient presented two problems. First, there was an interval during the active phase of dilatation when it appeared as if she were developing secondary arrest. Rather than wait until it became fully evolved (that is, until 2 hours had elapsed without further progress), the physician rightfully proceeded to evaluate the cephalopelvic relationship clinically to resolve his concerns in this regard. This is appropriate if we recognize that bony disproportion is a common concomitant of arrested labor. The physician was comfortable here in being able to provide evidence that the pelvis appeared adequate for this fetus. Moreover, no precedent inhibitory factor could be identified, such as sedation or anesthesia.

Indeed, as one examines the dilatation pattern in retrospect, it is possible that the apparent absence of progress was not real. If we can assume an error in each recording of as much as 0.5 cm in either direction, it is possible to construct a perfectly normal dilatation pattern from these data. This modified pattern is shown in Figure 70, illustrating the likelihood that the interval between noon and 2:30 P.M. constituted the acceleration phase of this

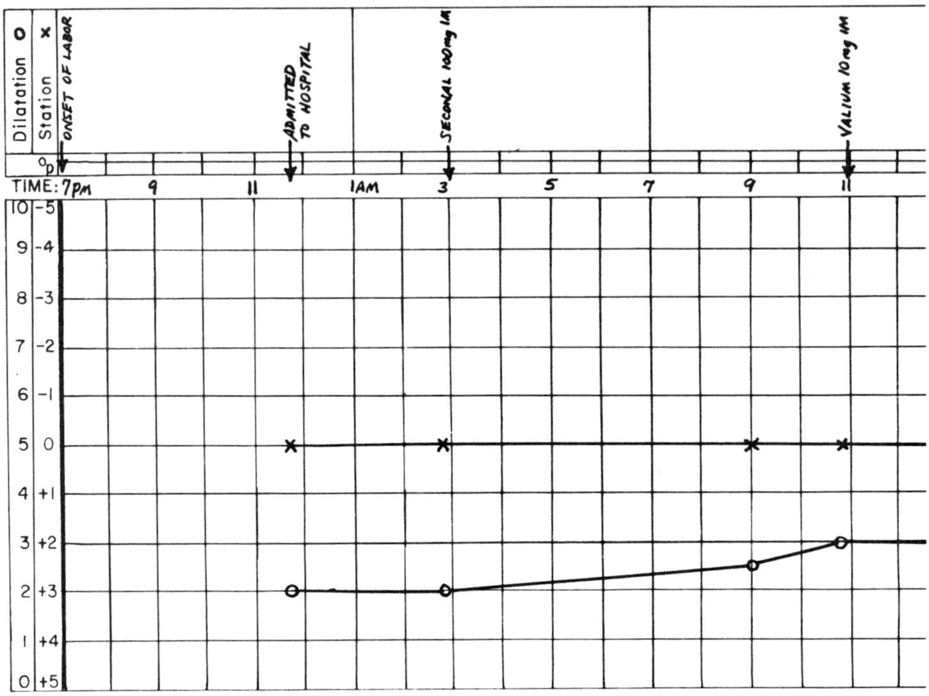


*Fig. 71.* Labor pattern of Patient SG, Case #2.

labor. Sources of error in constructing labor graphs and means for correcting or compensating for them have been discussed in Chapter 20.

The second problem is more critical, namely, protracted descent. This case represents an example of one in which the dilatation pattern gives no advanced clue as to what the descent pattern will do; whereas the maximum slope of dilatation here was 6.0 cm per hour, the maximum slope of descent was just 1.0 cm per hour. The issue of prolonged second stage never arose, however, because active descent began from an initial low station (+2). Thus, enough time was allowed to elapse for spontaneous delivery to occur. Under other circumstances, one can appreciate growing concern on the part of the physician as the second-stage duration exceeds 2 hours (clearly an uncritical limit that should not provide justification for intervention, as discussed in Chapter 24). With evidence of no disproportion, continuing progress in descent, even though occurring very slowly, should support a conservative approach, allowing labor to evolve until delivery occurs.

In this case, there was clear documentation that the fetal condition remained good, despite the cord patterns that were seen. It is imperative that the status of the fetus be closely watched under these circumstances. Advancing fetal station must be periodically confirmed by abdominal examination (see Chapter 20) to ensure that we are not misinterpreting cranial molding for descent. While positional dystocia might be an attractive hypothesis to

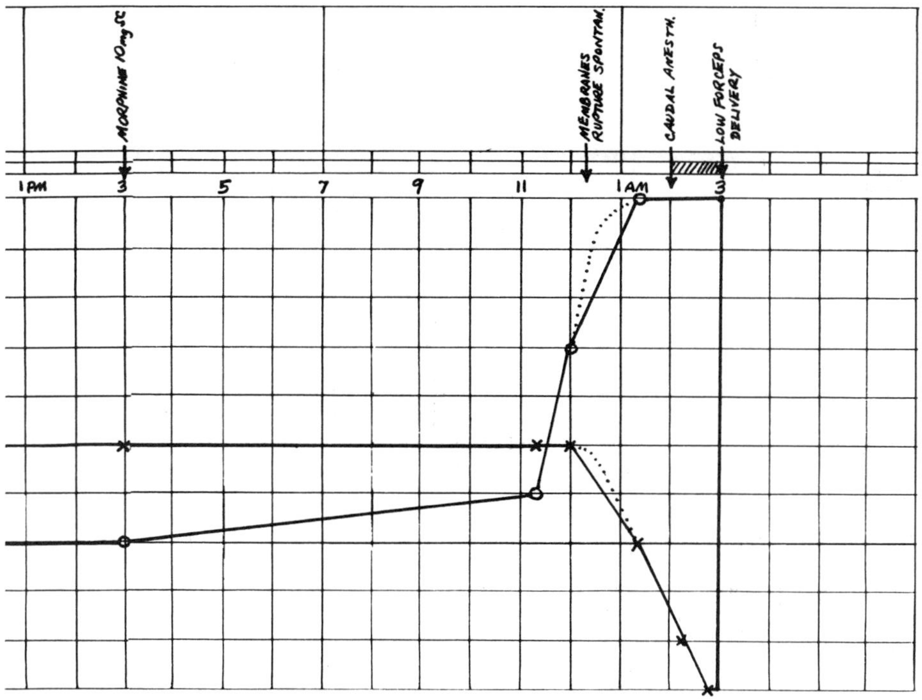


explain this disordered labor, we should note that its course was not corrected when the position spontaneously corrected itself as a consequence of internal rotation.

## Case #2

SG, a 27-year-old nullipara at 37 weeks' gestational age, began labor at 7:00 P.M. with intact membranes. She was short in stature (5 feet, 3 inches) and light in weight (104 pounds). When admitted to hospital nearly 5 hours later, her cervix was 2 cm dilated and 90 percent effaced; the fetus was in vertex presentation at station 0, position undetermined. Contractions recurred at 3- to 4-minute intervals, lasted 35 to 40 seconds, and were of moderate intensity. Although she slept intermittently during the night, the contractions were noted to continue at 3- to 6-minute intervals. Periodic examinations (Fig. 71) revealed minimal progress, the cervix advancing to no more than 3 cm by 3:00 P.M. the next day. Twenty hours having elapsed, the diagnosis of prolonged latent phase was made and the patient was given 10 mg of morphine sulfate subcutaneously. She slept soundly with no perceptible contractions to the observers for 8 hours.

When she awoke she was having strong uterine contractions at 3-minute intervals, lasting 55 to 60 seconds. Her cervix was 4 cm dilated and 100 per-

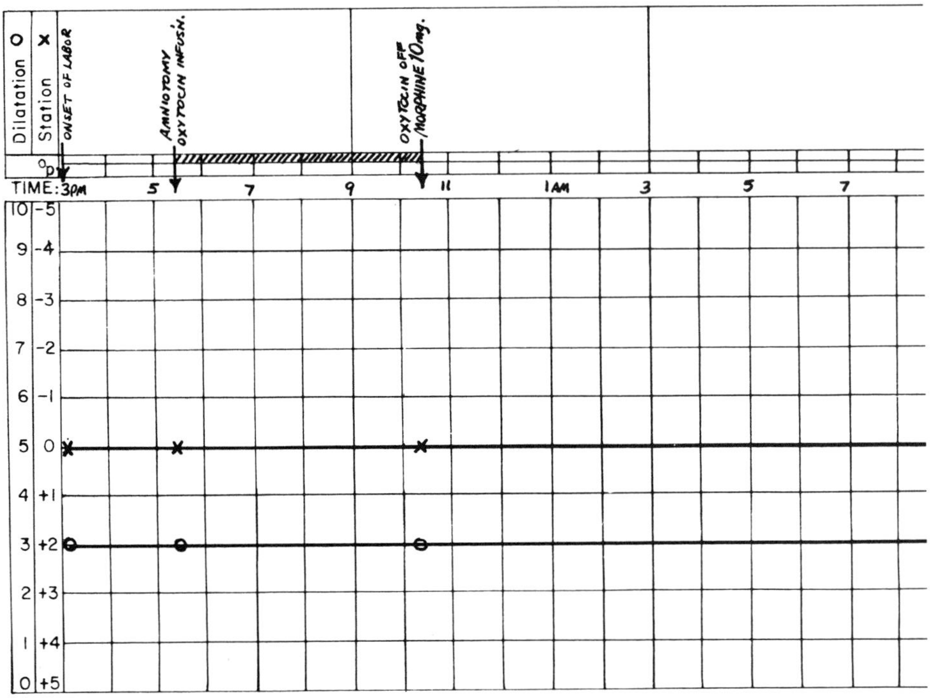


*Fig. 72.* Labor pattern of Patient RZ, Case #3.

cent effaced. The fetal station was unchanged. After 2 hours, the membranes ruptured spontaneously, the cervix reached full dilatation, and active descent was noted with the forward leading edge of the fetal presenting part at station +2. Less than 2 hours later, low forceps delivery was accomplished from the left occiput anterior position under caudal anesthesia. The baby weighed 2,400 g and was alert and responsive.

This is a straightforward case of prolonged latent phase, managed conservatively by means of therapeutic rest. Even though preterm, the use of morphine here did not adversely affect the neonate. Eleven hours elapsed from the time the medication was given to the time of birth. The physician astutely reduced the recommended dosage because of the patient's small stature and thin frame. The patient clearly benefited from the rest, having been thoroughly exhausted by her 20 hours of unavailing uterine contractions. When she awoke, the latent phase had already been terminated and she progressed rapidly in the active phase and second stage thereafter.

Since there was no urgency here, rest was certainly a much more appropriate choice for management than uterotonic stimulation. If the patient had been in false labor, the use of the narcotic would have demonstrated this fact by stopping the labor completely. This is an especially useful differential diagnostic tool.

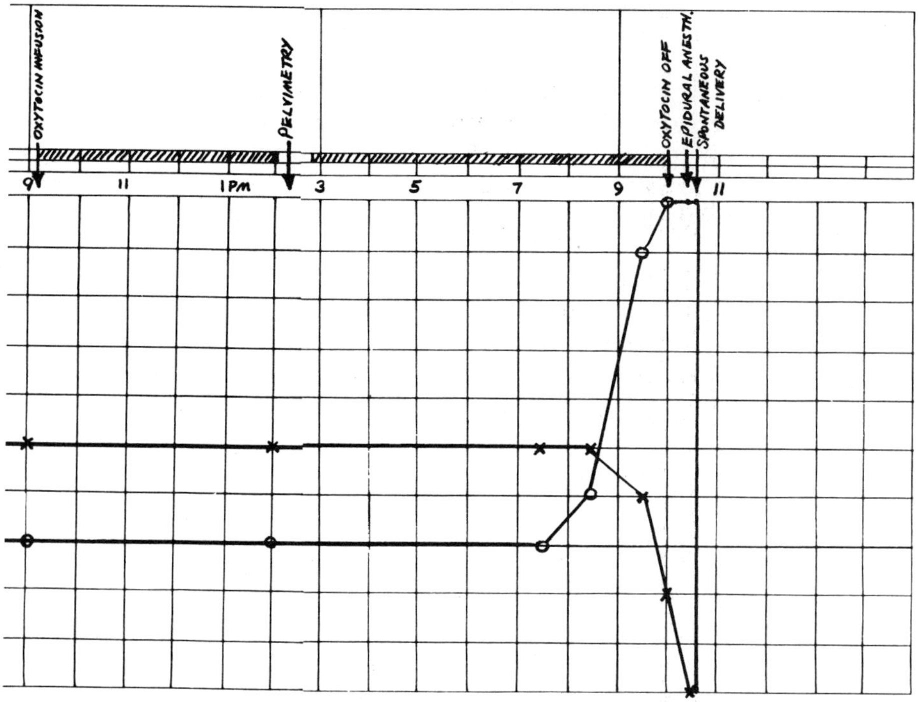


## Case #3

RZ, a 21-year-old nullipara at term, was admitted to the hospital at 11:00 A.M. with mild, irregular contractions. She weighed 177 pounds, and was 5 feet, 11 inches tall. The cervix was 3 cm dilated and 90 percent effaced; the vertex presented at station 0. Contractions became regularized at about 6- to 8-minute intervals by 3:00 P.M. Since no progress at all had been made by 5:30 P.M., the membranes were ruptured artificially and oxytocin infusion was begun. It was continued at ever-increasing dosages for 5 hours, yielding moderate uterine contractions at about 3- to 5-minute intervals, lasting 35 to 45 seconds. The cervix and station remained unchanged. At 10:30 P.M., 10 mg of morphine sulfate was administered. The patient slept intermittently during the next 8 hours, but was noted to have continuing contractions.

When she was reexamined at 9:00 A.M. the following morning, the cervix and station were the same as previously, contractions continuing as before. Again, oxytocin infusion was started. After 5 hours with no perceptible progress, radiographic pelvimetry was obtained. No cephalopelvic disproportion was found. Oxytocin was continued and, finally, at 8:30 P.M.—almost 36 hours after admission to the hospital—the patient entered the active phase of dilatation. Subsequently, rapid dilatation and descent evolved (Fig. 72), eventuating in a normal spontaneous delivery of a 2,750-g healthy infant under epidural anesthesia. Mother and baby did well.

Despite the fact that the results here were good, the case must be considered to represent unnecessary and inappropriate meddling. There does not seem to be any clear justification for the amniotomy and oxytocin infusion undertaken early in the course of the latent phase. Having failed to effect active dilatation by this means, the physician then proceeded to try to provide the patient with some rest. This was done about 12 hours after contractions began and within 8 hours of their regularization. The dose of morphine chosen was 10 mg, apparently inadequate for a patient of this size, because contractions continued. Although the patient was somewhat rested, her uterus was not; moreover, full advantage was not taken of the opportunity to provide her with appropriate supports in the form of fluid and electrolytes. The second attempt at uterotonic stimulation followed and in due course was successful, although the patient was thoroughly exhausted. Exposure to radiation here for pelvimetry appears to have been unnecessary.

Had the patient been allowed to evolve her own labor pattern without augmentation and without the complicating factor of amniotomy, she would eventually have declared herself. If the contractions subsided, false labor would have been obvious. If they progressed and she had entered the active phase, a normal labor pattern would have evolved. If she continued without progress for 20 hours, prolonged latent phase would exist. In each instance, the correct prescribed management program would have been clear. In this case, the situation was confused by the aggressive intervention. The potential hazards of uterotonic stimulation should be weighed before undertaking it in an otherwise normal situation. The problem here was created by the physician. That all turned out well is no reason to condone this course of action. The patient did not have an identifiable problem, nor could one be anticipated, until the physician created one. A long, difficult, and exhausting labor process was substituted for what might have been a much more benign course for the patient.

## Case #4

JJ, a 24-year-old nullipara (one prior abortion), was admitted at term 3 hours after the onset of uterine contractions. Her antepartum course to date had been benign. On admission at 10:00 P.M., the cervix was closed and 90 percent effaced; the fetus was in vertex presentation at station −1. Contractions were recurring at 3-minute intervals, lasting 50 seconds, and of moderate intensity. During the next 3 hours, the contractions increased in frequency, intensity, and duration. The cervix dilated to 1 cm, and the vertex was found to be in right occiput transverse position, advancing to station 0. Because of the patient's anxiety and discomfort, a tranquilizer (Valium, 10 mg) was given. A peridural catheter was placed, but only a test dose of anesthetic agent administered.

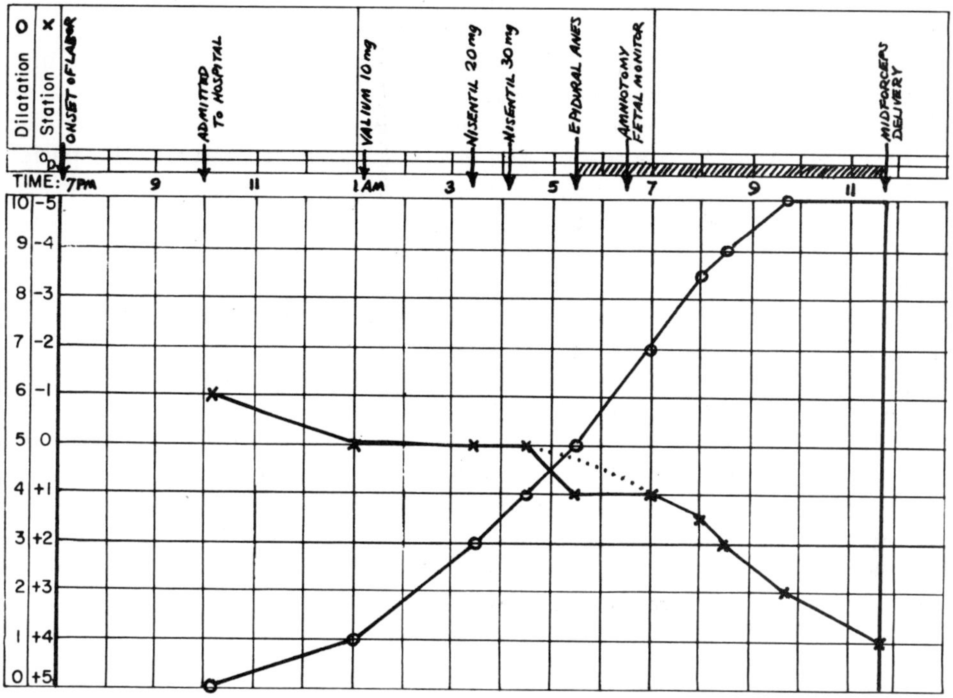


*Fig. 73.* Labor pattern of Patient JJ, Case #4.

By 3:30 A.M., active dilatation appeared to be in progress, the cervical os having reached 3 cm in diameter. Narcotic analgesics were administered for pain relief. Subsequent progress (Fig. 73) in dilatation occurred very slowly at an average rate of 1.2 cm/hr. A low level of epidural anesthesia (to dermatome thoracic-11) was administered at 5:30 A.M. This did not appear to affect the course of slow progression; neither did the amniotomy done at 6:30 A.M. for purposes of applying the fetal scalp electrode for internal fetal heart rate monitoring. Active descent approached maximum at about 8:00 A.M. and continued in a dilatory fashion thereafter. The patient was able to provide good expulsive efforts, and slow progressive descent was being made. At 11:45 A.M., the physician elected to terminate the labor by forceps delivery. The fetal position at that time was right occiput transverse, the station, +4. The fetal heart rate pattern was entirely normal. Delivery was accomplished with minimal difficulty (according to the physician) by Kjelland forceps rotation. The baby weighed 3,900 g and was in good condition, except for cephalhematoma and facial laceration. The mother sustained a left vaginal sulcus laceration requiring sutures.

This patient experienced both protracted active-phase dilatation and protracted descent. Optimally, she should have been managed with maximized support and minimized analgesia and anesthesia. Instead, she was given narcotic analgesics as well as epidural anesthesia. Contrary to expectations, however, neither affected the course of her labor. Most patients with protraction disorders subjected to these kinds of inhibitory influences would have their labor problems compounded by an arrest disorder. This patient was more fortunate in that the established course of dilatation and descent remained unshaken. When she entered her second stage, slow, progressive descent was being made. At the time the physician chose to effect delivery, the patient had been in second stage for only 2 hours. He appears to have used this arbitrary duration to elect to terminate the labor, without overriding justification. The fetus was in good condition and the labor process was continuing uninterruptedly.

There seems to be no acceptable rationale for undertaking potentially traumatic midforceps rotation and delivery on an elective basis at this time. Had the patient been allowed to continue to evolve the descent mechanism, she might eventually have delivered spontaneously. The benefits of interrupting this process, if any benefits do exist other than convenience, appear to be far outweighed by the risks. This case represents an example of the kinds of hazards—in trauma, morbidity, mortality and long-term developmental defects—that may accrue to infants subjected to this aggressive approach. Such observations apply especially to instrumental delivery undertaken in patients with protraction disorders.

## Case #5

RL is a 30-year-old nullipara at term. She began labor at 2:00 A.M. Her cervix was 4.5 cm dilated and 100 percent effaced when she was admitted at 5:00 A.M., but the fetal station was −3. Because of appropriate concerns over the possibility of cephalopelvic disproportion in this nullipara with unengaged fetal presenting part in labor, radiographic cephalopelvimetry (Ball technique) was done. It revealed no numerical deficit, but showed the fetus to be in left occiput posterior position and somewhat deflexed. Slow progressive cervical dilatation occurred (Fig. 74) at a rate of 1.0 cm/hr. The fetus descended to station 0 by 9:00 A.M., at which time amniotomy was performed and an internal monitor placed. The cervix approached near full dilatation (but was not fully retracted) by 11:00 A.M.; the fetal station was +1, fetal position, left occiput anterior. Epidural anesthesia was initiated and maintained over the next 3 hours. During this time, there was no further advancement in cervical dilatation or in fetal descent. At 1:30 P.M., late deceleration patterns were evident on the fetal heart rate monitor tracing. Fetal scalp blood sample was tested for pH; it was 7.30. The patient was subjected to cesarean section at 3:00 P.M. for fetal distress and clinical cephalopelvic disproportion. The baby weighed 3,050 g and had moderate caput and molding. Its neonatal course was complicated by hyperbilirubinemia, but it did well with phototherapy. The mother's postoperative course was uneventful.

A correct degree of concern was exhibited over the possibility that cephalopelvic disproportion was reflected in the unengaged fetal head in this nulliparous parturient. Having objectively ruled out disproportion by radio-

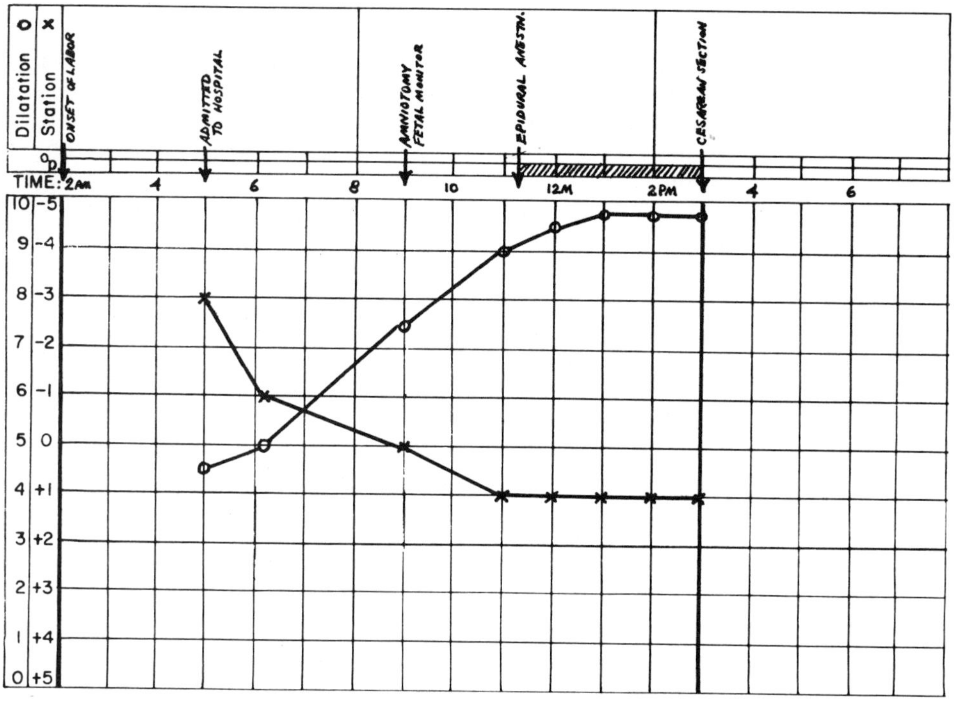


*Fig. 74.* Labor pattern of Patient RL, Case #5.

graphic cephalopelvimetry, the physician was faced with an abnormally evolving labor, characterized at first by a pattern of protracted active-phase dilatation, later complicated by protracted descent, and finally compounded twice more by prolonged deceleration phase and arrest of descent. Here, one may have anticipated that the use of peridural anesthesia would effectively inhibit this desultory labor, perhaps arresting further progress. When this actually did eventuate, it would have been appropriate to allow the anesthesia effect to abate. This might have demonstrated whether or not it were possible for the patient to resume her prearrest course—that is, to achieve full cervical dilatation and retraction while simultaneously resuming the prearrest slow rate of descent. Failing this, uterotonic stimulation might have yielded the same result. Neither was undertaken here, and the physician erroneously used the opportunity of the appearance of transient fetal heart rate abnormalities to rationalize abdominal delivery. Of the several options available in this case, abatement should have been considered first, uterotonic stimulation second (provided careful dynamic cephalopelvic assessment verified the absence of disproportion), and cesarean section last. There is no place for operative vaginal delivery in these specific circumstances. Poor immediate and long-term results strongly support this contention (see Chapter 23).

## Case #6

JB is a 19-year-old nullipara who had had one prior abortion. She was admitted to the hospital at 41 weeks' gestational age with ruptured membranes, not in labor. Her cervix was 3 cm dilated and 70 percent effaced; the fetal vertex was at station −2. Labor began 26 hours later. Neither the cervix nor the station had changed in the interim. The course of dilatation (Fig. 75) was rapid, full cervical dilatation having been achieved in 5 hours. The descent curve maintained an abnormally slow maximum rate of 0.7 cm/hr. Conduction anesthesia had been instituted, but was allowed to abate in an obvious effort to avoid inhibiting the abnormally protracted descent. Internal fetal heart rate monitoring revealed recurrent episodes of variable (cord compression) patterns, but periodic scalp blood samples showed stable pH determinations between 7.25 and 7.29. After 3.5 hours of second stage, midforceps delivery was accomplished from station +3 in the direct occiput posterior position (delivered as such) under caudal anesthesia. The baby weighed 3,650 g and was depressed at birth with low 1- and 5-minute Apgar Scores. The baby's head was moderately molded. The baby did well after prolonged resuscitation. In addition to the episiotomy, the mother sustained extensive vaginal lacerations, resulting in marked hemorrhage. Her postpartum course was complicated by infected perineal hematoma and endometritis.

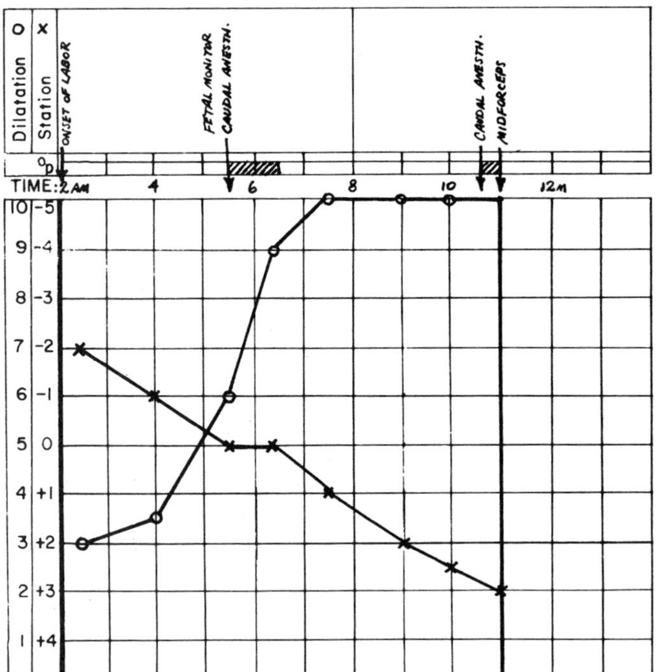


*Fig. 75.* Labor pattern of Patient JB, Case #6.

This labor pattern is unusual in that active descent appears to have begun at the onset of the active phase, or even before. Usually, of course, descent does not reach its maximum until the deceleration phase of dilatation. When it begins this early, it is usually a good prognostic sign. Here, however, it advanced at an abnormally slow rate, and this rate persisted unremittingly into the second stage. Because descent had begun from such a high station, it follows that it should be expected to take many hours for the fetal head to reach the perineum at the predetermined rate it had embarked upon. Essentially ignored in the management of this nullipara was that the fetal station was so high early in labor; the cephalopelvic relationships should certainly have been investigated. We have already addressed ourselves to the lack of justification for undertaking midforceps operation in a patient with protracted descent, and this need not be repeated here once more. As long as progress was still being made in descent and neither fetus nor mother was in any jeopardy, the labor should have been allowed to continue even though the second stage was already so prolonged. Clearly, the unfortunate traumatic result is not acceptable.

## Case #7

> LS, a 30-year-old nullipara with one prior abortion, was at 38 weeks' gestational age when her membranes ruptured and contractions began. When admitted to the hospital 2.5 hours later, her cervix was 4 cm dilated, and the fetal station was at the level of the ischial spines. The course of cervical dilatation proceeded rapidly (Fig. 76), but descent was slow. Caudal anesthesia was instituted when the cervix reached 9 cm of dilatation, but was allowed to abate when it became clear that the labor pattern was that of protracted descent. The second stage was entered 6.5 hours after the onset of labor. The patient was supported emotionally and physically. Management was entirely expectant, continuous slow descent being carefully monitored by vaginal and abdominal examinations. The patient was very cooperative, providing appropriate expulsive efforts over long periods of time, with intervening intervals of rest. Finally, a 2,950-g healthy infant was spontaneously delivered under caudal anesthesia. Both mother and baby did well.

Here is an example of the kind of disordered labor which, under other circumstances, might readily have been subjected to the trauma of instrumental intervention. Despite the very long second stage, the delivery process was flawlessly uncomplicated. Slow steady progress in descent was carefully watched. As long as real progress in descent was being made—as opposed to the impression of progress that is associated with molding only—the labor was allowed to continue. No inhibitory factors were allowed to compound the problem by arresting the descent; when it was realized that protracted descent was present, the caudal anesthesia was properly allowed to abate. If the descent process had arrested subsequently, one would not have to won-

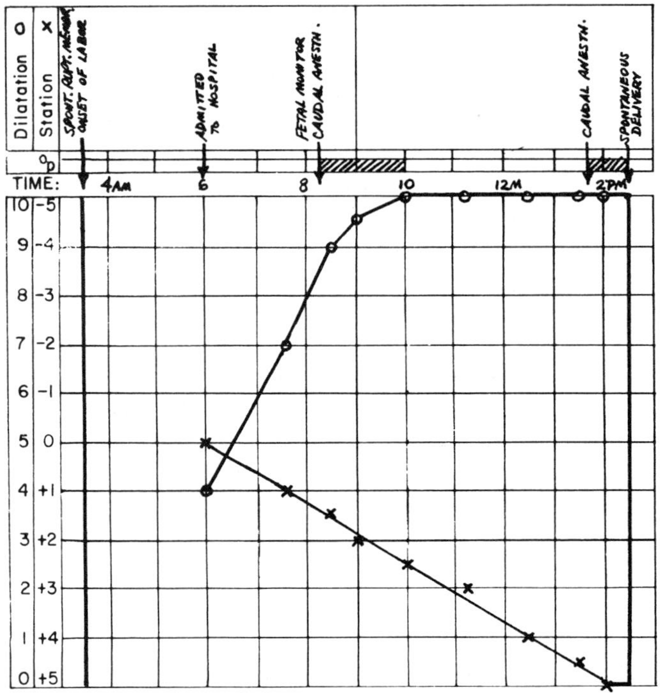

*Fig. 76.* Labor pattern of Patient LS, Case #7.

der whether the arrest might be due to the anesthesia. By allowing the anesthetic effect to wear off (or not giving it in the first place), one reduces the complexity of the problem in terms of ascertaining underlying etiology.

## Case #8

MF, a 20-year-old nullipara 2 weeks beyond term, was admitted to the hospital 3 hours after the onset of regular uterine contractions. Her antepartum course had been entirely unremarkable. Her cervix was found to be 4 cm dilated, and the fetal head was presenting at station −1. About 1 hour later (Fig. 77), the cervix had advanced to 5.5 cm and the vertex reached station 0. At that time amniotomy was done for purposes of applying a fetal scalp electrode and inserting an intrauterine catheter for monitoring. Progress in cervical dilatation continued at a rate of 1.0 cm/hr. Six hours after the onset of labor, epidural anesthesia was administered; the cervix by this time had reached 8 cm of dilatation, but the fetal head remained between station 0 and +1.

During the next 2 hours, it became obvious that no further progress was being made. Accordingly, the epidural anesthesia was allowed to abate. The capacity of the pelvis was checked with reference to the fetal head and the ability of the fetus to descend in the birth canal during contractions

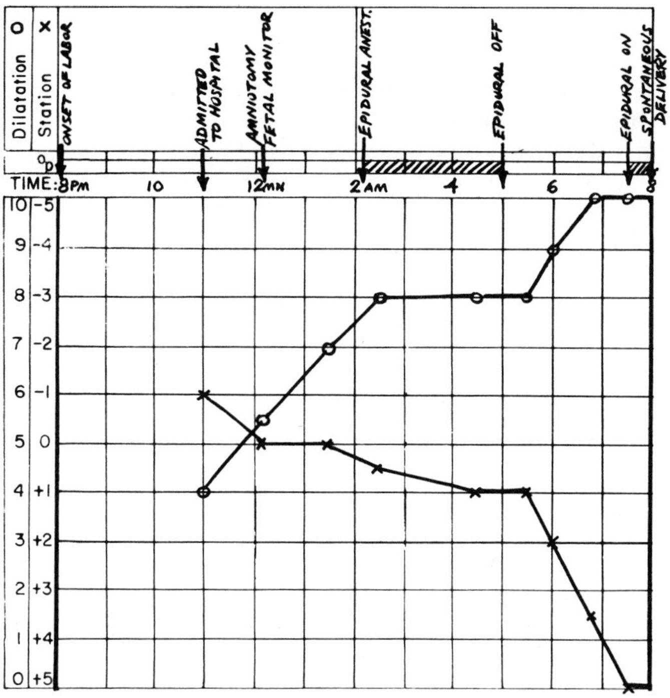


*Fig. 77.* Labor pattern of Patient MF, Case #8.

with added Kristeller pressure; radiographic pelvimetry was also undertaken. Cephalopelvimetry clearly demonstrated the pelvis to be adequate for this fetus. Both fetal heart rate and uterine contractile patterns remained good.

Within 1 hour of the abatement of epidural anesthesia, further dilatation occurred and the second stage was soon reached. Meanwhile, this was accompanied by active descent at a rate of 2.0 cm/hr. The patient made good expulsive efforts. When the fetal head reached the perineum, the epidural anesthesia was reinstituted, and spontaneous delivery followed shortly thereafter over a median episiotomy. The baby weighed 4,100 g and was in excellent condition. Both mother and baby did well subsequently.

When first observed, this patient was experiencing an abnormal active-phase progression (or at best, one on the borderline of normal limits). Contrary to some physicians' expectations, the amniotomy done here for purposes of labor surveillance did not enhance labor progression. Indeed, it would be unusual if it had done so. If anything, progress in dilatation after the amniotomy was somewhat slower than it had been earlier, but this is perhaps well within the limits of error. Nevertheless, when the epidural anesthesia became effective, arrest of dilatation followed secondarily.

Quite properly, the physician allowed the anesthesia effect to abate, while simultaneously assessing the cephalopelvic relationships. Without any form of uterotonic stimulation, subsequent events demonstrated a resumption of active dilatation after the arrest. The postarrest slope of dilatation was 2.0 cm/hr, implying a good prognostic outlook. We now know that the postarrest slope of the dilatation curve with oxytocin stimulation is a useful prognostic index: if it is the same as or greater than the prearrest slope, the outlook is good for vaginal delivery. For this to have occurred in this case even without uterotonic impetus suggests an even brighter forecast. Additional support for this optimism came in the form of the rapidly progressive descent pattern.

This patient represents one who was managed quite properly by a physician who diagnosed the specific disorder of secondary arrest of dilatation. He knew the kinds of etiologic factors associated with this type of abnormal labor pattern. On this basis, he proceeded to evaluate for such causative factors and to make suitable corrections for them.

## Case #9

MK is a 22-year-old nullipara who began spontaneous labor at 41 weeks' gestational age. She did not appear at the hospital for examination until nearly 11 hours had elapsed. When first seen, the cervix was 2.5 cm dilated and the fetal head was dipping into the pelvis at station −2. Since there was justifiable concern over the possibility of cephalopelvic disproportion in this case, as suggested by the unengaged fetal presenting part—especially because she had previously been assessed as having a small gynecoid pelvis—radiographic cephalopelvimetry was undertaken by the Ball technique. This revealed a midplane deficit of about 150 cc, signifying borderline disproportion, based on the numerical relationship between the capacity of the interspinous plane and the volume of the fetal head.

With this information known, the patient was allowed to labor. Progress occurred slowly at first (Fig. 78). Amniotomy was undertaken for monitoring purposes. Latent phase progress continued until the seventeenth hour after the onset of labor. At this time, the physician undertook to administer oxytocin infusion. This was done electively; that is, without clear indication or justification. The active phase of dilatation was entered during the next 2 hours, with ensuing rapid advancement of cervical dilatation to 8 cm at a maximum slope of 2.0 cm/hr; the fetus descended to station +1. Subsequently, all progress ceased.

The pelvis was assessed carefully to ascertain whether or not there was additional compensatory space available for further descent of the fetus in this birth canal. At the height of a contraction, it was quite apparent that Kristeller pressure did not advance the station at all. It was recognized that the fetal head was essentially fixed in the pelvis and tightly wedged at this station. The oxytocin infusion was discontinued and a cesarean section undertaken. A 3,700-g infant was delivered in good condition by a low flap, transverse incision procedure. Some difficulty was encountered in dislodging the head from the pelvis and it was necessary to apply some pressure by intravaginal manipulation. The mother's postoperative course was uneventful.

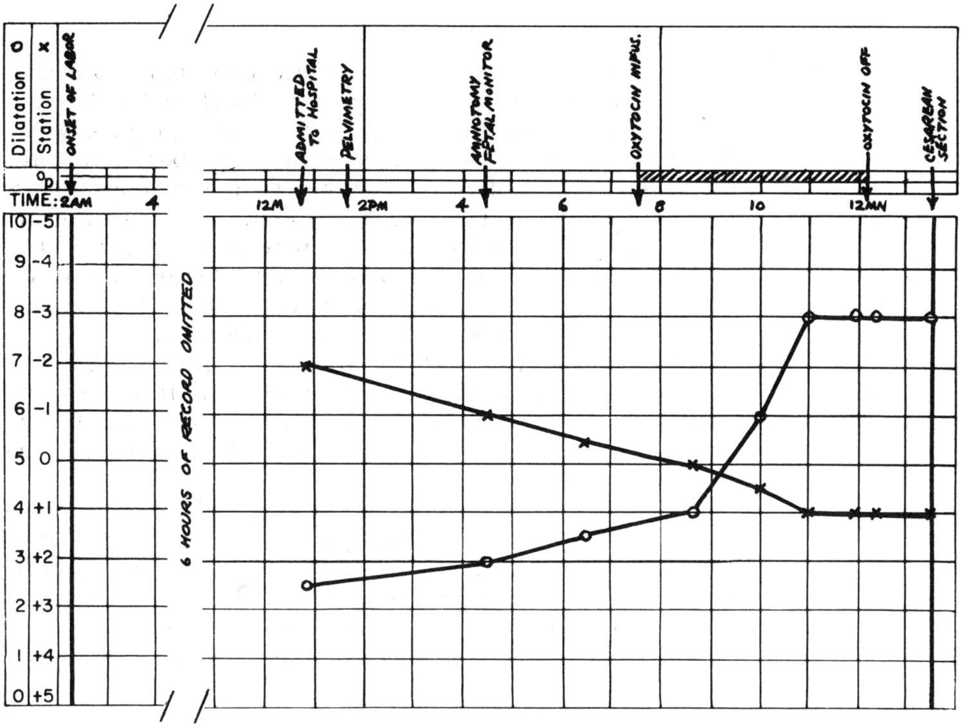


*Fig. 78.* Labor pattern of patient MK, Case #9.

This case represents an interesting example of a patient with clinical evidence of cephalopelvic disproportion who was properly allowed to evolve her labor. Not all nulliparas with unengaged fetal presenting part in early labor will require cesarean section. Indeed, more than 60 percent should be expected to deliver vaginally without difficulty. As labor evolved here, it seemed likely that the latent phase would be prolonged. However, technically, the latent phase was still within acceptable limits when the oxytocin infusion was initiated.

One could argue here against uterotonic stimulation in that it tends to obtund the value of the dilatation and descent curves as diagnostic indices. The spontaneously evolving curve, as we have seen, helps the obstetric attendant to follow labor progression and to identify abnormalities as they arise. It is sometimes possible to overcome or mask an abnormal pattern through the use of oxytocin. Such was not the case here, fortunately.

In actuality, we recognize that an arrest pattern developing during the course of oxytocin infusion, particularly arrest of descent, carries a dire prognosis. Under these circumstances, cesarean section is almost always indicated because of concurrent underlying, insurmountable fetopelvic disproportion. The cesarean section done here was clearly indicated for this reason.

## Case #10

LD is a 23-year-old secundigravida who had previously delivered a 10-pound, 7-ounce infant. The prior delivery was complicated by shoulder dystocia, and the baby was severely depressed at birth. The current pregnancy had been essentially uneventful until the patient went into labor during the 42nd week of pregnancy. Shortly after contractions began, she noted leakage of amniotic fluid. She arrived at the hospital 5 hours later with cervical dilatation of 2.5 cm and fetal station at −1. Progress was rapid at first (Fig. 79), dilatation reaching 8 cm within the hour. Because she was a multipara who had previously delivered a large infant, she was taken to the delivery room, and preparations were made for vaginal delivery.

Thirty minutes later, the cervix was 9 cm dilated and the fetal head, in position left occiput transverse at station +1. A good contractile pattern continued and 1 hour later, only an anterior lip of cervix remained, but no further descent had occurred. After still another hour, it was apparent that the cervix was becoming edematous.

At this time, the patient was returned to her labor bed. She was examined periodically over the next 5 hours and finally reached second stage when the cervix became fully dilated and fully retracted above the fetal presenting part. The fetal head had apparently descended to station +3, but no further advance could be made, despite good expulsive efforts.

Accordingly, after 2 hours of second stage, Simpson forceps were applied

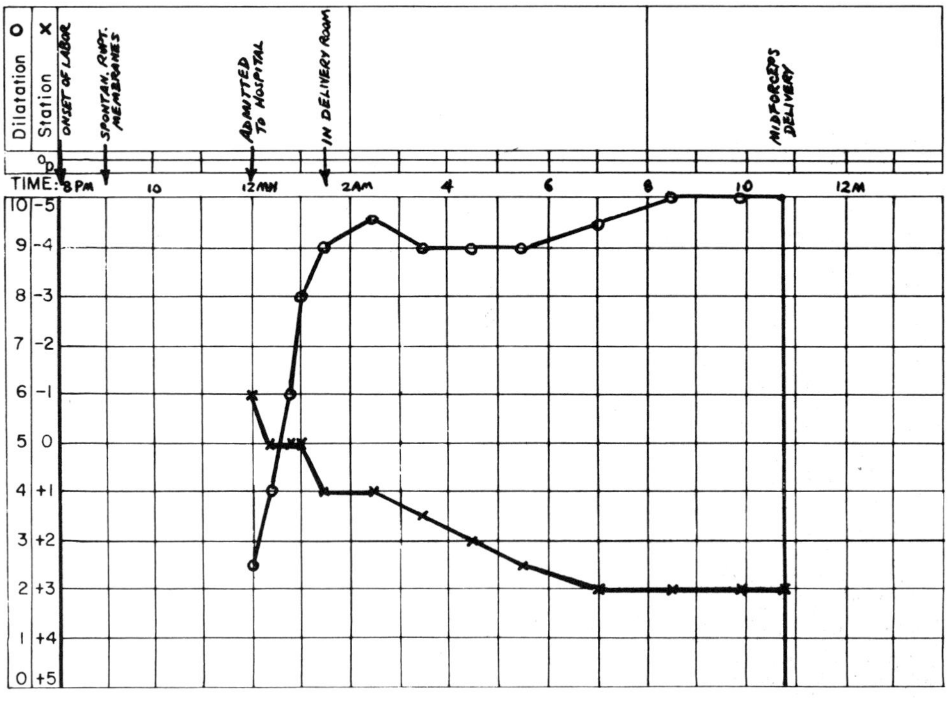


*Fig. 79.* Labor pattern of Patient LD, Case #10.

> to the fetal head in the left occiput transverse position under pudendal block anesthesia. After the head was delivered over the perineum, severe shoulder impaction was recognized. Extreme difficulty was encountered in the delivery of the shoulders and, ultimately, an essentially moribund 5,450-g (12-pound) baby was born over an intact perineum. The mother did well, but the baby required intensive resuscitation, including intubation and closed-chest cardiac massage. It survived to develop severe brain damage, probably the result of the prolonged period of hypoxia it suffered during the procedures undertaken to effect disimpaction of its shoulders.

This case, salvaged from another institution and another era of obstetric care, represents perhaps the worst form of obstetric mismanagement. Merely because this patient had previously delivered a large infant, she was assumed to be capable of repeating the performance easily, thus the term "treacherous multipara." It was unanticipated that this second fetus might be much larger than her first. Her pelvis, although obviously capacious and able to accommodate a large infant weighing 10.5 pounds, was in retrospect not adequate for this one.

Under other circumstances, one might argue that shoulder dystocia is not predictable on the basis of the foregoing labor pattern, and indeed, this is generally true. We have seen many instances of severe shoulder dystocia occurring after perfectly normal dilatation and descent patterns. Here, however, at least three different serious signals should have alerted the physician to the events that were forthcoming: (1) the marked prolongation of the deceleration phase, associated with progressively increasing edema of the cervix, (2) the protracted descent pattern reaching a maximum slope of 0.5 cm/hr, and (3) the arrest of descent at station +3.

To allow such a labor to continue for so long without a thorough and objective evaluation of the cephalopelvic relationships would be unthinkable today. Moreover, even after this degree of neglect, it is still likely that this infant would not have been damaged had it been delivered abdominally rather than by the vaginal route. As soon as it was recognized that the deceleration phase was prolonged (beyond 1 hour), assessment of the fetal head and pelvis would have revealed the insurmountable degree of disproportion that was likely present here. A cesarean section undertaken at that time would undoubtedly have had a happier outcome.

# Glossary

*Aberrant labor.* Specific disorder of labor based on disturbed dilatation or descent patterns. See *Dysfunctional labor.*

*Acceleration phase.* (1) Initial portion of the active phase of the dilatation pattern, characterized by upward changing slope from the negligible slope of the preceding latent phase to the maximum slope of the phase following. (2) Also the initial part of active descent.

*Active phase.* That portion of the first stage of labor extending from the upswing of the dilatation curve (at the end of the latent phase) to the beginning of second stage, when the cervix reaches full dilatation and complete retraction.

*Amniotomy.* Surgical rupture of the chorioamniotic membranes.

*Apgar Score.* Index for assessment of newborn infant, usually specified at 1 and 5 minutes of age, according to five criteria: heart rate, respiration, reflex irritability, muscle tone, and color.

*Arrest disorder.* One of four specifically defined labor dysfunctions, including secondary arrest of dilatation, prolonged deceleration phase, arrest of descent, and failure of descent.

*Arrest of descent.* Abnormal labor pattern characterized by cessation of progressive descent for at least 1 hour, usually diagnosed in the second stage.

*Asynchrony of uterine activity.* Uterine fibrillation; uncoordinated contractility pattern without suitably oriented propagation or polarization to effect efficient labor progression.

*Bishop Score.* Index of inducibility, based on prelabor soft-tissue conditions including dilatation, consistency, effacement, and position of the cervix, as well as the station of the fetus.

*Bony dystocia.* Cephalopelvic disproportion, implying verification by adequate trial of labor.

*Cardinal movements.* Passive adaptation of the fetal presenting part to the maternal pelvic architecture during descent, including flexion, internal rotation, extension, restitution, and external rotation.

*Cephalopelvic disproportion.* Condition in which pelvic capacity is inadequate to accommodate fetal head dimensions, as assessed digitally in labor or by appropriate radiologic cephalopelvimetric techniques.

*Cervical dilatation.* (1) Measurement of the dimension of the cervical os, usually based on digital estimates. (2) The process by which the cervix passively opens in response to the centrifugal forces of uterine contractions.

*Cervical dilatation at the onset of labor.* The degree of prelabor dilatation achieved, sometimes considerable in association with uterine overdistention (hydramnios or multiple pregnancy) or incompetent cervix.

*Cervical dilatation at onset of active phase.* The dilatation attained when the dilatation pattern begins its upswing; since it is a variable and unpredictable value, one cannot assume the active phase has been entered merely because a certain amount of dilatation exists.

*Cervical dystocia.* A rare condition in which the cervix is pathologically altered (for example, by scarification) so that it cannot dilate in response to the uterine contractions of labor; false labor or prolonged latent phase of benign origin may be mistaken for this.

*Cervimetric data.* Compilation of objective information on the course of cervical dilatation with elapsed time in labor, including mean values for durations of latent, active, and deceleration phases and second stage, as well as maximum slope of dilatation; more recently, descent pattern data are also included, most pertinently the mean maximum slope of descent.

*Contractility pattern.* Evaluation of intensity, frequency, and duration of uterine contractions, generally not useful for determining whether the labor is true or false, normal or abnormal.

*Deceleration phase.* Terminal portion of the active phase of dilatation, extending from the end of the phase of maximum slope to the beginning of the second stage; "transition," occurring at a time when the descent process reaches its maximum rate of progress.

*Depressed neonate.* Newborn infant with low Apgar Score at 1 or 5 minutes of age; it is usually the result of hypoxic or traumatic insult, but may also be due to transient analgesic or anesthetic effect.

*Descent pattern.* Graphic depiction of the progressive changes in fetal station with elapsed time in labor, usually traced in conjunction with the dilatation pattern in the same labor.

*Dilatation curve, graph, pattern.* Portrayal of the labor process in first stage by plotting estimates of cervical dilatation against elapsed time in labor on a square-ruled graph.

*Dilatational division of labor.* Functional division of the labor phenomenon during which most cervical dilatation takes place, congruent with phase of maximum slope.

*Dilatory progress.* Vague term to designate abnormally slow labor progression.

*Dissociation between contractions and progression.* Paradoxical relationship in which the processes of dilatation and descent appear to be unaffected by altered uterine contractility, or in which the course of labor progression changes despite an unaltered contraction pattern.

*Dysfunctional labor.* One of nine identifiable abnormal labor patterns, including prolonged latent phase, protracted active-phase dilatation, protracted descent, secondary arrest of dilatation, prolonged deceleration phase, arrest of descent, and failure of descent; also precipitate dilatation and precipitate descent.

*Dyskinetic labor.* Disordered uterine contractility. See *Asynchrony of uterine activity.*

*Dystocia, dystocic labor.* Nonspecific term applied to disordered labor, usually designated according to the impeding factor thought to be causative in the fetus (for example, positional dystocia), the pelvis (for example, bony dystocia), or the uterus (for example, inertial dystocia).

*Effacement of cervix.* Process by which cervical canal is taken up, usually completed before labor begins in nulliparas.

*Engagement.* Descent of the fetal presenting part into the pelvis so that the biparietal diameter is at or below plane of pelvic inlet, with forward leading edge at or below station 0, the plane of the ischial spines; generally accomplished well before labor in nulliparas.

*Failure of descent.* Abnormal labor pattern in which the descent that is expected to have begun by the time the dilatation curve reaches the deceleration phase fails to do so.

*Failure to progress.* A nondescript term that does not distinguish among such widely disparate conditions as prolonged latent phase, secondary arrest of dilatation, arrest of descent, and failure of descent.

*False labor.* A self-limited condition in which ineffectual uterine contractions, indistinguishable from contractions of true labor, fail to achieve cervical dilatation, fetal descent, and evacuation of the gravid uterus, usually diagnosable by hindsight only.

*Faulty presentation.* Fetal malpresentation, including face, brow, compound, oblique, and transverse lie.

*Fetal death.* Stillbirth, death in utero of a viable fetus (generally at or beyond 28 weeks) prior to delivery.

*Fetal dystocia.* Disturbed labor, ostensibly due to abnormally large fetal dimensions.

*Fetal monitoring.* Continuous surveillance of fetal wellbeing by recording instantaneous beat-to-beat heart rate, either by external (ultrasound, phono-, or abdominal wall electrocardiograph) or internal (fetal scalp electrode) means; usually done together with simultaneous uterine contraction pattern monitoring.

*Fetopelvic disproportion.* See *Cephalopelvic disproportion*

*First stage of labor.* Interval from onset of regular perceived uterine contractions to full cervical dilatation, encompassing latent plus active phases of dilatation.

*Full cervical dilatation.* The degree of cervical opening necessary to permit the fetus to exit from the uterus, designated 10 cm at term by convention only.

*Functional divisions of labor.* The three segments into which all labors can be partitioned on the basis of the constant interrelationship of the normal dilatation and descent patterns, namely, preparatory, dilatational, and pelvic divisions.

*Functional dystocia.* Nonspecific term used to describe "inert" labors, suggesting poor or absent progress based on ineffective uterine action.

*Graphic analysis of labor.* Method for following individual labors in progress by tracing dilatation and descent curves, and for studying homogeneous groups of labors to ascertain the effects of various factors on the course of labor.

*Hypertonic labor.* Rare disordered contractility pattern in which the uterus (teleologically) appears to be overcompensating for some obstructive factor by becoming hyperactive.

*Hypertonus.* Abnormally increased basal tonus, above normal levels of 8 to 12 mm Hg.

*Hypotonic labor.* Abnormal contractility pattern in which poor or absent progress in dilatation or descent is attributed to inefficient uterine activity, often mistakenly.

*Idiopathic functional dystocia.* Another cryptic term for the equally nebulous condition of uterine inertia.

*Inert labor.* Antiquated catch-basket term for abnormal labor; uterine inertia.

*Inertial dystocia.* Disordered labor ostensibly due to ineffective contractions.

*Labor pains.* Lay term for uterine contractions, generally decried today because of its emphasis on the discomfort of labor.

*Latent phase.* First part of the first stage of labor, from the onset of contractions to the upswing of the dilatation curve.

*Limits of normal.* Objective cut-off designations for the purposes of defining specific labor abnormalities, based on the 95th percentiles of the distribution of the several component durations and slopes of the dilatation and descent patterns.

*Malposition, fetal.* Variants of fetal position, including persistent occiput transverse and posterior, as well as problems in deflexion, attitude, and synclitism.

*Malpresentation, fetal.* Abnormal fetal presentation, including face, brow, compound, oblique, and transverse lie.

*Maternal exhaustion.* State in which laboring patient has become extremely weak as a result of a long, slowly progressive or nonprogressive labor without adequate rest, usually with associated fluid and electrolyte imbalance.

*Mechanisms of labor.* See *Cardinal movements.*

*Mechanical dystocia.* Nonspecific labor disorder believed to be based on an obstructive aspect.

*Midforceps delivery.* Potentially traumatic instrumental delivery in which forceps are applied before the fetal head has crowned (that is, is visible between contractions without spreading the labia), or is not in an occiput anterior position.

*Myometrial dysfunction.* Disordered labor believed based on ineffectual uterine contractions; uterine dysfunction.

*Neonatal death.* Death of a liveborn infant within 28 days of delivery.

*Operative delivery, intervention.* Euphemism for forceps delivery of all varieties.

*Pelvic contraction.* Cephalopelvic disproportion based primarily on markedly diminished pelvic dimension(s).

*Pelvic division of labor.* Functional division encompassing both deceleration phase and second stage, during which the fetus negotiates the pelvis and undergoes the classic cardinal movements.

*Pelvic dystocia.* Disordered labor thought to be due to the bony obstruction of pelvic contraction.

*Perinatal mortality.* Combined stillbirth and neonatal death rates based on total deaths among viable births (28 weeks of intrauterine life to 28 days of extrauterine life).

*Perineal phase.* Terminal portion of the descent curve, usually not graphable, during which caudad advancement stops and the fetal head extends forward over the perineum as it is delivered.

*Persistent occiput transverse, posterior position.* Malposition of fetal head due to failure of internal rotation mechanism, in second stage, usually associated with deflexion as well.

*Phase of maximum slope.* Midportion of active phase of dilatation, during which most cervical dilation is accomplished in a linear manner.

*Phase of labor.* Separate and identifiable component parts of the dilatation and descent curves, including latent, acceleration, maximum slope, and deceleration phases.

*Polysystole.* Contractility pattern characterized by excessively frequent contractions, sometimes associated with poor relaxation between them. See *Uterine tetany.*

*Precipitate delivery.* Rapid, uncontrolled delivery over an unprepared, unsterile field.

*Precipitate descent.* Specific labor aberration with abnormally rapid descent pattern, generally exceeding 5 cm/hr in nulliparas or 10 cm/hr in multiparas.

*Precipitate dilatation.* Excessively rapid dilatation pattern, defined in a manner similar to precipitate descent.

*Precipitate labor.* A nonspecific term referring to a short labor, usually less than 3 hours in duration.

*Precipitous labor.* A misnomer for precipitate labor.

*Premature rupture of membranes.* Spontaneous rupture of the chorioamniotic membranes before the onset of labor at any gestational age; variously defined by duration before labor begins at 1, 6, 12, and 24 hours.

*Preparatory division of labor.* Early functional division of labor encompassing latent and acceleration phases, during which myometrial contractions are undergoing orientation, coordination, and polarization, and the cervix is being changed subtly in preparation for later active dilatation.

*Primary dysfunctional labor.* Confusing term originally meant to be synonymous with protracted active-phase dilatation pattern, but still used widely to designate ill-defined condition of primary uterine inertia.

*Primary uterine inertia.* Abnormal labor of uncertain definition, not distinguishing between such different disorders as prolonged latent phase and the two protraction disorders.

*Prolonged deceleration phase.* One of the specific arrest disorders, characterized by deceleration phase duration exceeding 3 hours in nulliparas or 1 hour in multiparas.

*Prolonged labor.* Uncritical definition of abnormal labor based on total duration exceeding an arbitrary limit, such as 24 or 30 or 36 hours.

*Prolonged latent phase.* Dysfunctional labor pattern defined by abnormal duration of the latent phase, beyond 20 hours in nulliparas or 14 hours in multiparas.

*Protracted active-phase dilatation.* Serious labor disorder with abnormally slow maximum rate of dilatation in the active phase, less than 1.2 cm/hr in nulliparas or 1.5 cm/hr in multiparas.

*Protracted descent.* Aberration similar to protracted dilatation, with slope of descent less than 1.0 cm/hr in nulliparas or 2.0 cm/hr in multiparas.

*Second stage of labor.* Interval from full cervical dilatation and retraction to delivery of the baby.

*Secondary arrest of dilatation.* Important labor abnormality, with documented cessation of progressive cervical dilatation in the active phase for at least 2 hours.

*Secondary uterine inertia.* Nebulous term used to designate disordered labors of various and perhaps widely disparate types.

*Soft-tissue dystocia.* See *Cervical dystocia.*

*Station, fetal.* Index of location of the fetal presenting part with reference to the plane of the ischial spines (station 0), in centimeters, using a minus sign to indicate that the forward leading edge is above the spinous plane, and a plus sign for below the spines.

*Trial of labor.* Assessing labor progression under selected circumstances, based on use of an extrapolation of the dilatation (or descent) curve for purposes of prescribing the expected course of labor once the active phase of dilatation (or descent) has been documented.

*Uterine tetany.* Prolonged period of uterine contractility without intervening relaxation, usually defined as exceeding 90 seconds in duration; it may occur spontaneously, but is more often found associated with abruptio placentae or overstimulation by uterotonic agents.

# References


Abroms IF, Bresnan, MJ, Zuckerman JE, Fischer EG, Strand R: Cervical cord injuries secondary to hyperextension of the head in breech presentations. Obstet Gynecol 41:369, 1973

Alexopoulos KA: The importance of breech delivery in the pathogenesis of brain damage: End results of a long-term follow-up. Clin Pediatr 12:248, 1973

Alfonsi PL, Massi GB: Effetti degli anestètici sulla contrattilità uterina. Riv Ostet Ginecol 18:37, 1963

Alvarez H, Poseiro JJ, Pose SV, Sica-Blanco Y: Effects of the anesthetic blockage of the spinal cord on the contractility of the pregnant human uterus. XXI Int Cong Physiol Sci. Buenos Aires, 1959

Alver EC, White CW, Weiss JB, Heerdegen DK: An effect of succinylcholine on the uterus: Clinical observations. Am J Obstet Gynecol 83:795, 1962

Anderson DG: Arrested occiput posterior position. Clin Obstet Gynecol 8:867, 1965

Anderson GG, Hobbins JC, Cordero L, Speroff L: Clinical use of prostaglandins as oxytocin substances. Ann NY Acad Sci 180:499, 1971

Anderson GG, Hobbins JC, Speroff L: Intravenous prostaglandins $E_2$ and $F_{2\alpha}$ for the induction of term labor. Am J Obstet Gynecol 112:382, 1972

Anderson GG, Schooley GL: Comparison of uterine contractions in spontaneous and oxytocin- or $PGF_{2\alpha}$-induced labors. Obstet Gynecol 45:284, 1975

Auer ES, Simmons JM: The floating fetal head in the primipara at term. Am J Obstet Gynecol 58:291, 1949

Baillie J, Meehan FP, Tyack AJ: Treatment of premature labour with orciprenaline. Br Med J 4:154, 1970

Baird D: Social factors in obstetrics. Lancet 1:1079, 1949

Baird D: Environment and childbearing. Proc R Soc Med 46:53, 1953

Bakr SA, Robertson DNS: Pregnancy and labor in paraplegic patients. Int J Gynaecol Obstet 11:69, 1973

Ball RP: Roentgen pelvimetry and fetal cephalometry. Surg Gynecol Obstet 62: 798, 1936a

Ball RP: Pelvicephalometry. Am J Obstet Gynecol 32:249, 1936b

Ball RP: Cephalopelvimetry. In Glasser O (ed): Medical Physics. Chicago, Year Book Medical, 1950, vol II

Ball RP, Marchbanks SS: Roentgen pelvimetry and fetal cephalometry: A new technique. Radiology 24:77, 1935

Barber HRK, Graber EA, Orlando A: Augmented labor. Obstet Gynecol 39:933, 1972

Barden TP: Effect of ritodrine on human uterine motility and cardiovascular responses in term labor and early postpartum state. Am J Obstet Gynecol 112: 645, 1972

Barnafi L, Croxatto H: The in vitro effect of progesterone and estrogens on the oxytocin response of rat uterus. Acta Physiol Lat Am 13:26, 1963

Barnes AB: Prophylaxis in labor and delivery. New Engl J Med 294:1235, 1976

Batson GA: Cyanotic congenital heart disease and pregnancy. J Obstet Gynaecol Br Commonw 81:549, 1974

Baumgarten K: Librium und Valium in der Schwangerschaft und unter der Geburt. Wien Klin Wochenschr 75:263, 1963

Bayley N: Comparisons of mental and motor test scores for ages 1–15 months by sex, birth order, race, geographical location, and education of parents. Child Development 36:379, 1965

Beazley JM: Induction of labor with prostaglandins: Summary of present status. J Reprod Med 9:469, 1972a

Beazley JM: Use of partograms in labour. Proc R Soc Med 65:700, 1972b

Beazley JM, Gillespie A: Double-blind trial of prostaglandin $E_2$ and oxytocin in induction of labour. Lancet 1:152, 1971

Bedrosian L, Gamble JJ: Uterine tetany and fetal distress coincidental with administration of sparteine sulfate: Report of a case. Obstet Gynecol 21:400, 1963

Belizan JM, Diaz AG, Abusleme C, Poseiro JJ, Caldeyro-Barcia R: Effects of orciprenaline on uterine contractility and maternal heart rate. Obstet Gynecol 46:385, 1975

Bengtsson LP: The endocrine control of myometrial contractility in the uterus of the pregnant rabbit. Am J Obstet Gynecol 74:484, 1957

Bengtsson LP: Physical methods of measurement in obstetrics and gynaecology. J Obstet Gynaecol Br Commonw 69:1044, 1962

Berde B, Saameli K: Effect of bradykinin on uterine activity. Nature 191:83, 1961

Berger M: Die Wirkung von Librium in heher Desierung auf den Uterus. Gynaecol 152:292, 1961

Bieniarz J, Burd L, Motew M, Scommegna A: Inhibition of uterine contractility in labor. Am J Obstet Gynecol 111:874, 1971

Birnberg CH, Abitbol MM: Refined relaxin and length of labor: A preliminary report. Obstet Gynecol 10:366, 1957

Bishop EH: Dangers attending elective induction of labor. JAMA 166:1953, 1958

Bishop EH: Pelvic scoring for elective induction. Obstet Gynecol 24:266, 1964

Bishop EH, Vollman R: Duration of labor and fetal outcome. Compendium, Collaborative Study on Cerebral Palsy, Mental Retardation, and Other Neurological and Sensory Disorders of Infancy and Childhood. Washington DC, June 13, 1963

Bisset GW, Walker JM: The effects of nicotine, hexamethonium and ethanol on the secretion of the antidiuretic and oxytocic hormones of the rat. Br J Pharmacol 12:461, 1957

Bonica JJ: Obstetric analgesia and anesthesia. NY State J Med 70:2079, 1970

Borell U, Fernström I: The mechanism of labour. Radiol Clin North Am 5:73, 1967

Boros HH, Priver MS: Ethchlorvynol as a sedative in labor. Am J Obstet Gynecol 89:1016, 1964

Bosomworth P, Sikora F, Welch CM: Fetal ECG and obstetrical blood loss with halothane anesthesia. Anesthesiology 23:140, 1962

Boysen H: Sparteine sulfate and rupture of the uterus: Report of a case. Obstet Gynecol 21:403, 1963

Brenner WE, Bruce RD, Hendricks CH: The characteristics and perils of breech presentation. Am J Obstet Gynecol 118:700, 1974

Bromage PR: Continuous lumbar epidural analgesia for obstetrics. Can Med Assoc J 85:1136, 1961

Browne PJ, Browne, JCMcL: Postgraduate Obstetrics and Gynaecology, 3rd ed. Washington, Butterworths, 1964

Brummer HC: Interaction of E prostaglandins and Syntocinon on the pregnant human myometrium. J Obstet Gynaecol Br Commonw 78:305, 1971

Burke L, Rubin HW, Berenberg AL: The significance of the unengaged vertex in a nullipara at thirty-eight weeks' gestation. Am J Obstet Gynecol 76:132, 1958

Burnhill MS, Danezis J, Cohen J: Uterine contractility during labor studied by intra-amniotic fluid pressure recordings. Am J Obstet Gynecol 83:572, 1962

Buxton CL: A Study of Psychophysical Methods for Relief of Childbirth Pain. Philadelphia, Saunders, 1962

Bygdeman M, Eliasson R: Effect of progesterone and oestrone on the motility and reactivity of the pregnant human myometrium in vitro. J Reprod Fertil 7:47, 1964

Calder A, Embrey MP: Prostaglandins and the unfavorable cervix. Lancet 2:1322, 1973

Caldeyro-Barcia R: Uterine contractility in obstetrics. Deux Cong Int Gynecol Obstet 1:65, 1958

Caldeyro-Barcia R: Contractility of the pregnant human uterus and controlling factors. Symposium on function of the pregnant uterus. XXI Int Cong Physiol Sci, Buenos Aires, 1959

Caldeyro-Barcia R: Factors controlling the actions of the pregnant human uterus. In Kowlessor, M (ed): Fifth Conference on Physiology of Prematurity. New York, Josiah Macy Jr Foundation, 1960.

Caldeyro-Barcia R, Alvarez H: Abnormal uterine action in labor. J Obstet Gynaecol Br Emp 59:646, 1952

Caldeyro-Barcia R, Heller H: Oxytocin. New York, Pergamon, 1961

Caldeyro-Barcia R, Pose SV, Alvarez H: Uterine contractility in polyhydramnios and the effects of withdrawal of the excess of amniotic fluid. Am J Obstet Gynecol 73:1238, 1957

Caldeyro-Barcia R, Poseiro JJ, Alvarez H, Tost P: The action of chlorpromazine on uterine contractility and arterial pressure in normal and toxemic pregnant women. Am J Obstet Gynecol 75:1088, 1958

Caldeyro-Barcia R, Sica-Blanco Y, Poseiro JJ, Gonzales-Panizza VH, Mendez-Bauer C, et al: A quantitative study of the action of synthetic oxytocin on the pregnant human uterus. J Pharmacol Exp Ther 121:18, 1957

Caldwell WE, Moloy HC: Anatomical variations in the female pelvis and their effect in labor with a suggested classification. Am J Obstet Gynecol 26:479, 1933

Caldwell WE, Moloy HC, Swenson PC: The use of roentgen ray in obstetrics. Am J Roentgenol Ther Nucl Med 41:305, 505, 719, 1939

Calkins LA: The length of labor: III. The first stage: Labor pains and consistency of cervix. Am J Obstet Gynecol 27:349, 1934
Calkins LA: On predicting the length of labor: I. First stage. Am J Obstet Gynecol 42:802, 1941
Calkins LA: Second stage of labor—the descent phase. Am J Obstet Gynecol 48: 798, 1944
Calkins LA: The importance of the firm cervix in prolonged labor. Am J Obstet Gynecol 67:801, 1954
Calkins LA: Normal Labor. Springfield, Charles C Thomas, 1955a
Calkins LA: Breech presentation. Am J Obstet Gynecol 60:977, 1955b.
Calkins LA: Abnormal Labor. Springfield, Charles C Thomas, 1958
Calkins LA, Irvine JH, Horsley GW: Variation in the length of labor. Am J Obstet Gynecol 19:294, 1930
Calkins LA, Litzenberg JC, Plass ED: The length of labor. Am J Obstet Gynecol 22:604, 1931
Campbell RE: Pregnancy and labor complicated by myomatous tumors of the uterus. Am J Obstet Gynecol 26:1, 1933
Campbell C, Phillips OC, Frazier TM: Analgesia during labor: A comparison of pentobarbital, meperidine, and morphine. Obstet Gynecol 17:714, 1961
Carroll JJ, Hudson PW: Chlorpromazine and promethazine in obstetrics. Can Anaesth Soc J 2:340, 1955
Carsten ME: Regulation of myometrial composition, growth and activity. In Assali NS (ed) : Biology of Gestation. New York, Academic, 1968
Castaño-Almendral JL, Arto-Medrano F: Intravenous high doses of orciprenaline (Alupent) in women during labor. Int J Gynaecol Obstet 12:204, 1974
Chen HY, Wei PY: Facial presentation and pelvic type. J Int Coll Surg 34:756, 1960
Chertok L: Psychosomatic methods of preparation for childbirth: spread of the methods, theory, and research. Am J Obstet Gynecol 98:698, 1967
Chik L, Hirsch VJ, Sokol RJ, Rosen MG: Temporal characterization of intrauterine pressure data. Am J Obstet Gynecol 120:496, 1974
Christhilf SM Jr, Monias MB, Riley RA Jr, Sheehan JC: Chlorpromazine in obstetric analgesia. Obstet Gynecol 15:625, 1960
Cibils LA, Pose SV, Zuspan FP: Effect of l-norepinephrine infusion on uterine contractility and cardiovascular system. Am J Obstet Gynecol 84:307, 1962
Cibils LA, Spackman TJ: Caudal anesthesia in first-stage labor: Effect on uterine activity and cardiovascular system. Am J Obstet Gynecol 84:1042, 1962
Cohen WR: Influence of the duration of second stage labor on perinatal outcome and puerperal morbidity. Obstet Gynecol 49:266, 1977
Collier MC, Savage RS: Gompertz curve fit. Hewlett-Packard HP-65 Library, StatPac 2-07A, 1975
Cooper K, Moir JC: Paracervical nerve block: A simple method of pain relief in labour. Br Med J 1:1372, 1963
Corbit JD Jr, First SE: Clinical comparison of phenazocine and meperidine in obstetric analgesia. Obstet Gynecol 18:488, 1961
Cowett RM, Oh W: Foam stability predictions of respiratory distress in infants delivered by repeat cesarean section. N Engl J Med 295:1222, 1976
Crawford JS: Place of halothane in obstetrics. Br J Anaesth 34:386, 1962
Crichton D: A reliable method of establishing the level of the fetal head in obstetrics. S Afr Med J 48:784, 1974

Crödel W: Wehenmessung durch die Bauchdecke. Arch Gynaekol 132:23, 1929

Crödel W: Uterusarbeitmessung oder Tokergometrie. Geburtshilfe Gynaekol 97:138, 1930

Csapo A: The mechanism of myometrial function and its disorders. In Bowes K (ed): Modern Trends in Obstetrics and Gynaecology. London, Butterworths, 1955

Csapo A: Progesterone "block." Am J Anat 98:273, 1956

Csapo A: Function and regulation of the myometrium. Ann NY Acad Sci 75:790, 1959

Csapo A: Facts and themes about parturition. Eleventh Annual Meeting of the American College of Obstetricians and Gynecologists. New York, April 22, 1963a

Csapo A: Model experiments and clinical trials in the control of pregnancy and parturition. Am J Obstet Gynecol 85:359, 1963b

Csapo A: The diagnostic significance of the intrauterine pressure. Obstet Gynecol Surv 25:403, 515, 1970

Csapo A, Sauvage JP, Pulkkinen MO, Wood EC: The relationship between placental location, uterine activity, and the duration of labor. Int J Gynaecol Obstet 8:811, 1970

Curran JT, MacGregor J, Kern J: The foetal ballistocardiograph. Second World Congress on Ballistocardiography and Cardiovascular Dynamics. Oporto, Portugal, 1969

Daels J: Uterine contractility patterns of the outer and inner zones of the myometrium. Obstet Gynecol 44:315, 1974

Danforth DN, Buckingham JC, Roddick JW: Connective tissue changes incident to cervical effacement. Am J Obstet Gynecol 80:939, 1960

Danforth DN, Veis A, Breen M, Weinstein HG, Buckingham, JC, et al: The effect of pregnancy and labor on the human cervix: Change in collagen, glycoproteins, and glycosaminoglycans. Am J Obstet Gynecol 120:641, 1974

Davis CD, Curi JFJ: A comparative clinical study of a prepared childbirth program. Conn Med 32:113, 1968

Davis CD, Morrone FA: An objective evaluation of a prepared childbirth program. Am J Obstet Gynecol 84:1196, 1962

Davis, DS: Empiric Equations and Nomography. New York, McGraw-Hill, 1943

Davis JE, Frudenfeld JC, Frudenfeld K, Webb AN: Paracervical block for pain relief in labor. Obstet Gynecol 19:195, 1962

Dede JA, Friedman EA: Face presentation. Am J Obstet Gynecol 87:515, 1963a

Dede JA, Friedman EA: Management of the face presentation. Bull Sloane Hosp 9:118, 1963b

De Kornfeld TJ, Pearson JW, Lasagna L: Methotrimeprazine in the treatment of labor pain. N Engl J Med 270:391, 1964

DeVoe K Jr, Rigsby WC, DeVoe SJ, Lewis GW, McDaniels BA: Effect of sparteine sulfate on uterine contractility. Am J Obstet Gynecol 105:304, 1969a

DeVoe SJ, DeVoe K Jr, Rigsby WC, McDaniels BA: Effect of meperidine on uterine contractility. Am J Obstet Gynecol 105:1004, 1969b

DiFrancesco G: L'importanza dell'indagine tocografica nell'uso di farmaci in travaglio di parto. Milan, 1963

DiFrancesco G, Ferrero A, Rossi GD: Effetti rilascianti prodotti dalla succinilcolina sulla muscolatura liscia uterina (Rilievi tocografici). Atti Accad Med Lombarda 17:1, 1962

Dill LV, Maiden RM: Further studies on the electrical potentials of the human uterus in labor. Am J Obstet Gynecol 56:213, 1948

Dodek SM: A new method for graphically recording the contractions of the parturient human uterus. Surg Gynecol Obstet 55:45, 1932

Dodek SM: External hysterographic studies of the effect of certain analgesics and anesthetics upon the parturient human uterus. Anesth Analg 13:8, 1934

Duignan NM, Studd JWW, Hughes AO: Characteristics of normal labour in different racial groups. Br J Obstet Gynaecol 82:539, 1975

Duncan C, Hindman JF, Mayberger HW: Chloroform as an obstetrical anesthetic: A report of 18,302 cases. Am J Obstet Gynecol 72:1004, 1956

Duncan SLB, Ginsburg J, Morris NF: Comparison of pentazocine and pethidine in normal labor. Am J Obstet Gynecol 105:197, 1969

Dunn, LJ, Van Voorhis L, Napier J: Term breech presentation: A report of 499 consecutive cases. Obstet Gynecol 25:170, 1965

du Vigneaud V, Ressler C, Swan JM, Roberts CW, Katsoyannis PG: The synthesis of oxytocin. J Am Chem Soc 76:3115, 1954

du Vigneaud V, Ressler C, Swan JM, Roberts CW Katsoyannis PG, et al: The synthesis of an octapeptide amide with the hormonal activity of oxytocin. J Am Chem Soc 75:4879, 1953a

du Vigneaud V, Ressler C, Trippett S: The sequence of amino acids in oxytocin, with a proposal for the structure of oxytocin. J Biol Chem 205:949, 1953b

Eastman NJ: Editorial comments on a paper by Garrett. Obstet Gynecol Surv 16:185, 1961

Eastman NJ, Hellman LM: Williams Obstetrics, 13th ed. New York, Appleton, 1966

Eckerling B, Goldman JA, Gano B: The combined intravenous use of Pethidine, Phenergan and Lorfan for analgesia in obstetrics. Obstet Gynecol 14:331, 1959

Effer SB, Bértola RP, Vrettos A, Caldeyro-Barcia R: Quantitative study of the regularity of uterine contractile rhythm in labor. Am J Obstet Gynecol 105:909, 1969

Eichner E, Waltner C, Goodman M, Post S: Relaxin the third ovarian hormone: Its experimental use in women. Am J Obstet Gynecol 71:1035, 1956

Elliot DF, Horton EW, Lewis GP: Actions of purse bradykinin. J Physiol 153:473, 1960

Embrey MP: The effect of acetylcholine on the intact human uterus. J Obstet Gynaecol Br Emp 65:531, 1958

Embrey MP: PGE compounds for induction of labour and abortion. Ann NY Acad Sci 180:518, 1971

Epstein BS, Coakley CS, Barter RH, Chamberlain G: New developments in epidural anesthesia for obstetrics. Am J Obstet Gynecol 106:996, 1970

Eskes TKAB: Effect of morphine upon uterine contractility in late pregnancy. Am J Obstet Gynecol 84:281, 1962

Evans JA, Chastain GM, Phillips JM: The use of local anesthetic agents in obstetrics. South Med J 62:519, 1969

Fabre M: Une méthode d'hystérographie externe. Bull Soc Obstet Gynecol 16:68, 1913

Felton DJC, Goddard BA: Effect of suxamethonium chloride on uterine activity. Lancet 1:852, 1966

Fetchko AM, Weber JE, Carroll JH, Thomas GJ: Intravenous alcohol used for preinduction analgesia in obstetrics. Am J Obstet Gynecol 62:662, 1951

Filler WW Jr, Hall WC, Filler NW: Analgesia in obstetrics: the effect of analgesia on uterine contractility and fetal heart rate. Am J Obstet Gynecol 98: 832, 1967

Finney DJ: Probit Analysis. Cambridge, England, Cambridge University Press, 1952

Flowers CE: Trilene, an adjunct to obstetrical anesthesia and analgesia. Am J Obstet Gynecol 65:1027, 1953

French TA: Repository tubocurarine in obstetrics. Obstet Gynecol 12:550, 1958

Frey E: Die Bedeutung der Wehentafel für die Physiologie und Pathologie der Geburt beim vorzeitigen Blasensprung. Schweiz Med Wochenschr 59:613, 1929

Frey E: Hat die Bestimmung der Wehenkontraktionsdauer eine klinische Bedeutung. Schweiz Med Wochenschr 60:558, 1930

Frey E: Der Hysterotonograph. Zentralbl Gynaekol 57:545, 1933

Frey E, and Fehr A: Die Höchstwehenzahlen und die Höchstwehenkontraktionsdauer, welche bei Erstgebärenden mit vorzeitigem Blasensprung bei Länslagen noch zur Spontangeburt führen. Z Geburtshilfe Gynaekol 96:468, 1929

Friedman EA: Graphic analysis of labor. Am J Obstet Gynecol 68:1568, 1954

Friedman EA: Primigravid labor: A graphicostatistical analysis. Obstet Gynecol 6:567, 1955a

Friedman EA: Graphic appraisal of labor: A study of 500 primigravidae. Bull Sloane Hosp 1:42, 1955b

Friedman EA: Cervimetry: An objective method for the study of cervical dilatation in labor. Am J Obstet Gynecol 71:1189, 1956a

Friedman EA: Labor in multiparas: A graphicostatistical analysis. Obstet Gynecol 8:691, 1956b

Friedman EA: Trial of labor: Formulation, application, and retrospective clinical evaluation. Obstet Gynecol 10:1, 1957a

Friedman EA: Synthetic oxytocin: Critical evaluation in labor and postpartum. Am J Obstet Gynecol 74:1118, 1957b

Friedman EA: Graphic analysis of labor. Bull Am Coll Nurse-Midwifery 4:94, 1959

Friedman EA: Uterine inertia. Trans N Engl Obstet Gynecol Soc 15:129, 1961

Friedman EA: Management of the prolonged latent phase of labor. Bull Sloane Hosp 8:77, 1962

Friedman EA: The study of labor by graphic analysis, with discussion of the action of Tocosamine in labor. Bull Middlesex Gen Hosp 8:1, 1963a

Friedman EA: Management of secondary arrest of dilatation. Bull Sloane Hosp 9:18, 1963b

Friedman EA: The value of preparation for childbirth: A forum. Mod Med 31: 288, 1963c

Friedman EA: The introduction of objectivity to the management of abnormal labor. Bull Sloane Hosp 10:121, 1964

Friedman EA: Dysfunctional labor in clinical practice. Ob/Gyn Digest 7:23, 1965a

Friedman EA: The effect of amniotomy during labor in multiparas (Letter). Obstet Gynecol 25:140, 1965b

Friedman EA: Effects of drugs on uterine contractility. Anesthesiology 26:409, 1965c

Friedman EA: Abnormal labor. Hosp Med 2:30, 1965d

Friedman EA: Use of labor pattern as a management guide. Hosp Topics 46:57, 1968

Friedman EA: Stimulation and induction of labor. Chicago Med 72:127, 1969a

Friedman EA: A rational view of dysfunctional labor. In Reid DE, Barton TC (eds): Controversy in Obstetrics and Gynecology. Philadelphia, Saunders, 1969b

Friedman EA: An objective method of evaluating labor. Hosp Pract 5:82, 1970

Friedman EA: Functional divisions of labor. Am J Obstet Gynecol 109:274, 1971

Friedman EA: An objective approach to the diagnosis and management of abnormal labor. Bull NY Acad Med 48:842, 1972

Friedman EA: Obstetric infection in labor. In Charles D, Finland M (eds): Obstetric and Perinatal Infections. Philadelphia, Lea & Febiger, 1973a

Friedman EA: Dysfunctional labor. In Rovinsky JJ (ed): Davis' Gynecology and Obstetrics. New York, Harper & Row, 1973b

Friedman EA: Patterns of labor as indicators of risk. Clin Obstet Gynecol 16:172, 1973c

Friedman EA: The Management of Disordered Labor. New York, Medcom, 1974a

Friedman EA: Failure to progress in labor. Contemp Obstet Gynecol 4:41, 1974b

Friedman EA: Partograms and nomograms of cervical dilatation in management of primigravid labor (Editorial note). In Greenhill JP (ed): Year Book of Obstetrics and Gynecology. Chicago, Year Book, 1975a

Friedman EA: Disordered labor: Objective evaluation and management. J Family Pract 2:167, 1975b

Friedman EA: Evaluation and management of pelvic dystocia. Contemp Obstet Gynecol 7:155, 1976a

Friedman EA: A prerecorded program for the Ball pelvimetry technique. Am J Obstet Gynecol 126:477, 1976b

Friedman EA, Hunt HB, Sachtleben MR: Disordered labor: Simplified method for recognition. Ob/Gyn Digest 17:12, 1975

Friedman EA, Kroll BH: Computer analysis of labour progression. J Obstet Gynaecol Br Commonw 76:1075, 1969

Friedman EA, Kroll BH: Computer analysis of labor progression: II. Distribution of data and limits of normal. J Reprod Med 6:20, 1971a

Friedman EA, Kroll BH: Computer analysis of labor progression: III. Pattern variations by parity. J Reprod Med 6:179, 1971b

Friedman EA, Kroll BH: Computer analysis of labor progression: IV. Diagnosis of secondary arrest of dilatation. J Reprod Med 7:176, 1971c

Friedman EA, Kroll BH: Use of the computer in the analysis of labor progression. Ninth Annual Symposium on Biomathematics and Computer Sciences in the Life Sciences. Houston, 1971d.

Friedman EA, Kroll BH: Computer analysis of labor: V. Effects of fetal presentation and position. J Reprod Med 8:117, 1972

Friedman EA, Little WA: Evaluation of the management of the twin delivery. Bull Sloane Hosp 4:39, 1958

Friedman EA, Little WA: Significance of the placental site. Compendium, Collaborative Study on Cerebral Palsy, Mental Retardation and other Neurological and Sensory Disorders of Infancy and Childhood. Washington DC, 1963

Friedman EA, Niswander KR, Bayonet-Rivera NP, Sachtleben MR: Relation of prelabor evaluation to inducibility and the course of labor. Obstet Gynecol 28:495, 1966

Friedman EA, Niswander KR, Bayonet-Rivera NP, Sachtleben MR: Pre-labor status evaluation: II. Weighted score. Obstet Gynecol 29:539, 1967

Friedman EA, Niswander KR, Sachtleben MS, Nemore J: Dysfunctional labor: VIII. Relative accuracy of clinical and graphic diagnostic methods. Obstet Gynecol 33:145, 1969a

Friedman EA, Niswander KR, Sachtleben MR, Naftaly N: Dysfunctional labor: X. Immediate result to infant. Obstet Gynecol 33:776, 1969b

Friedman EA, Niswander KR, Sachtleben MR: Dysfunctional labor: XI. Neurological and developmental effects on surviving infants. Obstet Gynecol 33:785, 1969c

Friedman EA, Niswander KR, Sachtleben MR: Effect of diazepam on labor. Obstet Gynecol 34:82, 1969d

Friedman EA, Niswander KR, Sachtleben MR, Ashworth M: Dysfunctional labor: IX. Delivery outcome. Am J Obstet Gynecol 106:219, 1970

Friedman EA, Sachtleben MR: Caudal anesthesia: The factors that influence its effect on labor. Obstet Gynecol 13:442, 1959

Friedman EA, Sachtleben MR: Dysfunctional labor: I. Prolonged latent phase in the nullipara. Obstet Gynecol 17:135, 1961a

Friedman EA, Sachtleben MR: Dysfunctional labor: II. Protracted active phase dilatation in the nullipara. Obstet Gynecol 17:566, 1961b

Friedman EA, Sachtleben MR: Dysfunctional labor: III. Secondary arrest of dilatation in the nullipara. Obstet Gynecol 19:576, 1962a

Friedman EA, Sachtleben MR: The determinant role of initial cervical dilatation on the course of labor. Am J Obstet Gynecol 84:930, 1962b

Friedman EA, Sachtleben MR: Dysfunctional labor: IV. Combined aberrant dilatation patterns in the nullipara. Obstet Gynecol 20:761, 1962c

Friedman EA, Sachtleben MR: Dysfunctional labor: V. Therapeutic trial of oxytocin in secondary arrest. Obstet Gynecol 21:13, 1963a

Friedman EA, Sachtleben MR: Dysfunctional labor: VI. Abnormal progress in the multipara. Obstet Gynecol 22:478, 1963b

Friedman EA, Sachtleben MR: Amniotomy and the course of labor. Obstet Gynecol 22:755, 1963c

Friedman EA, Sachtleben MR: The effect of uterine overdistention on labor: I. Multiple pregnancy. Obstet Gynecol 23:164, 1964a

Friedman EA, Sachtleben MR: The effect of uterine overdistention on labor: II. Hydramnios. Obstet Gynecol 23:401, 1964b

Friedman EA, Sachtleben MR: Relation of maternal age to the course of labor. Am J Obstet Gynecol 91:915, 1965a

Friedman EA, Sachtleben MR: Dysfunctional labor: VII. A comprehensive program for diagnosis, evaluation, and management. Obstet Gynecol 25:844, 1965b

Friedman EA, Sachtleben MR: Station of the fetal presenting part: I. Pattern of descent. Am J Obstet Gynecol 93:522, 1965c

Friedman EA, Sachtleben MR: Station of the fetal presenting part: II. Effect on the course of labor. Am J Obstet Gynecol 93:530, 1965d

Friedman EA, Sachtleben MR: Station of the fetal presenting part: III. Interrelationship with cervical dilatation. Am J Obstet Gynecol 93:537, 1965e

Friedman EA, Sachtleben MR: Prognostic significance of the labor pattern in multiparas. Am J Obstet Gynecol 98:466, 1967

Friedman EA, Sachtleben MR: Influence of placental weight on labor. Obstet Gynecol 33:404, 1969a

Friedman EA, Sachtleben MR: Preterm labor. Am J Obstet Gynecol 104:1152, 1969b

Friedman EA, Sachtleben MR: Station of the fetal presenting part: IV. Slope of descent. Am J Obstet Gynecol 107:1031, 1970a

Friedman EA, Sachtleben MR: Station of the fetal presenting part: V. Protracted descent patterns. Obstet Gynecol 36:558, 1970b

Friedman EA, Sachtleben MR: High risk labor. J Reprod Med 7:52, 1971

Friedman EA, Sachtleben MR: Oral prostaglandin $E_2$ for induction of labor at term. Obstet Gynecol 43:178, 1974

Friedman EA, Sachtleben MR: Preinduction priming with oral prostaglandin $E_2$. Am J Obstet Gynecol 121:521, 1975a

Friedman EA, Sachtleben MR, Green W: Oral prostaglandin $E_2$ for induction of labor at term: II. Comparison of two low-dosage regimens. Am J Obstet Gynecol 123:671, 1975b

Friedman EA, Sachtleben MR: Station of the fetal presenting part: VI. Arrest of descent in nulliparas. Obstet Gynecol 47:129, 1976

Friedman EA, Sachtleben MR, Bresky PA: Dysfunctional labor: XII. Long-term effects on infant. Am J Obstet Gynecol 127:779, 1977

Friedman EA, Taylor MB: A modified nomographic aid for cephalopelvimetry. Am J Obstet Gynecol 105:1110, 1969; 106:884, 1970

Friedman EA, Von Micsky LI: Electronic cervimeter: A research instrument for the study of cervical dilatation in labor. Am J Obstet Gynecol 87:789, 1963

Fuchs A-R: Effect of intra-amniotic administration of progesterone and 6-methyl-17-acetoxy-progesterone on oxytocin-induced labor in rabbits. Acta Endocrinol 46:235, 1964

Fuchs F: Endocrinology of labor. In Fuchs F, Klopper A (eds): Endocrinology of Pregnancy. New York, Harper & Row, 1971

Fuchs F, Fuchs A-R, Poblete VF Jr, Risk A: Effect of alcohol on threatened premature labor. Am J Obstet Gynecol 99:627, 1967

Garrett WJ: Uterine overdistention and the duration of labour. Med J Aust 47:376, 1960

Geisendorf W: Le nombre des contractions dans l'accouchement dirigé. Gynecol Obstet 35:355, 1937

Gillespie A: Prostaglandin-oxytocin enhancement and potentiation and their clinical application. Br Med J 1:150, 1972

Glick E, Craig WSR, Trussell RR: Curve of labor as a screening device: Early recognition of protracted labor. Obstet Gynecol 38:69, 1971

Glick E, Trussell RR: The curve of labour used as a teaching device in Uganda. J Obstet Gynaecol Br Commonw 77:1003, 1970

Gluck L, Kulovich MV, Borer RC Jr, Brenner PH, Anderson GG, et al: Diagnosis of the respiratory distress syndrome by amniocentesis. Am J Obstet Gynecol 109:440, 1971

Goldfarb WS: Myometrial response: Activity of isolated strips of myometrium from the pregnant human uterus at term. Obstet Gynecol 3:248, 1954

Graham FK, Ernhart CB, Thurston D: The relationship of neonatal apnea to the development at three years. Res Publ Assoc Res Nerv Ment Dis 39:159, 1962

Grandin DJ: A review of 445 pregnancies complicated by fibromyomas. Am J Obstet Gynecol 57:532, 1949

Gready TG Jr, Estrada WJ, Haden J: Intramuscular perphenazine in labor: A study of 700 patients. Am J Obstet Gynecol 77:412, 1959

Greenhill JP: Analgesia and Anesthesia in Obstetrics. Springfield, Charles C Thomas, 1962

Greenhill JP, Friedman EA: Soft-tissue dystocia. Hosp Med 4:73, 1968

Greenhill JP, Friedman EA: Biological Principles and Modern Practice of Obstetrics. Philadelphia, Saunders, 1974

Gruenwald P, Minh HN: Evaluation of body and organ weights: II. Weight of body and placenta of surviving and of autopsied infants. Am J Obstet Gynecol 82:312, 1961

Hall DG, McGaughey HS Jr, Corey EL, Thornton WN Jr: The effects of magnesium therapy on the duration of labor. Am J Obstet Gynecol 78:27, 1959

Hall, JE, Kohl SG, O'Brien F, Ginsberg M: Breech presentation and perinatal mortality: A study of 6,044 cases. Am J Obstet Gynecol 91:665, 1965

Hallet RL: The conduct of labor and results with continuous caudal anesthesia. Am J Obstet Gynecol 66:54, 1953

Halliday EC, Heyns O: The activity of the gravid uterus. J Obstet Gynaecol Br Emp 49:309, 1952

Harer WB: Chlorpromazine in normal labor. Obstet Gynecol 8:1, 1956

Harer WB: Tranquilizers in obstetrics and gynecology: Studies with Trilafon. Obstet Gynecol 11:273, 1958

Harkins JL, Van Praagh IG, Irwin NT: A clinical evaluation of intravenous dimenhydrinate in labor. Can Med J 91:164, 1964

Harris JS, Gillespie EC: Development of methods for studying human uterine contractions in pregnancy. Obstet Gynecol Surv 5:1, 1950

Harris VG: Relation between placental site and length of gestation. Br J Obstet Gynaecol 82:581, 1975

Harrison KA, Ibeziako PA: Maternal anaemia and fetal birthweight. J Obstet Gynaecol Br Commonw 80:798, 1973

Healy TEJ: Suxamethonium and intrauterine pressure. Br J Anaesth 43:1156, 1971

Hendricks CH: Use of isoxsuprine for the arrest of premature labor. Clin Obstet Gynecol 7:687, 1964a

Hendricks CH: Patterns of fetal and placental growth: The second half of pregnancy. Obstet Gynecol 24:357, 1964b

Hendricks CH: Unpublished data, cited in Danforth DN: Textbook of Obstetrics and Gynecology. New York, Hoeber, 1966

Hendricks CH, Brenner WE, Gabel RA, Kerenyi T: In Barnes AC (ed): Progesterone. Augusta, Michigan, Brook Lodge Press, 1961

Hendricks CH, Brenner WE, Kraus G: Normal cervical dilatation pattern in late pregnancy and labor. Am J Obstet Gynecol 10:1065, 1970

Hendricks CH, Quilligan EJ, Tyler CW, Tucker GJ: Pressure relationships between the intervillous space and the amniotic fluid in human term pregnancy. Am J Obstet Gynecol 77:1028, 1959

Hershenson BB, Isaac SJ, Romney SL, Reid DE: A new sedative (antipsychomotor) drug useful in labor: Preliminary report. N Engl J Med 251:216, 1954

Hillis DS: Diagnosis of contracted pelvis. Ill Med J 74:131, 1938

Hogaki M: Analysis of the intrauterine pressure during labor based on simulation. Acta Obstet Gynecol Jpn 16:165, 1969

Hon EH, Paul RH: Quantitation of uterine activity. Obstet Gynecol 42:368, 1973

Hughes EC (ed): Obstetric-Gynecologic Terminology. Philadelphia, Davis, 1972

Hunter CA: Uterine motility studies during labor: Observation on bilateral sympathetic nerve block in the normal and abnormal first stage of labor. Am J Obstet Gynecol 85:681, 1963

Hutchinson HT, Nichols MM, Kuhn CR, Vasicka A: Effects of magnesium sulfate on uterine contractility, intrauterine fetus, and infant. Am J Obstet Gynecol 88:747, 1964

Ince JGH, Young M: The bony pelvis and its influence on labour: A radiobiological and clinical study of 500 women. J Obstet Gynaecol Br Emp 47:130, 1940

Ingleman-Sundberg A, Lindgren L: Intrauterine measurement of pressure during labour. J Obstet Gynaecol Br Emp 62:629, 1955

Inmon WB: A study of the effect of hydroxyzine hydrochloride on labor and delivery. Am J Obstet Gynecol 86:853, 1963

Israel SL, Groeber WR Jr: Relaxin: A persistent challenge. Obstet Gynecol 15:2, 1960

Jacobs JB: Management and outcome of labor in 742 women with borderline pelves. Am J Obstet Gynecol 43:267, 1942

Jacobson LJ, Johnson CE: Brow and face presentation. Am J Obstet Gynecol 84: 1881, 1962

Jeffcoate TNA, Baker K, Martin RH: Inefficient uterine action. Surg Gynecol Obstet 95:257, 1952

Jenssen H: The effect of paracervical block on cervical dilatation and uterine activity. Acta Obstet Gynecol Scand 52:13, 1973

Johansen K: Graphic records in labour. Br Med J 1:612, 1973

Johnson WL, Depp R, Hunter CA Jr: Comparison of spontaneous, oxytocin-stimulated and hypertonic saline-induced labor by different methods of record analysis. Am J Obstet Gynecol 107:268, 1970

Johnson WL, McGaughey HS, Scoggin WA, Wilson LA, Thornton WN: Effect of certain smooth muscle depressants on isolated human myometrial tissues. Am J Obstet Gynecol 86:296, 1963

Kaltreider DF: Effects of Height and Weight on Pregnancy and the Newborn. Springfield, Charles C Thomas, 1963

Kapp FT, Hornstein S, Graham VT: Some psychological factors in prolonged labor due to inefficient uterine action. Compr Psychiatry 4:9, 1963

Kappelman MD: Prochlorperazine in labor and delivery. Obstet Gynecol 19:118, 1962

Karim SMM: Effects of oral administration of prostaglandins $E_2$ and $F_{2\alpha}$ on the human uterus. J Obstet Gynaecol Br Commonw 78:289, 1971

Karim SMM, Sharma SD: Oral administration of prostaglandin $E_2$ for the induction and acceleration of labor. J Reprod Med 9:346, 1972

Karim SMM, Trussell RR, Patel RC, Hillier K: Response of pregnant human uterus to prostaglandin-$F_{2\alpha}$-induction of labour. Br Med J 4:621, 1968

Karim SMM, Trussell RR, Hillier K: Induction of labour with prostaglandin $F_{2\alpha}$. J Obstet Gynaecol Br Commonw 76:769, 1969

Kasius RV, Randall A, Tompkins WT, Wiehl DG: Maternal and newborn studies at Philadelphia Lying-In Hospital. Milbank Mem Fund Quart 36:335, 1958

Keetel WC, Diddle AW, Plass ED: Premature elective rupture of the membranes. Am J Obstet Gynecol 40:225, 1940

Kelly JV: The effect of intravenous estrogens on uterine motility. Am J Obstet Gynecol 82:1207, 1961

Kelly JV, Posse N: Hormone relaxin in labor: Tocometric studies of its effect on uterine contractions at term. Obstet Gynecol 8:531, 1956

Kepka A, Bieniarz J, Mutschler L, Shah N, Scommegna A: Uterine contractility data processing system. Am J Obstet Gynecol 123:246, 1975

King AG: Newer concepts of dry labor. JAMA 114:238, 1940

King EL: Occipitoposterior Positions. Springfield, Charles C Thomas, 1957

Klapholz H: A computerized aid to Ball pelvimetry. Am J Obstet Gynecol 121: 1067, 1975

Kobak AJ, Sadove MS: Combined paracervical and pudendal nerve blocks: Simple form of transvaginal regional anesthesia. Am J Obstet Gynecol 81:72, 1961

Kok FT, Wallenburg HCS, Wladimiroff JW: Ultrasonic measurement of cervical dilatation during labor. Am J Obstet Gynecol 126:288, 1976

Koller T: Versuch einer graphischen Darstellung des Geburtsverlaufes. Gynaecologia 126:227, 1948

Koller T, Abt K: Das vertikale Partogramm als zusätzliche Kontrolle des Geburtsverlaufes. Gynaecologia 130:419, 1950

Koller T, Abt K: Résultats de l'étude du "diagramme d'accouchement." Rev Franc Gynecol Obstet 47:163, 1952

Konzett H, Berde B, Cerletti A: Syntocinon, ein synthetisches uterus wirksames Hypophysenhinterlappenhormon. Schweiz Med Wochenschr 86:226, 1956

Korda AR, Lyneham RC, Jones WR: The treatment of premature labour with intravenously administered salbutamol. Med J Aust 1:744, 1974

Kornmesser JG, Nyboer J: Electrical and dynamic changes in uterine activity during labor (as measured by electrohysterograms and radiofrequency impedance plethysmograms) . Harper Hosp Bull 20:248, 1962

Krapohl AJ, Myers GG, Caldeyro-Barcia R: Uterine contractions in spontaneous labor: A quantitative study. Am J Obstet Gynecol 106:378, 1970

Kroc RL, Steinetz BG, Beach VL: The effects of estrogens, progestogens and relaxin in pregnant and nonpregnant laboratory rodents. Ann NY Acad Sci 75: 942, 1959

Kroenig W: Der Ersatz der inneren Untersuchung Kreissender durch die Untersuchung per rectum. Zentralbl Gynaekol 18:235, 1894

Kumar D, Goodno JA, Barnes AC: Studies in human myometrium during pregnancy: IV. In vitro progesterone-oxytocin relationship. Am J Obstet Gynecol 84:1111, 1962

Kumar D, Goodno JA, Barnes AC: In vitro effects of intravenous progesterone infusion on human gravid uterine contractility. Bull Johns Hopkins Hosp 113: 53, 1963a

Kumar D, Zourlas PA: Studies on human premature births: II. In vivo effect of nicotine on human uterine contractility. Am J Obstet Gynecol 87:413, 1963

Kumar D, Zourlas PA, Barnes AC: In vitro and in vivo effects of magnesium sulfate on human uterine contractility. Am J Obstet Gynecol 86:1036, 1963b

Kumar D, Zourlas PA, Barnes AC: In vivo effect of amyl nitrite on human pregnant uterus contractility. Am J Obstet Gynecol 91:1066, 1965

LaCroix GE: Monitoring of labor by an external tokodynamometer. Am J Obstet Gynecol 101:111, 1968

Laird MD, Hogan M: An elective program on preparation for childbirth at the Sloane Hospital for Women. Am J Obstet Gynecol 72: 641, 1956

Lamaze F: Painless Childbirth: Psychoprophylactic Method. London, Burke, 1958

Landesman R, Campbell, WL, Wilson KH: Uterine relaxant properties of bradykinin in vitro. Obstet Gynecol 22:102, 1963

Landesman R, deSouza JA, Coutinho EM, Wilson KH, de Souza MB: The inhibitory effect of diazoxide in normal term labor. Am J Obstet Gynecol 103: 430, 1969

Landesman R, Wilson KH: Relaxant effect of diazepam on uterine muscle. Obstet Gynecol 26:552, 1965

Landesman R, Wilson KH, Coutinho EM, Klima IM, Marcous RS: The relaxant action of ritodrine, a sympathomimetic amine, on the uterus during term labor. Am J Obstet Gynecol 110:111, 1971

Langreder W: Geburtshilfliche Messungen. Bibl Gynaecol 20:9, 1959

Ledger WJ: Monitoring of labor by graphs. Obstet Gynecol 34:174, 1969

Lee DT: The effects of diazepam (Valium) on labour. Can Med Assoc J 98:446, 1968

Lee JG: Transvaginal pudendal nerve block: A new technique. Am J Obstet Gynecol 77:419, 1959

Lekprasert V: Monitoring of labour by graph. J Med Assoc Thai 55:647, 1972

Leonard RF: Evaluation of selection tendencies of patients preferring prepared childbirth. Obstet Gynecol 42:371, 1973

Liepmann W: Die Grössenbestimmung des äusseren Muttermundes in der Geburt, ein Vorschlag für Unterricht und Praxis. Zentralbl Gynaekol 45:1289, 1921

Liggins GC, Vaughn GS: Intravenous infusion of salbutamol in the management of premature labour. J Obstet Gynaecol Br Commonw 80:29, 1973

Lindgren L: The influence of uterine motility upon cervical dilatation in labor. Am J Obstet Gynecol 117:530, 1973

Lindgren L, Holmlund D: Friction between the foetal head and the cervix during labour. Acta Obset Gynecol Scand 48:479, 1969a

Lindgren L, Holmlund D: Friction between the fetal head and uterine wall during normal labor and lower uterine spasm. Am J Obstet Gynecol 103:939, 1969b

Lindgren CL, Smyth CN: Measurement and interpretation of the pressure upon the cervix during normal and abnormal labour. J Obstet Gynaecol Br Commonw 68:901, 1961

Little WA: The significance of the placental position in utero. Am J Obstet Gynecol 90:328, 1964

Little WA, Friedman EA: The twin delivery: Factors influencing second twin mortality. Obstet Gynecol Surv 13:611, 1958a

Little WA, Friedman EA: Anesthesia for the twin delivery. Anesthesiology 19: 515, 1958b

Little WA, Friedman EA: Significance of the placental position: A report of the Collaborative Study of Cerebral Palsy. Obstet Gynecol 23:804, 1964

Lóránd S: Über einen neuen Wehenzeichnenden Apparat (Tokograph). Zentralbl Gynaekol 57:554, 1933

Lóránd S: Erfahrungen mit dem modifixierten Tokograph. Monatschr Geburtshilfe Gynaekol 103:137, 1936

Margolis K: Behaviour of the cervix and the presenting vertex in labour in blacks and Indians of Natal. S Afr Med J 48:791, 1974

Matthews AEB: Double-blind trials of promazine in labour. Br Med J 2:423, 1963

McElin TW, Horton BT: The administration of histamine during pregnancy: Apparent lack of a clinical oxytocic effect with small doses. Am J Med Sci 218: 432, 1949

McGarry J, Pearson JF: Time of onset and duration of labour in women with cardiac disease. Lancet 1:483, 1973

McGaughey HS Jr, Corey EL, Eastwood D, Thornton WN Jr: Effect of synthetic anesthetics on the spontaneous motility of human uterine muscle in vitro. Obstet Gynecol 19:233, 1962

McGaughey HS Jr, Corey EL, Thornton WN Jr: An evaluation of the action of relaxin on isolated human uterine muscle and cervical tissues in vitro. Am J Obstet Gynecol 75:23, 1958

Meltzer RM, Sachtleben MR, Friedman EA: Brow presentation. Am J Obstet Gynecol 100:255, 1968

Miller FC, Yeh S-Y, Schifrin BS, Paul RH, Hon EH: Quantitation of uterine activity in 100 primiparous patients. Am J Obstet Gynecol 124:398, 1976

Miller JR, Stoelting VK: Halothane in obstetric anesthesia. Anesthesiology 26: 256, 1965

Miller JR, Stoelting VK, Stander RW, Watring W: In vitro and in vivo responses of the uterus to halothane anesthesia. Anesth Analg 45:583, 1966

Moir DD: Anesthesia for caesarean section: An evaluation of a method using low concentrations of halothane and 50 per cent of oxygen. Br J Anaesth 42:136, 1970

Moloy HC, Steer CM: A new method of quantitative estimation of cephalopelvic disproportion. Am J Obstet Gynecol 60:1135, 1950

Moya F: Obstetric anesthesia: General principles. Bull Sloane Hosp 6:41, 1960

Moya F: General anesthesia in obstetrics. J Int Fed Gynaecol Obstet 1:195, 1963

Müller P: Untersuchungen über die Verkürzung der Vaginalportion in den letzten Monaten der Gravidität. Beitr Geburtshilfe Gynaekol 5:191, 1868

Müller P: Über die Prognose der Geburt bei engem Becken. Arch Gynaekol 27: 311, 1886

Munson ES: Effects of anesthetics on uterus and labor. In Schnider SM, Moya F (eds): The Anesthesiologist, Mother and Newborn. Baltimore, Williams and Wilkins, 1974

Munson ES, Maier WR, Caton D: Effects of halothane, cyclopropane and nitrous oxide on isolated human uterine muscle. J Obstet Gynaecol Br Commonw 76:27, 1969

Murphy DP: Uterine Contractility in Pregnancy. Philadelphia, Lippincott, 1947

Myers GG, Krapohl AJ, Varner J: Fourier series analysis of amniotic fluid contraction waves. Obstet Gynecol 30:327, 1967

Nisbet R, Boulas SH, Kantor HI: Diazepam (Valium) during labor. Obstet Gynecol 29:726, 1967

Niswander KR: Effects of diazepam on meperidine requirements of patients during labor. Obstet Gynecol 34:62, 1969

Niswander KR, Friedman EA, Hoover DB, Pietrowski H, Westphal MC: Fetal morbidity following potentially anoxigenic obstetric conditions: I. Abruptio placentae. Am J Obstet Gynecol 95:838, 1966a

Niswander KR, Friedman EA, Hoover DB, Pietrowski H, Westphal MC: Fetal morbidity following potentially anoxigenic obstetric conditions: II. Placenta previa. Am J Obstet Gynecol 95:846, 1966b

Niswander KR, Friedman EA, Hoover DB, Pietrowski H, Westphal MC: Fetal morbidity following potentially anoxigenic obstetric conditions: III. Prolapse of the umbilical cord. Am J Obstet Gynecol 95:853, 1966c

Niswander KR, Friedman EA, Hoover DB, Pietrowski H, Westphal MC: Fetal morbidity following potentially anoxigenic obstetric conditions: IV. Occult prolapse of the umbilical cord. Am J Obstet Gynecol 95:1099, 1966d

Niswander KR, Friedman EA, Bayonet-Rivera NP: Prelabor pelvic score as a predictor of birth weight. Obstet Gynecol 29:256, 1967

Niswander KR, Patterson RJ: Hazards of elective induction of labor. Obstet Gynecol 22:228, 1963

Norris PR: The action of cardiac glycosides on the human uterus. J Obstet Gynaecol Br Commonw 68:916, 1961

Norton HI, Weingarten M, McDonough ET: Chlorpromazine (phenothiazine derivative) in obstetric sedation. Am J Obstet Gynecol 71:1251, 1956

Notelovitz M: Graphic records in labour. Br Med J 1:50, 1973

Nyboer J, Kornmesser JG: Electrical impedance of the abdomen during maternal labor. Ann NY Acad Sci 170:801, 1970

O'Driscoll K, Jackson RJA, Gallagher JT: Active management of labour and cephalopelvic disproportion. J Obstet Gynaecol Br Commonw 77:385, 1970

O'Driscoll K, Stronge JM, Minogue M: Active management of labour. Br Med J 3:135, 1973

Olson RO, Riva HL: Evaluation of phenazocine with meperidine as an analgesic agent during labor by the double blind method. Am J Obstet Gynecol 88:601, 1964

Oppenheim BE, Griem ML, Meier P: Effects of diagnostic x-ray exposure on human fetus: Examination of evidence. Radiology 114:529, 1975

Ovadia L, Halbrecht I: Neuroleptanalgesia: A new method of anesthesia for normal childbirth. Harefuah 72:143, 1967

Persianinov LS, Davydov SN: A radiotelemetric study of uterine activity in labour. Acta Obstet Gynecol Scand 50:269, 1971

Peterson WF, Richey TW: Routine vaginal examinations during labor: Comparative study with bacteriologic analysis. Ill Med J 122:35, 1962

Pettit AV, Garland LH, Dunn RD, Shumaker P: Correlation between the shape of the female pelvis and the clinical course of labor. West J Surg 44:1, 1936

Phillips OC, Lyons WB, Campbell C, Frazier TM: Trilafon analgesia during labor. Obstet Gynecol 15:182, 1960

Philpott RH: Graphic records in labour. Br Med J 4:163, 1972

Philpott RH, Castle WM: Cervicographs in the management of labour in primigravidae: I. The alert line for detecting abnormal labour. J Obstet Gynaecol Br Commonw 79:592, 1972a

Philpott RH, Castle WM: Cervicographs in the management of labour in primigravidae: II. The action line and treatment of abnormal labour. J Obstet Gynaecol Br Commonw 79:599, 1972b

Pinto RM, Fisch L, Schwarcz RL, Montuori E: Action of estradiol 17-$\beta$ upon uterine contractility and the milk-ejecting effect in the pregnant woman. Am J Obstet Gynecol 90:99, 1964a

Pinto RM, Votta RA, Montuori E, Baleiron H: Action of estradiol 17-$\beta$ on the activity of the pregnant human uterus. Am J Obstet Gynecol 88:759, 1964b

Pitkin RM, Goddard WB: Paracervical and uterosacral block in obstetrics: A controlled double-blind study. Obstet Gynecol 21:737, 1963

Pittinger CB, Morris LE, Keettel WC: Vaginal deliveries during profound curarization. Am J Obstet Gynecol 65:635, 1953

Plentl AA, Friedman EA: Sparteine sulfate: A clinical evaluation of its use for the induction of labor. Am J Obstet Gynecol 85:200, 1963

Plentl AA, Friedman EA, Gray MJ: Sparteine sulfate: A clinical evaluation of its use in the management of labor. Am J Obstet Gynecol 82:1332, 1961

Pollock GB, Spitzer JJ, Mason DJ: Promazine for obstetrical sedation-analgesia. Obstet Gynecol 15:504, 1960

Pose SV, Cibils LA, Zuspan, FP: Effect of l-epinephrine infusion of uterine contractility and cardiovascular system. Am J Obstet Gynecol 84:297, 1962

Poseiro JJ, Sica-Blanco Y, Cibils LA, Negreiros de Paiva CE, Burnhill MS: Effects of relaxin on uterine contractility, response to oxytocin and cervical dilatability. XXI Int Cong Physiol Sci, Buenos Aires, 1959

Posner AC, Friedman S, Posner LB: Modern trends in the management of face and brow presentation. Surg Gynecol Obstet 104: 485, 1957

Potter N, MacDonald RD: Obstetric consequences of epidural analgesia in nulliparous patients. Lancet 1:1031, 1971

Pritchard JA, MacDonald PC: Williams Obstetrics, 15th ed. New York, Appleton, 1976

Read GD: Childbirth Without Fear. New York, Harper and Brothers, 1959

Reich AM: Paravertebral lumbar sympathetic block in labor. Am J Obstet Gynecol 61:1263, 1951

Reich AM: Paravertebral sympathetic block anesthesia in labor: Its benefits and accomplishments. Obstet Gynecol 1:672, 1953

Reier CE, Moster WG: Effects of neuromuscular blocking agents on uterine contractions in vitro. Am J Obstet Gynecol 108:610, 1970

Renaud R, Irrmann M, Gandar R, Flynn MJ: The use of ritodrine in the treatment of premature labour. J Obstet Gynaecol Br Commonw 81:182, 1974

Reynolds SRM: Uterine contractility and cervical dilation. Proc R Soc Med 44: 695, 1951

Reynolds SRM: Physiology of the Uterus, 2nd ed. New York, Hafner, 1965

Reynolds SRM, Harris JS, Kaiser IH: Clinical Measurement of Uterine Forces in Pregnancy and Labor. Springfield, Charles C Thomas, 1954

Reynolds SRM, Heard OO, Burns P: Recording uterine contraction patterns in pregnant women: Application of the strain-gage in a multi-channel tokodynamometer. Science 106:427, 1947

Ries D: Über die innere Untersuchung Kreissender durch den Mastdarm. Zentralbl Gynaekol 18:404, 1894

Robertson DNS, Guttmann L: The paraplegic patient in pregnancy and labour. Proc R Soc Med 56:381, 1963

Rossier AB, Ruffieux M, Ziegler WH: Pregnancy and labour in high traumatic spinal cord lesions. Paraplegia 7:210, 1969

Rothman ED, Bentley WG, Floyd WS: The use of relaxin (Cervilaxin) in accelerating the first stage of labor. Am J Obstet Gynecol 78:38, 1959

Rotter CW, Whitaker JL, Yared J: The use of intravenous dramamine to shorten the time of labor and potentiate analgesia. Am J Obstet Gynecol 75:1101, 1958

Rouchy R, Blondeau P, LeCannelieu R, Creze J, Grosieux P: Le diazepam par voie intraveineuse en obstétrique. Presse Med 74:312, 1966

Rovinsky JJ, Miller JA, Kaplan S: Management of breech presentation at term. Am J Obstet Gynecol 115:497, 1973

Rübsamen W: Die externe Hysterographie als klinischexperimentelle Testmethod für die Bestimmung der Wertigkeit von Wehenmitteln. Arch Gynaekol 112:459, 1920

Sadove MS, Balagot RC, Branion JM, Kobak AJ: Report on the use of a new agent, phenazocine, in obstetric analgesia. Obstet Gynecol 16:448, 1960

Sakaguchi M, Nakajima A: Electrical activity of the human uterus in labor. Am J Obstet Gynecol 108:992, 1970

Sakaguchi M, Nakajima A: Electromyogram of the human uterus in labor. J Appl Physiol 35:423, 1973

Sala NL, Schwarcz RL Jr, Althabe O Jr, Fisch L, Fuente O: Effect of epidural anesthesia upon uterine contractility induced by artificial cervical dilatation in human pregnancy. Am J Obstet Gynecol 106:26, 1970

Sandmire HF, Austin SD: Paracervical block anesthesia in obstetrics. JAMA 187:775, 1964

Savage D: Chlorpromazine ("Largactil") as analgesic in labour: Report of 127 controlled cases. Br J Anaesth 27:346, 1955

Scheer K, Nubar J: Variation of fetal presentation with gestational age. Am J Obstet Gynecol 125:269, 1976

Schifrin BS: Fetal heart rate patterns following epidural anaesthesia and oxytocin infusion during labour. J Obstet Gynaecol Br Commonw 79:332, 1972

Schulman H, Ledger WJ: Practical applications of the graphic portrayal of labor. Obstet Gynecol 23:442, 1964

Schulman H, Romney SL: Variability of uterine contractions in normal human parturition. Obstet Gynecol 36:215, 1970

Scommegna A, Burd L, Goodman C, Bieniarz J: The effect of pregnenolone sulfate on uterine contractility. Am J Obstet Gynecol 108:1023, 1970

Scott JR, Rose NB: Effect of psychoprophylaxis (Lamaze preparation) on labor and delivery in primiparas. N Engl J Med 294:1205, 1976

Scott RS, Wallace KH, Badley DN, Watson BH: Use of dimenhydrinate in labor. Am J Obstet Gynecol 83:25, 1963

Seitchik J, Chatkoff ML: Intrauterine pressure wave form characteristics in hypocontractile labor before and after oxytocin administration. Am J Obstet Gynecol 123:426, 1975

Senties L, Arellano G, Casellas A, Ontiveros E, Santos J: Effects of some vasopressor drugs upon uterine contractility in pregnant women. Am J Obstet Gynecol 107:892, 1970

Shaaban AH, Youssef AF: Effect of autonomic drugs on uterine action in labour. Gaz Egypt Soc Gynaecol Obstet 9:107, 1959

Shabanah EH, Toth A, Maughan GB: The role of the autonomic nervous system in uterine contractility and blood flow: I. The interaction between neurohormones and sex steroids in the intact and isolated uterus. Am J Obstet Gynecol 89:841, 1964a

Shabanah EH, Toth A, Maughan GB: The role of the autonomic nervous system in uterine contractility and blood flow: II. The role of the parasympathetic neurohormone acetylcholine in uterine motility and blood flow. Am J Obstet Gynecol 89:860, 1964b

Sicuranza BJ, Tisdall LH, Leen WM, Palmeri T: The planes of Hodge as an index of the progress of labor. J Reprod Med 5:132, 1970

Siener H: Cervical dynamometry: A new method in obstetrical research. Am J Obstet Gynecol 89:579, 1954

Siener H: Ein Gerät zur Registrierung der Muttermundseröffnung unter der Geburt (Zervixwehenschreiber). Zentralbl Gynaekol 78:2069, 1956

Siener H: Studien über das Verhalten des Muttermundes während der Eröffnungsperiode. Arch Gynaekol 18:556, 1957

Siener H: First stage of labor recorded by cervical tocometry. Am J Obstet Gynecol 86:303, 1963

Simeckova M, Shaw W, Pool E, Nichols EE: Numorphan in labor: A preliminary report. Obstet Gynecol 16:119, 1960

Slate WG, Mengert WF: Effect of the relaxing hormone on the laboring human uterus. Obstet Gynecol 15:409, 1960

Smyth CN: Measurement of the forces and strains of labour and the action of certain oxytocic drugs. Comptes-Rendus du Congrès International de Gynécologie et d'Obstétrique. Geneva, SA George, 1954

Smyth CN: Biomechanics of uterine action. Lancet 1:208, 1973

Snow DL, Sattenspiel E: Report on oxymorphone in obstetrics. Am J Obstet Gynecol 83:23, 1962

Snyder FF: Obstetric Analgesia and Anesthesia. Philadelphia, Saunders, 1949

Sogolow SR, Friedman EA: Fetopelvic disproportion in the multipara. Obstet Gynecol 29:848, 1967

Soiva I, Castrén O, Ruponen S: Tocographic studies with Librium and Valium. Ann Chir Gynaecol Fenn 53:141, 1964

Sokol RJ, Nussbaum RS, Chik L, Rosen MG: Computer diagnosis of labor progression: I. Development of an on-line interactive digital computer program for the diagnosis of normal and abnormal dilatation patterns. J Reprod Med 11:149, 1973a

Sokol RJ, Nussbaum RS, Chik L, Rosen MG: Computer diagnosis of labor progression: II. Application of an on-line interactive program in 45 high-risk labors. J Reprod Med 11:154, 1973b

Sokol RJ, Walker R, Nussbaum RS, Rosen MG, Chik L: Computer diagnosis of labor progression: III. Dysfunctional labor patterns in the very elderly gravida. Am J Obstet Gynecol 119:767, 1974a

Sokol RJ, Nussbaum RS, Chik L, Rosen MG: Computer diagnosis of labor progression: IV. An on-line interactive digital computer subroutine for evaluating descent of the fetal presenting part during labor. J Reprod Med 13:177, 1974b

Sokol RJ, Nussbaum RS, Chik L, Rosen MG: Computer diagnosis of labor progression: V. Subroutine for evaluating station and descent of the fetal presenting part. J Reprod Med 13:183, 1974c

Sokol RJ, Roux JF, McCarthy S: Computer diagnosis of labor progression: VI. Fetal stress and labor in the occipitoposterior position. Am J Obstet Gynecol 122:253, 1975

Sokol RJ, Stojkov J, Chik L, Rosen MG: Normal and abnormal labor: I. A quantitative assessment and survey of the literature. J Reprod Med 18:47, 1977

Sokol RJ, Zador I, Rosen MG: Slowing of active labor associated with internal fetal monitoring. Am J Obstet Gynecol 124:764, 1976

Spellacy WN, Gall SA: Prostaglandin $F_{2\alpha}$ and oxytocin for term labor. J Reprod Med 9:300, 1972

Sprague LD: Predelivery sedation with promazine: A clinical evaluation. Obstet Gynecol 9:633, 1957

Stander RW: An approach to quantitative analysis of intrauterine pressure data. Obstet Gynecol 27:110, 1966
Steer CM: The electrical activity of the human uterus in normal and abnormal labor. Am J Obstet Gynecol 68:867, 1954
Steer CM, Hertsch GJ: Electrical activity of the human uterus in labor. Am J Obstet Gynecol 59:25, 1950
Stein S, Paxson NF: Use of a monoamine oxidase inhibitor in obstetrics. Am J Obstet Gynecol 85:507, 1963
Stewart RH: Phenothiazine derivatives in labor and delivery: A study of four drugs. Obstet Gynecol 17:701, 1961
Stipp CG: The primigravida in labor with high fetal station. Am J Obstet Gynecol 104:267, 1969
Stoelting VK: Fluothane in obstetric anesthesia. Anesth Analg 43:243, 1964
Studd J: Partograms and nomograms of cervical dilatation in management of primigravid labour. Br Med J 4:451, 1973
Studd J, Clegg DR, Sanders RR, Hughes AO: Identification of high risk labours by labour nomogram. Br Med J 2:545, 1975
Studd J, Duignan N: Graphic records in labour. Br Med J 4:426, 1972
Talbert LM, McGaughey HS, Corey EL, Thornton WN: Effects of anesthetic and sedative agents commonly employed in obstetric practice on isolated human muscle. Am J Obstet Gynecol 75:16, 1958
Taubert HD, Haskins AL: Intravenous infusion of progesterone in human females: blood levels obtained and effect on labor. Obstet Gynecol 22:405, 1963
Theobald GW: The separate release of oxytocin and antidiuretic hormone. J Physiol 149:443, 1955
Thoms H: Variations in the female pelvis in relation to labor. Surg Gynecol Obstet 60:680, 1935
Thoms H, Foote WR, Friedman I: The clinical significance of pelvic variations. Am J Obstet Gynecol 38:634, 1939
Thoms H, Karlovsky ED: Two thousand deliveries under a training for childbirth program: A statistical survey and commentary. Am J Obstet Gynecol 68:279, 1954
Todd WD, Steer CM: Term breech: Review of 1,006 term breech deliveries. Obstet Gynecol 22:583, 1963
Tunstall MD: The muscle relaxants in obstetrics. Br J Anaesth 35:535, 1963
Tuppy H: The amino-acid sequence in oxytocin. Biochim Biophys Acta 11:449, 1953
Van Auken WBD, Tomlinson DR: An appraisal of patient training for childbirth. Am J Obstet Gynecol 66:100, 1953
Vanden Driessche R, Draps H, Schoysman R, Riva G: La chlorpromazine dans l'analgésie obstétricale: Étude experimentale et clinique. Bull Féd Soc Gynéc Obstet 6:453, 1954
Van Liere EJ, Bell WE, Mazzocco TR, Northrup DW: Mechanism of action of nitrous oxide, ether and chloroform on the uterus. Am J Obstet Gynecol 90:811, 1964
Vartan CK: Breech presentation and delivery. Clin Obstet Gynecol 2:390, 1959
Vasicka A, Hutchinson HT, Eng M, Allen CR: Spinal and epidural anesthesia, fetal and uterine response to acute hypo- and hypertension. Am J Obstet Gynecol 90:800, 1964
Vasicka A, Kretchmer HE: The effect of prochlorperazine on uterine contractions: A clinical and experimental study. Obstet Gynecol 14:500, 1959

Vasicka A, Kretchmer HE: Effect of conduction and inhalation anesthesia on uterine contractions. Am J Obstet Gynecol 82:600, 1961

Vasicka A, Robertazzi R, Raji M, Scheffs J, Kosmowski J, Goei T: Fetal bradycardia after paracervical block. Obstet Gynecol 38:500, 1971

Vorherr H: Disorders of uterine functions during pregnancy, labor, and puerperium. In Assali NS, Brinkman CR III (eds) : Pathophysiology of Gestation. New York, Academic, 1972

Ware D, Haynes DM: A study of relaxin in primigravidas. Am J Obstet Gynecol 83:792, 1962

Weekes ARL, Flynn MJ: Engagement of the fetal head in primigravidae and its relationship to duration of gestation and time of onset of labour. Br J Obstet Gynaecol 82:7, 1975

Weinberg A, Scadron SJ: Value and limitations of pelvioradiography in management of dystocia, with special reference to midpelvic capacity. Am J Obstet Gynecol 52:255, 1946

Weiss RR, Tejani N, Israeli I, Evans MI, Bhakthavathasalan A, et al: Priming of the uterine cervix with oral prostaglandin $E_2$ in the term multigravida. Obstet Gynecol 46:181, 1976

White RL: Intravenous ethyl alcohol analgesia with pitocin induction of labor. Am J Obstet Gynecol 70:983, 1955

Wolf W: Der unzeitige Blasensprung. Stuttgart, Wissenschaftliche Verlagsgesellschaft, 1946, p 103

Wolf W: Discussion of Rydberg E: Geburtmechanismus. Arch Gynaekol 180:171, 1951

Wolfs G, Rottinghuis H: Electrical and mechanical activity of the human uterus during labour. Arch Gynaekol 208:373, 1970

Wood C, Elstein M, Pinkerton JHM: The effect of progestogens upon uterine activity. J Obstet Gynaecol Br Commonw 70:839, 1963

Woodbury RA, Hamilton WF, Torpin R: The relationship between abdominal, uterine and arterial pressures during labor. Am J Physiol 121:640, 1938

Zador I, Wolfson RN, Neuman MR: Ultrasonic measurement of cervical dilatation during labor. Ann Conf Engin Med Biol 16:187, 1974

Zambrana MA, Gonzalez Panizza VH, Santiso-Galvez R, Garcia de Paz H, Fernandez R, Arellano Hernandez G: Relación de la contractilidad espontaneo del útero con el progreso del parto. Tercer Congreso Uruguayo de Ginecotocologia 3:354, 1960

Zatuchni GI, Andros GJ: Prognostic index for vaginal delivery in breech presentation. Am J Obstet Gynecol 93:237, 1965

Zax M, Sameroff AJ, Farnum JE: Childbirth education, maternal attitudes, and delivery. Am J Obstet Gynecol 123:185, 1975

Zimmer K: Die Muttermundseröffnung bei den Schädellagen im Wegzeit-Diagramm. Arch Gynaekol 179:35, 1951

Zlatnick FJ, Fuchs F: A controlled study of ethanol in threatened premature labor. Am J Obstet Gynecol 112:610, 1972

Zourlas PA: In vitro and in vivo effects of sparine (promazine hydrochloride) on human uterine contractility. Am J Obstet Gynecol 88:770, 1964

Zuckerman H, Reiss U, Robinstein I: Inhibition of human premature labor by indomethacin. Obstet Gynecol 44:787, 1974

Zuspan FP, Cibils LA, Pose SV: Myometrial and cardiovascular responses to alterations in plasma epinephrine and norepinephrine. Am J Obstet Gynecol 84:841, 1962

# Index